Oxford Medical Publications
The Psychoimmunology of Cancer

The Psychoimmunology of Cancer
Second edition

Edited by

C. E. Lewis
Professor of Molecular and Cellular Pathology, Section of Pathology,
Division of Oncology and Cellular Pathology, University of Sheffield
Medical School, UK

R. M. O'Brien
Palliative Care Nurse, Sir Michael Sobell House, Oxford

and

J. Barraclough
Consultant in Psychological Medicine, Oxford Radcliffe Hospital
NHS Trust, Oxford

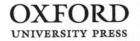

OXFORD
UNIVERSITY PRESS

OXFORD
UNIVERSITY PRESS

Great Clarendon Street, Oxford OX2 6DP

Oxford University Press is a department of the University of Oxford.
If furthers the University's objective of excellence in research, scholarship,
and education by publishing worldwide in

Oxford New York

Auckland Bangkok Buenos Aires Cape Town Chennai
Dar es Salaam Delhi Hong Kong Istanbul Karachi Kolkata
Kuala Lumpur Madrid Melbourne Mexico City Mumbai
Nairobi Sao Paulo Shanghai Taipei Tokyo Toronto

and an associated company in Berlin

Oxford is a registered trade mark of Oxford University Press
in the UK and in certain other countries

Published in the United States
by Oxford University Press Inc., New York

A catalogue record for this title is available from the British Library

Library of Congress Cataloging in Publication Data

The psychoimmunology of cancer / edited by J. Barraclough, R. M. O'Brien,
and C. E. Lewis.–2nd ed.

1. Cancer–Immunological aspects.   2. Cancer–Psychological aspects.
3. Psychoneuroimmunology.   I. Barraclough, Jennifer.   II. O'Brien, R. M.
(Rosalind M.)   III. Lewis, Claire E.

RC268.3 .P79 2001   616.99′4079—dc21   2001055171

ISBN 0 19 263060 1 (Hbk.)

10 9 8 7 6 5 4 3 2 1

Typeset by Integra Software Services Pvt. Ltd., Pondicherry, India
www.integra-india.com
Printed in Great Britain
on acid-free paper by Biddles Ltd., Guildford and King's Lynn

Preface

When the first edition of this book came out in 1994, the psychoimmunology of cancer was still emerging as a topic for serious scientific study. Now, less than ten years later, there is a huge academic literature about the relationships between psychological variables, the immune system, and cancer growth, accompanied by a lively popular interest.

Because the field has grown so large, this second edition contains less detailed description of individual research projects than the first. Instead, we have asked selected experts for broad critical reviews of different aspects. We hope the book will have a multidisciplinary appeal. Part I, which presents the biological background, will be of particular interest to those with technical knowledge of the relevant laboratory-based disciplines. Part II is more clinically oriented, and accessible to a wider audience. Whether psychotherapeutic interventions can help patients to live longer, as well as coping better, is obviously a question of key importance and several contributors consider the evidence on this. A new, speculative chapter on the spiritual context of immunity and cancer has also been added.

The psychoimmunology of cancer involves many complex issues, understanding of which remains far from complete. Our contributors, besides reviewing the current state of knowledge, offer some predictions for the future and ideas about further research.

Oxford J. B.
August 2001 C. E. L.
  R. O'B.

Contents

List of Contributors

J. Anderson   Institute of Rehabilitation, University of Hull, 215 Anlaby Road, Hull HU3 2PG, UK

D. L. Bellinger   Loma Linda University, Center for Neuroimmunology, Alumni Hall for Basic Sciences, Rm 321, 11021 Campus Street, CA 92354, USA

R. J. Booth   Department of Molecular Medicine, The University of Auckland, Private Bag 92019, Auckland, New Zealand

K. Calde   Department of Psychiatry and Behavioral Sciences, Stanford University School of Medicine, California, USA

C. Classen   Department of Psychiatry and Behavioral Sciences, Stanford University School of Medicine, Stanford, California 94305, USA

A. J. Cunningham   Ontario Cancer Institute, Toronto, Canada

A. G. Dalgleish   Division of Oncology, St George's Hospital Medical School, Cranmer Terrace, London SW17 0RE, UK

D. L. Felten   Susan Samueli Center for Complementary and Alternative Medicine, University of California, Irvine, College of Medicine, University Tower, Suite 620, 4199 Campus Drive, Irvine, CA 92612–5850, USA

B. Garssen   Helen Dowling Institute for Biopsychosocial Medicine, Rotterdam, the Netherlands

K. Goodkin   Helen Dowling Institute for Biopsychosocial Medicine, Rotterdam, the Netherlands; Department of Psychiatry and Behavioral Sciences, University of Miami School of Medicine, Miami, USA

J. L. Levenson   Department of Psychiatry, Medical College of Virginia, Virginia Commonwealth University, Richmond, Virginia 23298–0268, USA

D. Lorton   Hoover Arthritis Research Center, Sun Health Research Institute, PO Box 1278, Sun City, AZ 85372, USA

K. S. Madden   Department of Psychiatry, University of Rochester School of Medicine, 300 Crittenden Blvd, Rochester, New York 1464, USA

K. McDonald   Massey Cancer Center, Medical College of Virginia of Virginia Commonwealth University, Richmond, Virginia, USA

D. Spiegel   Department of Psychiatry and Behavioral Sciences, Stanford University School of Medicine, California 943405, USA

P. W. Szlosarek   ICRF Translational Oncology Laboratory,
                     St Bartholomew's and the Royal London School
                     of Medicine and Dentistry, Charterhouse Square,
                     London EC1M 6BQ, UK
S. ThyagaRajan   Susan Samueli Center for Complementary and
                     Alternative Medicine, University of California, Irvine,
                     College of Medicine, University Tower, Suite 620, 4199
                     Campus Drive, Irvine, CA 92612–5850, USA
L. Tran   Loma Linda University, Center for Neuroimmunology,
                     Alumni Hall for Basic Sciences, Rm 321, 11021 Campus
                     Street, CA 92354, USA
L. G. Walker   Institute of Rehabilitation, University of Hull, 215
                     Anlaby Road, Hull HU3 2PG, UK

PART I

Psychology, immunity, and cancer: the biological links

1

Psychoimmunology today: mechanisms mediating the effects of psychological status on the immune system

D. L. BELLINGER, S. THYAGARAJAN, D. LORTON,
K. S. MADDEN, L. TRAN, AND D. L. FELTEN

1 Introduction

Psychosocial factors and stressors can influence the health and well-being of an individual. These environmental stimuli are transduced by the brain into chemical signals that can affect the immune system. Behavioural conditioning studies reveal that the CNS also can detect alterations in immune responses and, subsequent to detection, is able to initiate a change in immune response upon re-exposure to the conditioned stimulus. The specific neural circuits in the brain that mediate these changes in immune function have been the focus of much research over the past ten years. However, these neural circuits are still not well defined, and the functional significance of brain–immune interactions under a variety of conditions is not fully understood.

However, it is clear that the neuroendocrine system and the autonomic nervous system (ANS) are important regulators of brain–immune interactions. The brain communicates with the immune system through nerves that distribute to lymphoid tissue. In addition to the traditional targets of autonomic nerves in the periphery such as cardiac muscle, smooth muscle, and exocrine (secretory) glands, the sympathetic nervous system (SNS) innervates hepatocytes, brown fat cells, and cells of the immune system. The autonomic circuitry consists of a two-neuron chain, where autonomic preganglionic neurons in the brain stem and spinal cord terminate on postganglionic neurons in autonomic ganglia distributed throughout the body. Axons from postganglionic neurons project to target tissue in the periphery. Preganglionic neurons are regulated directly by the cerebral cortex, limbic forebrain structures, specific regions of the hypothalamus, and brain stem autonomic and reticular nuclei. Additionally, there is some evidence suggesting that primary afferent fibres from dorsal root ganglion and vagal nerve fibres innervate lymphoid organs. Cells of the immune system possess specific receptors for catecholamines (CAs), acetylcholine, and neuropeptides. Neurotransmitters, contained in nerves that distribute to lymphoid organs, have been shown to alter immune function.

The second route through which the brain communicates with the immune system is via the neuroendocrine system. Neuroendocrine outflow from the brain is mediated by the release of pituitary hormones under the control of the hypothalamus, limbic forebrain, and brain stem circuitry, generally termed the hypothalamic–pituitary–endocrine target organ axis. Neurons from the magnocellular paraventricular nucleus (mPVN) and the supraoptic nucleus (SON) secrete oxytocin and arginine vasopressin (AVP) directly into the systemic circulation in the posterior pituitary. Neurons from a number of other hypothalamic nuclei secrete releasing or inhibitory factors into the hypophyseal portal blood at the median eminence, which in turn carries these hormones to the anterior pituitary to regulate the release of pituitary hormones, such as adrenocorticotropic hormone (ACTH), thyroid-stimulating hormone (TSH), follicle-stimulating hormone (FSH), luteinizing hormone (LH), growth hormone (GH), and prolactin (PRL). Apart from their many classic endocrine effects, pituitary hormones act as signal molecules through which the brain interacts with the immune system.

Cytokine regulation of sympathetic and neuroendocrine outflow has also been a major focus of research in the past ten years, particularly in regard to immune regulation of the hypothalamic–pituitary–adrenal (HPA) axis. Numerous studies have shown that alterations in neuroendocrine secretions are produced by interleukin 1 (IL-1), IL-2, tumour necrosis factor-α (TNF-α), IL-6, interferon-γ (IFN-γ), and many other immunoregulatory cytokines. These cytokines have potent effects on the secretion of the majority of hormones under neuroendocrine control. Clearly, there are several routes through which cytokines from cells of the immune system can interact with the nervous system. Receptors for a variety of cytokines have been demonstrated on both central and peripheral neurons, and on glia, making it possible for cytokines to signal the brain. Additionally, the synthesis and secretion of some cytokines have been reported in neurons and glia in certain brain regions.

This chapter reviews published findings that demonstrate innervation of lymphoid organs and functional studies that support a role for neurotransmitters present in these nerves in the modulation of the immune system. Next, a summary of research investigating the influence of the hypothalamic–pituitary–target tissue axis on immune function is presented. Finally, mechanisms through which immunological mediators regulate autonomic and neuroendocrine outflow are reviewed. The relevance of bidirectional communication between the nervous and immune systems to infectious diseases and cancer is discussed throughout the chapter.

2   Innervation of lymphoid organs

2.1   NORADRENERGIC SYMPATHETIC INNERVATION

2.1.1   Bone marrow

Nerve bundles supply the periosteum and enter the interior of the bone via the nutrient foramena to the medulla. These medullary bundles of myelinated and unmyelinated nerve fibres distribute along the branches of the nutrient artery. Some, but not all, of these nerves are noradrenergic (NA) (1), since some nerves remain after sympathectomy (2, 3). Within the marrow, the majority of NA nerves form dense plexuses along the vasculature (4–6). From these vascular plexuses, occasional nerve fibres branch into the surrounding parenchyma among haemopoietic cells in the marrow. Adrenergic receptors are present on granulocyte-macrophage progenitor cells and primitive progenitor cells (7, 8). Neurochemical measurements of CAs in murine bone marrow reveal on the order of 1–3 ng of norepinephrine (NE) per gram bone marrow tissue (9), one to two orders of magnitude lower than is generally reported in secondary lymphoid organs in rats (10, 11).

The presence of NA nerves adjacent to the vasculature suggests that NE may have vasomotor activity, controlling blood flow and volume within the bone marrow. Direct apposition between nerve terminals and a particular type of stromal cell, the periarterial adventitial cell (12), an important source of growth factors and adhesion molecules, suggests that efferent nerves may regulate haematopoiesis via modulation of factors released by these stromal cells (12, 13). Other findings are consistent with this hypothesis: (a) developmentally, NA nerves innervate the rat bone marrow when haemopoietic activity begins (14, 15); (b) NE and dopamine concentrations in mouse bone marrow exhibit diurnal rhythmicity (9) with a time course that correlates positively with the G2/M and S phase of the cell-cycle functions (9, 16); (c) inhibiting sympathetic outflow enhances myelopoiesis and exerts an inhibitory effect on lymphopoiesis (7, 17); and (d) Wu and colleagues (18) have utilized a three-dimensional bone marrow culture system to demonstrate that isoproterenol treatment of murine bone marrow cultures greatly enhances cell proliferation in the culture, and stimulates granulopoiesis in a dose-dependent fashion. In fact, isoproterenol is as effective as granulocyte colony-stimulating factor (G-CSF) in stimulating granulopoiesis, and synergized the stimulating effects of G-CSF.

NE appears to influence cell migration in the bone marrow (13). Transection of the femoral nerve or chemical sympathectomy decreases bone marrow cellularity due to mobilization of progenitor and mature cells (13). This effect is attributed to the bolus release of NE from damaged nerves (13). However, using neonatal chemical sympathectomy, surgical denervation of the hind limb, or electrical stimulation of the hind limb, Benestad et al. (19) could not confirm these findings. NE also mobilizes fat from the bone marrow (20). Finally, stimulation of the posterior hypothalamus causes a release of reticulocytes through activation of descending sympathetic innervation to the bone marrow (21). However, it is not yet clear whether the release of reticulocytes is due to a direct action of NE on these cells or to an indirect action of NE on the vasculature.

2.1.2 Thymus

NA fibres enter the thymus adjacent to large blood vessels as dense vascular plexuses. In these nerve plexuses, NA nerves travel in the capsule and interlobular septa, or continue with the vasculature into the cortex. NA nerve fibres exit the vascular plexuses to course along very fine septa into the cortical region, in close proximity to thymocytes and cells with yellow autofluorescence, a macrophage-like cell in the cortex. In the capsule and septa, NA nerve fibres course adjacent to mast cells (22, 23). At the corticomedullary junction, NA nerves are present along the medullary venous sinuses, which are continuous with the system of innervated vessels in the septa. NA fibres extend from these sinuses into the adjacent cortical region, and occasionally into the medullary parenchyma. Immunocytochemical staining for tyrosine hydroxylase (TH), the rate-limiting enzyme for the synthesis of NE, reveals that TH$^+$ nerves also course adjacent to corticomedullary macrophages and mast cells (22). Neurochemical analysis of CAs in the thymus indicates that almost all the CA-containing nerves are NA. It appears that not all of the NA nerve fibres are positive for PGP 9.5 (24), a general marker for nerve fibres, regardless of the neurotransmitter phenotypes (25).

One potential target of NA nerves in the thymus is the thymic epithelial cell, since CA-containing nerve fibres closely appose thymic epithelial cells (26), and they possess β_1- and β_2-adrenergic receptors (26). Close appositions between non-myelinated nerves containing dense core vesicles and myoid cells and fibroblasts have also been reported in the chick thymus (27). Without the presence of any diffusion barrier, it is likely that NE released from NA nerves can interact with thymocytes and other target cells in the thymus, particularly since extensive diffusion of NE from sympathetic postganglionic nerves is well documented in other peripheral target organs. The functional significance of NA innervation of the thymus is not clear. Experimental studies by Singh and Owen (28–33) suggest that NE exerts an effect on the maturation of thymocytes, since it inhibits proliferation and promotes differentiation of thymocytes *in vitro*. This effect is mediated through the activation of β-adrenergic receptors via adenosine 3′,5′-cyclic monophosphate (cAMP) as a second messenger (reviewed in 34, 35).

2.1.3 Spleen

Innervation of the spleen has been studied more widely than innervation of any other lymphoid organ. NA nerves enter the spleen as a dense plexus associated with the splenic artery and its branches beneath the capsule of the spleen. NA fibres from this subcapsular plexus plunge into the depths of the spleen along the trabeculae and its associated vasculature. NA plexuses follow the central arterioles and their branches into the white pulp of the spleen. NA nerve fibres exit this vascular plexus and travel into the surrounding periarteriolar lymphatic sheaths (PALS), regions composed primarily of T lymphocytes. In transgenic mice that overexpress nerve growth factor (NGF) in the skin and other epithelial structures, the marginal zone is hyperinnervated compared with control mice (36). Furthermore, concanavalin A (Con A)-induced proliferation is suppressed in splenocytes from NGF transgenic mice, suggesting that NGF-induced sympathetic hyperinnervation of the spleen has functional consequences on immune response (36).

In the PALS, TH⁺ nerves reside in close proximity to T lymphocytes of both the T-helper and T-cytotoxic/suppressor subsets. TH⁺ nerves also course along the marginal sinus adjacent to ED3⁺ macrophages, and in the marginal zone in close association with ED3⁺ macrophages and immunoglobulin (Ig)M⁺ B lymphocytes. Only an occasional TH⁺ nerve fibre is present among IgM⁺ B lymphocytes in the follicle.

Electron microscopic examination of sections stained immunocytochemically for TH (37) has revealed TH⁺ nerve terminals adjacent to smooth muscle cells of the central arteriole, and TH⁺ nerve terminals in direct contact with lymphocytes in the PALS. These terminals possess long, smooth zones of contact with lymphocyte plasma membranes, separated by as little as 6 nm. Similar close appositions are present at the marginal sinus and in the marginal zone between TH⁺ nerve terminals and lymphocytes and macrophages. No postsynaptic specializations are apparent; however, such CNS-type synaptic specialization is rarely found at any peripheral sympathetic neuroeffector junctions with any target cells. These TH⁺ profiles are not present in spleens denervated either by 6-hydroxydopamine (6-OHDA), a neurotoxin that destroys nerve terminals, or by ganglionectomy, or in immunocytochemically stained tissue sections incubated with goat anti-rabbit IgG (the secondary antibody) alone.

Strain differences have been used to explain differing results when studying neural–immune interactions in laboratory animals (38). This possibility was examined for NA innervation of the spleen using three mouse strains (BALB/cJ, C57Bl/6J, and DBA/2). Small but significant differences between these strains were demonstrated in total resting splenic NE content (BALB/cJ > C57Bl6J > DBA/2) and in resting NE concentration (C57Bl/6J > BALB/cJ > DBA/2). These findings may be due in part to differences in the size of the spleens from these murine strains (BALB/cJ > DBA/2 > C57Bl/6J). No diurnal differences were found in NE concentration of the spleen, but the expected diurnal pattern of plasma corticosterone (serving as a positive control) was observed in all strains.

2.1.4 Lymph nodes

Both fluorescent histochemical and immunocytochemical staining for NA sympathetic innervation of lymph nodes in rodents (34, 39–43) reveal dense plexuses of NA nerves along blood vessels at the hilus, the presumed point of entry of NA nerves. In lymph nodes, NA nerves travel in a subcapsular plexus or continue in vascular plexuses through the medullary cords. NA fibres distribute adjacent to many lymphoid cell types, and to both vascular and lymphatic channels in the medulla. These fibres continue along small vessels that course from the medulla into the paracortical regions, which are rich in T lymphocytes. Single NA profiles exit these vascular plexuses and travel in the paracortical parenchyma. NA fibres that contribute to subcapsular plexuses also course along small vessels into the cortex and give off individual fibres that project into the cortical parenchyma. Linear fibres that enter into T-lymphocyte compartments of the cortex and paracortex do not travel into the adjacent nodular regions and germinal centres where B lymphocytes predominate. Dopamine β-hydroxylase (an enzyme that converts the precursor, dopamine, to NE) nerve fibres have been demonstrated in lymph nodes from rats, guinea-pigs, mice, cats, pigs, and humans (44). In NGF transgenic mice where NGF is overexpressed by the skin, peripheral lymph nodes that drain the skin are more densely innervated compared with peripheral lymph nodes from control mice, and compared with mesenteric lymph nodes from transgenic and control mice (36). NGF concentration in peripheral lymph nodes is also elevated 13-fold. These findings suggest that NGF provides a trophic influence on sympathetic nerves in this genetic mouse model.

The compartmentalization of NA nerves in lymph nodes displays many similarities with NA innervation of the spleen, suggesting a common functional role in both organs. A role for NE in antigen processing, i.e. antigen capture and antigen presentation, is supported by studies showing reduced primary antibody responses in spleen and lymph nodes following sympathetic denervation (35). Egress of activated lymphocytes into the circulation from spleen and lymph nodes occurs following the infusion of CAs (34, 45, 46), suggesting an additional role for NE at these secondary lymphoid organs in lymphocyte trafficking.

2.1.5 SNS modulation of immune function

In vivo, investigators have used ablation of sympathetic NA innervation, infusion with adrenergic receptor agonists/antagonist, and sympathetic activation to examine the role of the SNS in modulating immune function (11). One of the most commonly used pharmacological means of examining SNS–immune system interactions is chemical sympathectomy, the destruction of peripheral sympathetic NA nerve fibres by treatment with 6-OHDA. 6-OHDA is a neurotoxin highly selective for NA nerve fibres that does not cross the blood–brain barrier (47). A single intraperitoneal injection rapidly depletes NE by 75–90 per cent in spleen and lymph nodes for more than 2 weeks (48).

Chemical sympathectomy has been demonstrated to alter a variety of immune parameters, including *in vivo* cellular proliferation in lymphoid organs, lymphocyte migration, natural killer (NK) cell activity, humoral immunity, and cell-mediated responses (reviewed in 11, 49). The 6-OHDA-induced effects are variable and are dependent on a variety of factors. For example, spleen cells from sympathectomized BALB/c and C57Bl/6 mice immunized with a protein antigen, keyhole limpet haemocyanin (KLH), proliferate more in response to KLH *in vitro*, and produce more IL-2 and IL-4 production (50). KLH-induced IFN-γ production and serum anti-KLH antibody titres increase only in C57Bl/6, but not BALB/c, sympathectomized mice (50, 51). Cell-mediated immunity, in the form of delayed-type hypersensitivity (DTH), is reduced in sympathectomized mice, in conjunction with reduced cytotoxic T-lymphocyte generation and IL-2 production by draining lymph node cells *in vitro* (52). Removal of sympathetic NA innervation can also influence autoimmune processes through modulation of T-cell activity (34, 42). These results suggest a complex role for NE and the SNS in modulation of a variety of immune parameters *in vivo*, depending on genetic and other factors, that may affect host resistance and susceptibility to disease.

An important role of the immune system is surveillance of the host for foreign agents, and a corresponding rapid mobilization of the appropriate leukocytes. The localization of sympathetic NA nerve fibres to the marginal zone in the spleen suggests that the SNS is a good candidate for regulating lymphocyte trafficking. Following physical exercise, exposure to mental or physical stressors, or following injection of epinephrine or isoproterenol, a rapid and transient leukocytosis occurs, consisting of increased NK cells, lymphocytes, and monocytes in the blood. All these effects are prevented by administration of β-adrenergic receptor antagonists (reviewed in 53). *In vitro*, β_2-adrenergic receptor stimulation reduces adhesion of T cells and NK cells to endothelial cells (54, 55), suggesting that cells in the marginal pool are less likely to attach firmly to the endothelium in the presence of CAs. Neither NE nor epinephrine alters expression of a variety of cell adhesion molecules, although affinity has not been examined. Understanding the mechanism underlying CA-induced changes in lymphocyte trafficking may help to provide the means by which cells can be mobilized or immobilized during local immune and inflammatory responses.

In vitro assessments of the effects of adrenergic agonists on cells of the immune system have been employed to eliminate the influence of altered lymphocyte migration and other potential confounding effects present *in vivo*. This approach has allowed the precise identification of targets of CAs and their function. For example, using highly purified lymphocyte populations, polyclonal B-cell proliferation and differentiation are enhanced by addition of β-adrenergic agonists *in vitro* (56, 57). T-cell proliferation in response to mitogen tends to be reduced, although cytotoxic T-cell generation is enhanced in the presence of β-adrenergic agonists (58, 59). T helper (Th) cell types might also influence the response to CAs. Th1 clones express β-adrenergic receptors, but Th2 clones do not. Functionally, β_2-adrenergic receptor stimulation inhibits anti-CD3-induced Th1, but not Th2, cytokine production (60). When Th1 clones are activated by anti-CD3 in the presence of the β_2-selective agonist terbutaline or NE, IL-2 production is reduced, but not IFN-γ (60). Clearly, the complexity of CA interactions with the immune system present *in vivo* is also apparent *in vitro*. This complexity is most probably due in part to heterogeneity present within the immune system, as well as differences in adrenergic receptor expression within lymphocyte populations (61).

Using a variety of experimental approaches, the immunomodulatory potential for CAs has been established, but a precise role for the SNS in modulating immune function has been difficult to define. As described briefly above, reports of CA influences on immune reactivity have revealed a complexity of interactions between the SNS and the immune system, so that a simple unidirectional definition of SNS modulation of immune reactivity is not possible. These data suggest that the SNS regulates effector immune responses through alterations in such functions as lymphocyte proliferation, cytokine production, and migratory behaviour; the net effect is dependent on genetic factors, such as Th dominance, and perhaps the nature of the activational signal received by lymphocytes. Investigations into the cellular and molecular basis of CA and immune system interactions may provide new revelations concerning how changes in the external environment are communicated to the immune system.

The role of SNS modulation of immune function in tumour development has not been investigated extensively, but several reports suggest that further investigations in this area could be fruitful. In rats administered the NK-cell-sensitive adenocarcinoma MADB106, β-adrenergic receptor agonist treatment increases lung retention of the cell line 24 hours after tumour cell injection, and lung metastases assessed 3 weeks after tumour cell injection (62). In these experiments, metaproterenol (MET), a β-adrenergic receptor non-selective agonist, is administered subcutaneously 1 hour prior to intravenous (i.v.) injection of MADB106. β-Blockade by treatment with the non-selective β-adrenergic antagonist, nadolol, prevents these effects. Furthermore, evidence suggests that reduced NK-cell activity contributes to the MET-induced increase in metastases. Peripheral blood NK-cell activity is decreased within 1 hour after MET administration, an effect that is blocked by the β-antagonists, propranolol and nadolol. NK-cell depletion by treatment of rats with anti-NKR-P1 antibody prevents the MET-induced increase in lung tumour retention, suggesting that MET acts by stimulating NK-cell β-adrenergic receptors. These results suggest that inhibition of NK-cell activity following sympathetic activation and CA release may promote tumour cell metastases.

By contrast, increased metastasis of Line 1 cells to the lung is observed in mice that are treated with 6-OHDA to remove sympathetic NA innervation.

This result suggests that an intact NA innervation can inhibit tumour metastases (63). The increased metastasis occurs only when 6-OHDA is administered prior to, but not following, Line 1 injection. No change in NK-cell activity is detected in sympathectomized animals, as assessed *in vivo* in the lungs, spleen, and liver, or by a standard *in vitro* assay. These results may indicate that non-immunological mechanisms are responsible for the increased metastases, e.g. 6-OHDA-induced changes in blood flow and vascular permeability in the lung. Further research is necessary to understand the influence of the SNS on tumour metastases, whether through immunological or non-immunological mechanisms.

2.1.6   Senescence and the NA innervation

With advancing age, the density of NA nerve fibres in all compartments of the rodent thymus increases progressively as the thymus continues to involute (64, 65). NA innervation is especially dense in the cortex and at the corticomedullary junction of the aged thymus. Dense tangles of NA nerve fibres engulf the vasculature and course as free fibres through the parenchyma of the cortex and paracortex. Free fibres often form long longitudinal arrays oriented parallel to the long axis of the thymic surface. The density of NA nerves in the medulla is not as markedly altered with advancing age, making the boundary between the cortex and medulla much more distinct than in younger animals. Neurochemical data also indicate that NA innervation increases in density with age because the full complement of nerve fibres is maintained in the increasingly diminishing thymic cortex as it involutes.

These studies reveal the remarkable ability of NA nerves to accommodate to the loss of cellularity in the cortex and conform to the changing geometry of the aged thymus. Even though there does not appear to be an increase in the total innervation of the aged thymus, the thymus becomes hyperinnervated with age by progressively shrinking in volume. The increased thymic NE concentration that occurs with advancing age suggests an increase in NE availability in the thymic cortex for interaction with remaining thymocytes and other target cells of the immune system. In the report by Josefsson *et al.* (66), they find that exposure of lymphocytes to catecholamines at concentrations as low as 10 nM decreases proliferation and differentiation. This catecholamine-dependent inhibition of T- and B-lymphocyte activity is mediated via an induction of a Bcl-2/Bax and Fas/FasL involved in apoptosis, suggesting a novel mechanism for regulation of lymphocyte activity (67). If similar regulatory mechanisms for proliferation exist in thymocytes, then perhaps sympathetic hyperinnervation and increased NE availability may promote apoptosis of thymocytes, contributing to the decrease in cellularity of the thymus with ageing.

With advancing age, NA innervation of spleens from F344 rats declines progressively, manifested as a decline in the density of fluorescent NA nerves and TH$^+$ nerves, and by a decline in splenic NE content, by 27 months of age

(68, 69). Age-resistant nerves reside near the hilus; the more extensive nerve depletion is apparent distal from the hilus. Additionally, an increase in circulating NE with age has been reported, which may be contributory to maintaining the NE content of the spleen at a level slightly higher than loss of nerve fibres would predict. In longitudinal studies, NA innervation of the spleen is maintained through 12 months of age, and then gradually begins to decline through 27 months of age (70). Double-label immunocytochemistry further reveals a gradual decline in the density of T lymphocytes in the PALS, and ED3[+] macrophages in the marginal zone that parallels the decline in NA innervation. In 12-month-old rats, the PALS and marginal zone are reduced as a result of this cell loss. At this time point, however, NA innervation of these compartments is still robust. NA nerves retract into the smaller lymphoid compartments to maintain their anatomical distribution within these shrinking lymphoid compartments, giving the appearance of hyperinnervation. By 17 months of age, a further loss of T lymphocytes and ED3[+] macrophages is apparent; at this time point there is also a decline in density of TH[+] nerves associated with these compartments. This parallel decline in the density of specific populations of cells of the immune system and in NA innervation continues through to 27 months of age.

Whether the loss in NA innervation is causally related to the reduced cellularity of T lymphocytes and macrophages in the spleen is not known. Preliminary studies by S. Y. Stevens (unpublished data) examining the ability of sympathetic nerves to innervate spleen fragments from young and old rats transplanted into the anterior chamber of the eye suggest that macrophages may be important for ingrowth and maintenance of sympathetic nerves. Additionally, macrophages synthesize NGF and other neurotrophic factors, consistent with a neuroprotective role for these cells in the spleen. Support for this hypothesis comes from preliminary studies from D. Lorton and colleagues (unpublished data) showing dramatically reduced immunoreactivity for NGF in the PALS and marginal zone of spleens from Lewis rats with experimental arthritis, in which NA sympathetic nerve fibre density declines as the disease progresses. In severe combined immunodeficient (SCID) mice, which are deficient in T and B lymphocytes, NA sympathetic innervation of the spleen is robust within a greatly diminished PALS (S. Y. Stevens, unpublished data). These findings suggest that T lymphocytes may not be critical in providing neurotrophic support necessary to maintain NA nerves in the spleen in these mice. Furthermore, NA innervation of the young adult murine spleen following lymphocyte depletion using hydrocortisone or cyclophosphamide does not decline acutely (71). Collectively, these findings suggest that NA denervation may not be compensatory to the loss of T lymphocytes in the white pulp of the spleen with age, although we cannot dismiss the possibility that it could, in conjunction with other ageing changes, be contributory. T and B lymphocytes express mRNA for NGF, making it possible, at least under some conditions, to provide trophic support to NA nerve fibres in lymphoid tissues.

The density of β-adrenoceptors on splenocytes increases in ageing F344 rats, consistent with upregulation of β-adrenoceptors in response to declining NE levels from an age-related loss of innervation (72). Alternatively, increased β-adrenoceptor expression on old splenocytes may reflect age-related changes in specific subsets of cells in the spleen. No difference in receptor affinity was detected in old rats. Some investigators have reported a dysfunction of β-adrenergic receptors with age, but studies from our laboratory do not entirely support a defect in NE signalling in splenocytes from F344 rats. First, if NE signalling is defective, we would predict that mechanisms important for regulating β-adrenoceptor density on splenocytes from old rats also would be defective. Enhanced β-adrenoceptor expression in the face of diminished NA innervation in ageing suggests that β-adrenoceptor surface expression and function is intact in F344 rats. Next, the density of β-adrenoceptor–adrenoceptor expression on splenocytes from old rats treated with 6-OHDA correlates well with the changes in splenic NE concentrations that occur from denervation and then subsequent reinnervation. However, once the reinnervation of the spleen is established, β-adrenoceptor–adrenoceptor density increases on splenocytes, as in untreated old animals. These findings suggest that old splenocytes respond appropriately to diminished NE concentrations in the spleen, but β-adrenoceptor expression becomes dysregulated at higher splenic NE concentrations.

Functional studies using sympathectomized young and old immunized rats indicate that old splenocytes are still responsive to NA stimulation (73). Sympathectomy followed by intraperitoneal (i.p.) immunization with KLH (150 μg/rat) increases serum IgM anti-KLH response in both young and old F344 rats. This effect is much greater in old rats than it is in young rats. Sympathectomy also enhanced serum IgG anti-KLH response in old rats, but not young animals. The ability of splenocytes from KLH-immune animals to respond to KLH *in vitro* was assessed to examine whether proliferative responses to KLH were altered with sympathectomy. Sympathectomy enhances KLH-induced proliferation by spleen cells from young and old rats (greater effect in old), suggesting that antigen-specific T- and B-cell proliferation are altered by sympathectomy. Sympathectomy elevates Con A-induced T-cell proliferation and lipopolysaccharide (LPS)/dextran sulfate (DxS)-stimulated B-cell proliferation in 17-month-old, but not in 3-month-old, immunized rats. Enhanced proliferation is not the result of enhanced IL-2 production, suggesting that other cytokines that regulate T-cell proliferation may be responsible for this sympathectomy-induced enhancement. These changes also do not result from alterations in the proportions of T and B cells in the spleen, since the percentages of these cells do not change after sympathectomy in either age group. Collectively, these findings suggest that NA sympathetic innervation in aged rats, though diminished compared with young rats, is capable of modulating immune reactivity. Elevated antibody production and lymphocyte proliferation following sympathectomy suggests that in immunized rats, sympathetic innervation may provide an inhibitory signal to humoral responses.

When effects of sympathectomy are observed in young rats, the effects are qualitatively similar to those seen in old rats, although less dramatic, suggesting that immunomodulatory effects of the SNS are similar in young and old rats. It is likely that compensatory mechanisms after NA nerve loss are more robust in young spleens compared with old spleens. The constant ratio of T or B cells suggest that sympathectomy-induced changes occur by mechanisms that directly alter the ability of lymphocytes to proliferate and/or produce antibody. In immunized rats, splenic T-cell proliferation is decreased following sympathectomy, an effect that is directionally opposite to that seen in non-immune rats, and in immunized mice. These findings suggest that immunomodulatory effects of SNS may depend on a variety of factors, including activational state of the immune system, lymphoid microenvironment, and species.

In rodents, an age-related decline in cell-mediated immune functions occurs concomitant with remodelling of sympathetic nerves in secondary lymphoid organs. Age-related immunological dysfunction is associated with an increased incidence of autoimmune and immune complex diseases, certain types of cancer, and viral and fungal infections. Alterations in T-cell-mediated immunity with advancing age include decreased T-cell-dependent humoral immune responses, delayed skin allograft rejection time, reduced intensity of delayed hypersensitivity, lowered resistance to tumour cell challenge, decreased graft-versus-host reactivity, decreased cytolytic immune response, decreased proliferative responsiveness of T cells to mitogens, altered cytokine production after stimulation, and reduce NK-cell activity. Immunological ageing appears to exhibit dynamic Th-cell alterations in cytokine profiles. In newborn mice and human infants cellular immunity is impaired but humoral immunity is strong, indicating a type 2 (Th2) dominant state. Soon after birth, the type 1 (Th1) state becomes dominant and persists in mice and humans until mid- to later life, at which time a dominant Th2 profile tends to emerge again.

The age-related shift from Th1 to Th2 type of immunity has led some investigators to suggest that the increase in tumour incidence, the increased rate of infections, and the reappearance of latent viral infections may result from decreased cellular immune surveillance. Individual variances in dysfunction that can result from this switch in Th cytokine profile could contribute to remodelling of NA nerves in primary and secondary lymphoid tissue. If altered sympathetic innervation of lymphoid organs contributes to the age-related decline in cell-mediated immunity, then it is conceivable that changes in lifestyle to reduce stress and improve coping strategies, or intervention with adrenergic agents, could be used to drive immune responses back towards Th1 type of immunity in the elderly, or towards the arm of immunity that is most effective in combating a particular disease.

2.2.1 Bone marrow

To date, neurotransmitter-specific nerves innervating the bone marrow, other than NA sympathetic nerves, have not been identified. The localization of peptidergic nerves with immunocytochemistry in the bone marrow has been hampered by the difficulty of preserving antigenicity with standard decalcification methods used in the tissue preparation of bone. Recently, immunocytochemistry for PGP 9.5 (a general neuronal marker), TH, and neuropeptide Y (NPY) has been performed in rat bone marrow (6). NPY$^+$ profiles have a distribution similar to that of TH$^+$ nerves, travelling adjacent to the vasculature and in the parenchyma among haemopoietic and lymphopoietic cells in the marrow. The overlapping distribution of NA- and NPY-containing nerves suggests that these neurotransmitters are co-localized in nerves that innervate bone marrow.

PGP 9.5 staining reveals a greater density of nerve profiles associated with the vasculature and in the marrow parenchyma than is seen with TH or NPY staining, indicating the presence of non-NA sympathetic nerve fibres (6). In support of these findings, several investigators (74–76) have reported substance P (SP)$^+$ and calcitonin gene-related peptide (CGRP)$^+$ nerves in the bone marrow. The distribution of these two types of nerves is similar, although CGRP$^+$ fibres are more numerous, suggesting a co-localization of SP with some CGRP$^+$ nerves (74). Varicose, winding fibres are present among haemopoietic cells of the bone marrow and generally do not course along the vasculature. Long, non-varicose fibres course along the bone trabeculae and in close relationship to blood vessels in the marrow. Ahmed *et al.* (77) measured SP and CGRP in bone, periosteum, and bone marrow, but its compartmentation in cellular and neural components was not investigated.

Although the function of these nerves in bone marrow is not clear, there are reports that SP is involved in the regulation of haematopoiesis either by direct interaction with primitive bone marrow stem cells and/or by modulation of cytokines that in turn regulate this process (78–84). Similarly, CGRP appears to modulate early B-lymphocyte differentiation by bone marrow cells (85).

With immunoelectron microscopy, Elhassan *et al.* (86) have demonstrated somatostatin (SOM) labelling in myelinated nerves of the periosteum, and in cells of the bone marrow. Measurements of SOM content using a radioimmunoassay indicate the highest concentrations of SOM in bone marrow, followed by periosteum and cortical bone. Involvement of SOM in nociception and in bone growth in the periosteum has been suggested since SOM inhibits cell growth *in vitro*. SOM$^+$ nerves in the bone marrow, however, have not been demonstrated.

2.2.2 Thymus

NPY$^+$ nerves (23, 87–89) provide the most extensive peptidergic innervation of the rodent thymus to date. The distribution of NPY$^+$ nerves overlaps with the NA innervaion of the thymus, and chemical sympathectomy by administration of the neurotoxin 6-OHDA destroys NPY-immunoreactive nerves in the rat thymus (88). NPY$^+$ fibres travel in bundles that enter the thymus through the capsule, or with surface arteries that extend along the thymic capsule and traverse the interlobular septa. In the septa, these fibres course adjacent to mast cells and macrophages (22, 87). From these subcapsular and arterial plexuses, NPY$^+$ nerves extend into superficial and deep cortical regions to arborize among thymocytes and other supportive cells of the thymus. The densest innervation occurs at the corticomedullary junction. NPY$^+$ profiles are also found in the medulla along the vasculature adjacent to the corticomedullary junction. A similar distribution of NPY$^+$ nerves has been described recently in the chicken thymus, but they are not as numerous as vasoactive intestinal polypeptide (VIP)$^+$ fibres (90). NPY$^+$ nerves closely appose macrophages and mast cells, similar to that described for NA nerves (22, 23).

The thymus also receives innervation from SP/tachykinin (TK)- and CGRP-containing nerve fibres (22, 23, 87, 89, 91–95). SP/TK$^+$ and CGRP$^+$ nerves enter the thymus along the capsule and travel in the interlobular septa, where they frequently reside adjacent to mast cells. An occasional nerve fibre exits from the interlobular septa to pass among immature thymocytes in the parenchyma of the cortex, or to enter the medulla. SP$^+$ and CGRP$^+$ fibres also course along blood vessels, particularly those of the corticomedullary boundary, and are found in close association with the large number of mast cells also present along these vessels (22, 94). SP/CGRP-containing nerves reside adjacent to mast cells in the capsule, interlobular septum, and at the corticomedullary junction (22, 92, 94). Free SP fibres are especially prominent at the corticomedullary junction, and form close associations with SP-positive cells in this region (95). They are also closely apposed to ED1$^+$ and ED3$^+$ macrophages in the capsule, interlobular septum, cortex, and corticomedullary junction (22, 94).

Weihe *et al.* (87) suggest that TK and CGRP serve a sensory function. Treatment with capsaicin, a neurotoxin specific for small non-myelinated afferent nerves when administered in low concentrations, depletes SP in the thymus (96). These findings indicate that SP resides in neural compartments in the thymus, and support a sensory origin for SP. The distribution of CGRP$^+$ nerves in the thymus closely overlaps the distribution of SP$^+$ staining. Based on neurochemical measurements of SP and CGRP using radioimmunoassay following capsaicin treatment, these two peptides do not appear to be co-localized in the thymus (97). However, using anterograde tracing methods from the C2–C4 dorsal root ganglia of the guinea-pig, nerve fibres stain positive for both the tracer and for SP or CGRP. These studies further indicated that SP- and CGRP-immunoreactive nerves remain in the ipsilateral thymus, and are, at least in part, primary sensory afferents arising from cervical dorsal root ganglia (98).

While VIP⁺ nerves have not yet been reported in bone marrow, they have been demonstrated in other primary lymphoid organs, including the thymus and bursa fabricii of birds. VIP⁺ nerve fibres have been described in the rodent (4, 23, 88, 99, 100) and chicken (90) thymus. VIP⁺ nerves have a different pattern of innervation than SP and CGRP. Most VIP⁺ fibres are present in the capsule and interlobular septa, often residing close to mast cells. Some VIP⁺ nerves are also seen along blood vessels at the corticomedullary junction, closely associated with perivascular mast cells and macrophages (22, 100), and as free fibres in the capsule, cortex, and medulla. This association of peptide-containing nerves with mast cells is similar to that described in mucosa of the gut (101), and may be a source of neuropeptide signals for regulation of mast-cell secretion. In the chicken thymus, VIP fibres were more abundant than NPY, SP, or CGRP nerves (90).

Measurable levels of SOM, as well as mRNA for SOM, exist in the thymus (102). With immunofluorescent staining, SOM⁺ cells are present in the medulla and at the corticomedullary junction. At least some of the SOM⁺ cells are thymocytes (102). Immunocytochemistry for SOM has not provided convincing evidence for SOM⁺ nerves in the thymus. In support of non-neural sources of SOM in the thymus, Geppetti et al. (96) found that SOM-like immunoreactivity was not affected by either capsaicin or 6-OHDA treatment.

Similarly, immunocytochemical staining for oxytocin, AVP, and associated neurophysins is present in epithelial cells, nurse cells, and other non-neural elements in the human thymus (103–106), but there is no evidence that these neuropeptides are present in nerves that innervate the thymus. Using nicotinamide adenine dinucleotide phosphate-diaphorase (NADPH-d) histochemistry to demonstrate the presence of nitric oxide (NO) in nerves of the chick thymus (107), since it co-localizes with nitric oxide synthase (NOS) (90), the enzyme responsible for the synthesis of NO, NADPH-d⁺ nerves were occasionally seen in the interlobular septa by embryonic day 18/19 in the chick thymus (107). By day 21, these nerves formed perivascular plexuses, and occasional fibres were present in the medullary parenchyma. Corticotrophin-releasing hormone (CRH)-containing nerves have been found recently in the thymus and spleen 12 and 24 hours after intraperitoneal injection of human recombinant IL-2 into Fischer 344 rats (D. L. Bellinger, unpublished observation).

2.2.3 Spleen

The distribution of NPY⁺ nerves (23, 108–110) closely parallels NA innervation of the spleen. NPY⁺ nerves travel along the capsular, trabecular, and venous systems, and along the arterial systems, including prominent innervation of the central arterioles in the white pulp. NPY⁺ nerves arborize into the surrounding PALS away from the central arteriolar plexuses; these fibres end among T lymphocytes. Additional NPY⁺ fibres extend along the marginal sinus and are scattered in the marginal zone, where they branch among IgM⁺ B lymphocytes and ED1⁺ (111) and ED3⁺ macrophages. Ultrastructural analysis of immunocytochemically-stained spleen sections revealed direct contacts between NPY⁺ terminals and lymphocytes, similar to those seen for TH⁺ terminals (108, 110).

Romano and colleague (108) have shown that destruction of sympathetic NA nerves with 6-OHDA eliminates NPY⁺ profiles in immunocytochemically-stained sections. By differential staining of consecutive tissue sections, they also showed direct co-localization of TH and NPY in some nerve fibres in the rat spleen. Studies of the bovine splenic nerve (112) demonstrated NE and NPY co-localized in large, dense core vesicles with enkephalins. Immunofluorescence staining also supports co-localization of these neurotransmitters in some nerves along the large blood vessels near their entry into the bovine spleen. NE and NPY co-localize in vascular and trabecular nerves of spleens from cats (113) and pigs (114), where NPY is believed to mediate vasoconstriction and possibly play a neuromodulatory role, enhancing the action of NE on the vasculature.

SP-immunoreactive nerves innervate the vasculature of the pig and cat spleen, apparently to modulate vascular tone and blood volume (114, 115). In rodents, SP⁺ and CGRP⁺ nerves have been described along the vasculature and in lymphoid compartments of the spleen (23, 108–110, 116). SP⁺ and CGRP⁺ nerves (23, 91, 116) also appear to have overlapping distributions in the rat spleen, which differ from TH⁺, NPY⁺, or VIP⁺ nerve fibres. Overall, the spleen is more densely innervated by CGRP⁺ profiles. SP⁺ and CGRP⁺ nerves travel along the large venous sinuses and extend from these sinuses along the trabeculae. Numerous linear SP⁺ and CGRP⁺ nerves extend from the venous plexuses and trabeculae into the surrounding red pulp. SP⁺ and CGRP⁺ long, linear profiles occasionally travel through the marginal zone, and to a lesser extent, the PALS. SP⁺ fibres are sometimes present adjacent to large arteries near the hilus of the spleen, which is presumably their site of entry into the spleen.

Whether SP⁺ and CGRP⁺ nerves in the spleen represent sensory innervation is not clear. Very few myelinated fibres are reported in the splenic nerve (117, 118), and none is thus far described within the spleen itself. Tracing studies reveal very few labelled cells in sensory ganglia (119, 120). In a careful tracing study by Baron and Jänig (117), only 5 per cent of the fibres in the splenic nerve of the cat are sensory. Anterograde tracing of primary sensory afferents from thoracic dorsal root ganglia (T7–T12) also indicates the existence of sensory nerve fibres that contain SP and CGRP in the guinea-pig spleen (121). Physiological evidence of reflexes between the spleen and kidney indicates that some fibres are able to evoke reflex responses (reviewed in 5).

Lundberg *et al.* (115) reported VIP innervation of the splenic vasculature on which the nerves mediate vascular and volume control. These investigators did not further describe the distribution of these nerves in specific compartments of the spleen. Fried and colleagues (112) reported the presence of SP-, SOM-, and VIP-immunoreactive nerve profiles in the bovine splenic nerve that are not co-localized with NE. VIP was also described along the vasculature in the cat spleen (115). In the rat spleen, VIP⁺ nerves course along large arteries and central arterioles, and in the white pulp, venous/trabecular system, and red pulp (100). VIP innervation is more robust in Long–Evans hooded rats than in Fischer 344 rats (100). Surgical sympathectomy of the superior mesenteric–celiac ganglionic complex, the major source of sympathetic fibres to the spleen, does not alter splenic VIP content or the density of VIP⁺ nerves in the spleen (100).

Infusion of VIP results in vasodilation and increased splenic volume, suggesting that VIP may exert at least some of its effects directly on the vasculature. Similarly, we have found a sparse VIP innervation of the splenic vasculature (4, 23) and adjacent PALS, and relatively low VIP concentration in the rat spleen (122). VIP⁺ nerves course along the venous sinuses and trabeculae, in the red pulp, in the marginal zone, and along the central artery and in the adjacent PALS. The sparsity of VIP-immunoreactive fibres in the spleen is supported by the findings of Chevendra and Weaver (123) indicating that less than 1 per cent of the mesenteric neurons that innervate the spleen is immunoreactive for VIP. They also reported that no SOM⁺ neurons innervate the spleen, consistent with our efforts to stain for SOM in the spleen. VIP-immunoreactivity is also present in cells of the immune system, suggesting an additional source of VIP in the spleen (reviewed in 99). SOM also is present in cells of the spleen (102), and can be measured by radioimmunoassay (34.44±6.6 pg SOM per mg of protein in spleen) (102). SOM mRNA⁺ and SOM⁺ cells occur in clusters in the white pulp and are dispersed in the red pulp of the rat and chicken spleen. At least a subset of these cells are B lymphocytes (102). Again, SOM in nerves has not been revealed in the spleen.

A report by Schultzberg and colleagues (124) described IL-1-containing nerve fibres in the spleen, perhaps co-localized in sympathetic NA nerves. An early report by Felten *et al.* (4) indicates Met-enkephalin-containing nerves in the rodent spleen. Nohr *et al.* (125) have recently demonstrated proenkephalin opioid peptides in the porcine and bovine splenic nerves but were unable to find them in splenic nerves from rats, mice, hamsters, and guinea-pig. This study confirms earlier work by Fried and co-workers (112) who reported enkephalin-immunoreactive nerves in bovine spleen. In addition, Fried *et al.* (112) have provided evidence that enkephalin is co-expressed with NA and NPY in the splenic nerve. Nohr *et al.* (125) did not confirm the findings by Felten *et al.* (4) of enkephalin-containing nerves in the rat spleen. This discrepancy may be due to the use of antibodies with different specificities, or to strain differences. Enkephalin-containing nerves form a dense plexus along blood vessels in the spleen suggesting a functional role of opioid peptides in modulating vascular effector functions similar to those described for NPY and NE (125). In the PALS, numerous peri- and paravascular proenkephalin-immunoreactive fibres course in close apposition to lymphocytes and reticular cells. Proenkephalin-immunoreactive fibres also reside in the red pulp.

2.2.4 Lymph nodes

Immunoreactivity for NPY in nerves has been described in lymph nodes in a variety of mammalian species including rat (5, 23, 44, 126), mouse (44, 127), guinea-pig (44, 127), cat (44, 128), pig (44), beluga whale (109), and human (44). Studies from our laboratories have demonstrated NPY-immunoreactive nerve fibres in mesenteric, popliteal, and inguinal lymph nodes of the rat (5, 23). The distribution of NPY$^+$ nerves again appears to overlap NA innervation. NPY$^+$ nerves course along blood vessels in the hilus, medullary, and interfollicular regions of lymph nodes. Some NPY$^+$ fibres are present as linear profiles in the parenchyma in paracortical and cortical regions, where they end among fields of lymphocytes.

Immunoreactivity for SP and CGRP in nerves has been described in a variety of lymph nodes from many different mammalian species, including rat (5, 23, 44, 126), mouse (44, 127), guinea-pig (44, 127), cat (44, 128), pig (44), beluga whale (109), and human (44). In mesenteric, popliteal, and inguinal lymph nodes from the rat (5, 23), SP$^+$ and CGRP$^+$ nerves closely overlap in their distribution. These nerves are found in the hilus, beneath the capsule, at the corticomedullary junction, in medullary regions, and in internodal regions of the lymph nodes. SP$^+$ and CGRP$^+$ nerve fibres course along the vasculature or branch into the parenchyma among lymphocytes and accessory cells.

Immunoreactivity for VIP in nerves is found along the vasculature in internodal regions of the cortex, with meagre innervation of surrounding parenchyma, and along medullary cords (44, 128). VIP and PHI staining overlap in their distribution, and may be co-localized. These fibres generally are found in association with the vasculature. In the rat, VIP$^+$ nerves were found in mesenteric lymph nodes but not in popliteal lymph nodes (100).

Immunoreactivity for peptide histidine isoleucine (PHI), dynorphin A, enkephalin, and CCK in nerves has been described in lymph nodes. Dynorphin A$^+$ and CCK$^+$ profiles travel in the medulla of lymph nodes from the guinea-pig (129). In contrast to the spleen and thymus, SOM-immunoreactive cells are not found in lymph nodes (102), even though an SOM receptor may be present in these lymphoid organs in some sites (130). Popper *et al.*, however, could not detect SOM binding sites in mesenteric lymph nodes (128), suggesting regional difference in the cell composition of lymph nodes.

2.2.5 *Neuropeptides and immune function*

There is abundant evidence supporting modulation of immune responses by neuropeptides. Cells of the immune system possess receptors specific for neuropeptide found in nerves that innervate lymphoid tissue, including receptors for VIP, NPY, SP, SOM, and opioid peptides. Additionally, cells of the immune system contain many of the neuropeptides found in peripheral nerves. Neuropeptides can affect immune functions indirectly, since they are potent mediators of many vascular, smooth muscle, and secretory functions. Many neuropeptides recruit and activate mast cells to release an array of mediators, important mediators of inflammation, wound healing, and tissue repair.

NPY is most noted for synergizing effects of NE in the vasculature. In addition, NPY potently inhibits spontaneous activation of human granulocytes and macrophages, as well as *Mytilus edulis* immunocytes, in a concentration-dependent manner (131). NPY also inhibited the chemotactic response of these immunocytes to the chemoattractant, N-formylmethionylleucylphenylalanine (fMLP). Incubation of both human and invertebrate immunocytes in fMLP (10^{-9} M) causes 'activation' as noted by random locomotion (chemokinesis), an effect blocked by NPY. NPY at 10^{-9} to 10^{-12} M produced a significant dose-dependent suppression of NK-cell activity against K 562 target cells (132), an effect inhibited by rabbit anti-NPY anti-sera at 1:800 and 1:1600 dilutions. NPY (same concentration) also inhibited, in a dose-dependent fashion, NK activities of NK-enriched large granular lymphocytes against LAV-infected 8E5/LAV target cells. This effect was not due to direct toxicity of effector cells, since lymphocytes treated with NPY showed normal levels of ^{51}Cr release and their viability was comparable to that of untreated control cells.

NPY and peptide YY (10^{-12} to 10^{-8} M) stimulate several functions of resting peritoneal macrophages from BALB/c mice *in vitro*, including adherence to substrate, chemotaxis, ingestion of inert particle (latex beads) and foreign cells (*Candida albicans*), and production of superoxide anion measured by nitro-blue tetrazolium reduction. These effects are dose-dependent, with maximal stimulation of functions at 10^{-10} M (133), and are mediated via stimulation of protein kinase C (PKC). NPY upregulates the adhesiveness of human umbilical vein endothelial cells for ^{51}Cr-labelled human neutrophils or human monocytic U937 cell-line leukocytes ($0.01–1 \mu$) in a dose- and time-dependent manner (134). NPY also primes polymorphonuclear neutrophil oxidative metabolism, and causes a direct and dose-related increase in cytosolic calcium concentrations in these cells (135).

SP is involved in both acute hypersensitivity and delayed-type immune responses. At micromolar concentrations, SP evokes the release of histamine and leukotrienes from rat serosal or CT-type mast cells (136, 137). Elevated SP at local sites of inflammation in the patients with rheumatoid arthritis indicates that SP plays a role in chronic inflammation. In capsaicin-treated animals, the inflammatory responses to thermal, mechanical, and immunological stimulation is reduced. SP is a vasoactive peptide that increases blood flow and vascular permeability leading to vasodilatation and smooth muscle cell contraction (138, 139). *In vitro* studies have demonstrated that SP can release histamine and leukotrienes from mast cells, enhance phagocytosis, and promote polymorphonuclear leukocyte and mononuclear chemotaxis. SP stimulates human and guinea-pig monocyte chemotaxis *in vitro*, an effect blockable by D-amino acid analogues of SP, but not by antagonists of fMLP, suggesting SP specificity (140). SP also stimulates the synthesis of inflammatory mediators from macrophages activated by bacteria (141). Several other macrophage functions are evoked by SP, including downregulation of membrane-associated enzymes and the release of inflammatory products derived from the lipoxygenase and cyclooxygenase (COX) pathways (142), and stimulated production of IL-1, TNF-α, and IL-6 (143). SP-induced production of these cytokines may be important in the initiation of specific immune responses, and may play a role in inflammation, fever induction, and acute-phase protein production. SP-induced IL-6 synthesis is involved in B-lymphocyte maturation into antibody-producing cells, and in SP-induced enhancement of murine immunoglobulin synthesis. SP augments IgA, IgG$_3$, and IgG$_4$ production in IL-5 and TGF-β_2-stimulated purified human T and B cells, and blocks the inhibitory effect of IL-5 and TGF-β_2 on IgG$_1$ and IgM production (144). Except for IgM, these effects are blocked by SP receptor antagonists. In this culture, T and B cells expressed neurokinin-1 (NK1) receptors, and after co-stimulation, NK3 receptors. These effects were only present in T- and B-cell co-cultures after activation, and were dependent on co-stimulation by IL-5 and TGF-β_2.

SP, in nanomolar concentrations, stimulates human and murine T-lymphocyte proliferation (145, 146). SP increases the *in vitro* production of IgA in lymphocytes from spleen and Peyer's patches (146), an effect mediated by IL-6 release. SP receptors are present on T and B lymphocytes (147, 148). SP is present in eosinophils (149) from chronic granuloma in livers from mice infected with the parasite *Schistosomiasis mansoni*. During the late stages of certain inflammatory responses, SP and substance K promote tissue repair by enhancing the proliferation of smooth muscle cells, fibroblasts, and endothelial cells (150, 151) through SP receptor binding and subsequent increases in Ca^{2+}, suggesting phosphatidylinositol pathway activation (151).

A single class of SP-binding sites have been reported on guinea-pig macrophages using the low-specific activity [^{3}H]SP ligand with a K_d of approximately 19 nM (142). Functional studies indicate that quiescent and activated human monocytes express SP receptors, but these have not been fully characterized with binding studies. SP receptors are also present on a human B-lymphoblast cell line (IM-9) (152).

One of the principal activities of CGRP is vasodilatation. CGRP augments SP-induced microvascular permeability, promoting a greater cutaneous flare and wheal, but does not alter vascular permeability alone. CGRP inhibits the enzymatic degradation of SP, enhancing the activity of SP when they are released together. In immediate hypersensitivity reactions, CGRP has both indirect and direct effects on target tissues, activating and regulating tissue mast cells and basophils. CGRP suppresses mitogen- and antigen-induced proliferation of thymocytes, splenocytes, lymph node cells, and purified T lymphocytes (153–156), inhibits NK-cell activity (43, 157), and inhibits DTH and contact hypersensitivity response (158). CGRP also reduces antigen presentation by macrophages (158–160), and decreases macrophage antigen presentation, in part, by reducing expression of B7–2 (159, 160). CGRP-induced inhibition of antigen presentation was abrogated by anti-IL-10, suggesting that the response is mediated by IL-10, and is consistent with an increase in IL-10 production following treatment of macrophages with CGRP. CGRP also reduces macrophage IL-1, IL-12, and IFN-γ (159, 160) production. CGRP is chemotactic for CD4$^+$ and CD8$^+$ T cells, suggesting a role in lymphocyte trafficking.

A variety of human and rodent lymphoid cell lines possess VIP receptors, including Molt-4b, SUPT-1, and Jurkat T-cell lines, and Raji, Kakiki, Nalm6, U266, and SKW 6.4 B-cell lines (reviewed in 99). The binding sites on these cell lines are similar in their selectivity and/or molecular weight to that seen in normal tissue preparations. THP-1 monocyte/macrophage and murine T-lymphoblastic cell lines bear unusual VIP receptors in that the high-affinity receptors recognize helodermin with higher affinity than VIP and PHI (161, 162). VIP-binding sites are present on human monocytes, T cells, B cells, neutrophils, and erythrocytes (reviewed in 99). In rodents, VIP receptors have been reported on T lymphocytes and macrophages (163, 164).

VIP influences the regional distribution and trafficking of lymphocytes, particularly in gut-associated lymphoid tissue (GALT). Depending on the concentration, VIP either inhibits (10^{-7} to 10^{-9} M) or stimulates (10^{-12} to 10^{-14} M) mononuclear leukocyte migration in a sealed capillary migration test (165). In mice, transfer of labelled syngeneic lymphocytes after incubation with VIP *in vitro* downregulates VIP receptors on treated cells and decreases localization of the treated cells in mesenteric lymph nodes and Peyer's patches, with no change in migration of VIP-treated cells to other lymphoid or non-lymphoid compartments (166). Infusion of VIP into afferent lymphatics of popliteal lymph nodes in sheep increases intracellular cAMP in lymphocytes, and reduces egress of lymphocytes from the nodes, while agents such as SP that increase guanosine 3′,5′-cyclic monophosphate (cGMP) have an opposite effect on lymphocyte egress (167). Similarly, infusion of VIP into the superior mesenteric artery of the rat reduces lymphocyte migration through intestinal (especially Th cells) and mesenteric lymph nodes (particularly T-suppressor cells) without changing lymph flow (168). The change in CD4$^+$ T cells is consistent with the findings of Moore *et al.* (167) and Ottaway (166); the changes in CD8$^+$ are not. A selective decrease in the number of CD4$^+$ IgA$^+$ cells in GALT may diminish T-helper cell-driven inhibition of suppressor T-cell activity, promoting reduced antibody response to presentation of antigen (169). VIP stimulates *in vitro* chemotaxis of T lymphocytes from both CD4$^+$ and CD8$^+$ subsets (as well as monocytes, but not neutrophils), an effect more potent on unstimulated T cells than activated T cells. In these cells, VIP induces cell adhesion to intercellular adhesion molecule (ICAM) and vascular (VCAM) integrins, and to fibronectin (170, 171).

VIP (in concentrations ranging from 10^{-7} to 10^{-10} M) inhibits mitogen- and antigen-induced proliferation and decreases IL-2 and IL-4 production (but not IFN-γ) in rodent T lymphocytes from a variety of tissues (reviewed in 99). This effect can be blocked by co-incubation of VIP with dexamethasone at the time of mitogen stimulation (172). An 18-hour preincubation with low concentrations of VIP has no effect on proliferation, but makes these cells resistant to the effects of dexamethasone. An 18-hour preincubation with high concentrations of VIP increased proliferation, an effect blockable by dexamethasone. In contrast, VIP effects on mitogen-stimulated proliferation in human peripheral blood lymphocytes, and in cell lines, are not consistent (reviewed in 99).

VIP effects on antibody concentration are isotype- and tissue-specific (146, 173). VIP (10^{-8} M) increases the IgA response in mesenteric lymph nodes and spleen, but inhibits IgA synthesis in cells from Peyer's patches. IgM synthesis in Peyer's patches is increased by VIP, but is not affected by 10^{-8} M VIP in spleen and mesenteric lymph nodes. IgG synthesis is not altered in these lymphoid organs by VIP. These effects are believed to be T-cell mediated, and differences in organ responses may be related to differences in local T-cell subsets in these organs. In contrast, Neil *et al.* (174) found no effect of VIP on immunoglobulin production by splenic and liver granuloma cell preparations from *S. mansoni*-infected mice incubated with VIP for 4 hours. These differences may result from differences in B-cell subsets in the cultures, differences in antigen used to activate B cells, or may reflect the length of time that cells are cultured in the presence of VIP.

In human mononuclear cells from tonsillectomies for chronic tonsillitis in non-atopic children, VIP (10 pM to 10 nM) inhibits IL-4 stimulated IgE, IgG_2, and IgG_4 production (175), an effect that requires both T cells and monocytes and involves IL-4-induced isotype switching. VIP also inhibits spontaneous IgE and IgG4 production in human atopic tonsils (176). VIP stimulates IgA_1, IgA_2, and IgM production in sIgM$^+$ and sIgM$^-$, CD19$^+$ foetal B cells (sIgA$^-$) stimulated with anti-CD40 monoclonal antibody (177). Collectively, these studies indicate selective modulation of different antibody classes and subclasses by VIP that involves isotype switching, and that VIP effects on antibody response require both T cells and monocytes in the B-cell cultures.

The effects of VIP on NK-cell activity are variable depending on the source of NK cells, activational state, the target cells, whether cells are pre-incubated with VIP before but not during the assay, or whether VIP was present throughout the assay period (co-incubation), assay incubation time, and concentration of VIP. Continual presence of VIP in a 4-hour cytotoxicity assay produces a potent inhibition of NK-cell activity in human peripheral blood lymphocytes to K-562 target cells (10^{-6} M only; 10^{-10} to 10^{-8} M, optimal 10^{-8} M; 10^{-8} to 10^{-6} M) (178–180). Addition of $2',5'$-dideoxyadenosine (DDA), an inhibitor of adenylate cyclase, to the culture does not block VIP-induced inhibition of NK-cell activity (179).

In human peripheral blood lymphocyte cultures pre-incubated with VIP at 10^{-10} to 10^{-8} M for 30 to 60 minutes and washed before the assay, VIP-enhanced cytotoxicity of cells against the target occurs (179), blockable by DDA. van Tol and colleagues (181, 182) found that pre-incubation of VIP (10^{-8} M) stimulates cytotoxicity of human peripheral blood mononuclear cells, and lamina propria mononuclear cells from normal mucosa, against CaCo-2 human colon cancer cells but not against K-562 target cells. A decrease in NK-cell activity without a decrease in NK-cell number occurs in patients with inflammatory bowel disease (183), suggesting the possibility that a loss of VIP innervation in the gut may contribute to NK-cell dysfunction (184, 185).

VIP has a protective effect on inflamed lung tissue from injury caused by hydrochloric acid (186), xanthine/xanthine oxide (187), and toxic oxygen metabolites (188). Some effects of VIP are indirect, acting on vascular smooth muscle (vasodilator) and endothelial cells of the vasculature to change blood vessel diameter, plasma extravasation, and cell adhesion molecular expression (189). VIP does, however, directly influence accessory cells of the immune system. Micromolar concentrations of VIP inhibit superoxide anion (O_2^-) formation in fMLP-activated inflammatory cells (peripheral blood neutrophils and mononuclear cells) from healthy human subjects (188). A similar effect of VIP on O_2^- formation is seen in the human monoblastoid cell line, U937, peripheral blood eosinophils, and aveolar macrophage (188). VIP, in nanomolar concentrations, inhibits the respiratory burst of human monocytes in response to zymogen by a cAMP-mediated mechanism (190), while VIP at 10^{-7} M for 2 minutes primes respiratory bursts in human neutrophils induced by either phorbol myristate acetate or fMLP. The latter effect does not appear to be mediated through binding of VIP with VIP receptors.

VIP moderately inhibits antigen-induced release of histamine from guinea-pig lung (191) and peptidoleukotriene release from platelet-activating factor-stimulated rat lung tissue (192). This response (a response also seen in other mucosal sites) differs from that seen in rat peritoneal mast cells and in human skin where VIP evokes histamine release in a non-cytolytic manner (193–195).

SOM can have an indirect effect on immune function, particularly inflammation, by blocking the release of SP from peripheral nerve endings (136). SOM receptors are present on T cells, basophilic leukaemia cells, basophils, and mast cells, and can modulate several immune functions *in vitro*, including concentration-dependent modulation of spontaneous proliferation of murine splenocytes (196), inhibition of mitogen-stimulated proliferation of murine splenocytes (197), human T lymphocytes, and Molt-4b human lymphoblast cells (198), and reduction in colony-stimulating activity of murine splenocytes (199). SOM is also a major mediator of immediate hypersensitivity through its stimulation of leukocyte and monocyte chemotaxis (140), neutrophil phagocytosis (200), macrophages effector functions (142), and release of histamine and leukotrienes by basophils and mast cells (195, 201). At low concentrations, SOM inhibits IgE-dependent release of histamine from human basophils and rat basophilic leukaemia cells (201), but at higher concentrations SOM inhibits the immunological release of mediators from mucosal mast cells (202). In the parasitic disease *S. mansoni*, SOM modulates the amount of IgG_{2a} secreted in response to schistosome egg antigens in murine *S. mansoni*, and inhibits IFN release from macrophages in the inflamed liver and intestines via binding to SOM receptors on granuloma T cells (203, 204).

3 Neuroendocrine mediators of neural–immune modulation

Every hormone secreted or regulated by the pituitary gland has been shown to affect at least some parameters within the immune system. The earliest evidence indicating the importance of the neuroendocrine system on immune regulation comes from clinical studies in patients with neuroendocrine deficiencies, and from studies using laboratory animals in which the pituitary had been removed. Since these early observations, more sophisticated techniques have been used to determine the influence of pituitary hormones on immune function. Also, it has become clear that in addition to pituitary-derived hormones, cells of the immune system can synthesize and release most, if not all, of the pituitary hormones thus far identified. Early observations will not be reviewed here; instead, more recent literature demonstrating the effects of each of the pituitary hormones on the immune system will be described.

3.1 GROWTH HORMONE

Thymocytes and thymic epithelial cells, splenocytes, and lymph node cells synthesize GH-releasing hormone (GHRH) and GH, providing an extra-pituitary and extra-hypothalamic source, respectively, for these hormones. Since immunocytes possess receptors for these hormones (205, 206), these findings suggest that GHRH and GH released by cells of the immune system are involved in the autocrine/paracrine regulation of immune functions. The contribution made by GH and GHRH released from cells of the immune system to the modulation of immune function is not clear at present, but perhaps local release promotes macrophage activation, killing of bacteria and viruses, and local release of cytokines. The distribution of human (h)GH receptors are relatively high on CD20$^+$ B cells, while fewer receptors are expressed on CD3$^+$ T cells and CD16$^+$ NK cells. In the rat spleen, B cells, T helper cells, and macrophages are predominantly responsible for the secretion of GH, whereas T-suppressor cells and NK cells synthesize and secrete only minor quantities of GH (205). *In vivo* GH administration increases the release of thymocytes from the thymus, the percentage of CD3-bearing cells, the total thymocyte count, and the secretion of thymulin from thymic epithelial cells. *In vitro* addition of GH increases the secretion of thymulin from thymic epithelial cultures. Intraventricular infusion of MB-35 peptide, a fragment of thymosin component, and *in vitro* perfusion of the rat pituitaries with thymulin enhances pituitary GH production (207, 208). These findings demonstrate the involvement of GH and thymic hormones in the bidirectional regulation of neuroendocrine–immune system interactions.

The ontogeny of GH and GH-receptor expression in lymphoid organs varies depending upon the species and the lymphoid tissue examined. GH mRNA is predominantly distributed in the bone marrow and thymus, but not in the spleen or liver, of neonatal rats (209). GH-receptor expression in bovine foetal thymocytes is high during the early and mid-gestational period, and relatively low during the late-gestational period, but no changes in GH-receptor density occurs on splenocytes during gestation (210). The difference in GH-receptor density with gestation in the thymus may reflect a preference for maturation of thymocyte specific subsets bearing GH receptors, or in the homing pattern of GH-receptor-positive cells. Early expression of GH receptors in the bovine fetus is of relevance to humans, because the immune system in the human fetus attains early maturity as in cattle. The specific binding of radiolabelled-hGH and hGH-receptor mRNA expression in peripheral blood lymphocytes is low in newborns, and increases progressively with adulthood. mRNA expression for insulin-like growth factor-1 (IGF-1), IGF-2, and IGF-binding proteins (1–6) in newborn and adult thymus and lymph nodes, suggests that these hormones may influence heterogeneous functions in the thymus, and exert a paracrine effect on lymphocytes in lymph nodes (211). GH, IGF, and IGF-binding proteins in the thymus may influence the development of immunity through the induction of cytokines, the promotion of T-cell maturation, and enhanced adhesion and subsequent migration to target lymphoid organs, although the exact mechanisms have not been elucidated.

Numerous investigators have demonstrated a role for GH and IGF-1 in erythropoiesis, lymphopoiesis, and myelopoiesis (212). In normal and dwarf rodents, administration of GH or IGF-1 enhances the weight of the spleen and thymus. It also augments the number of $CD4^+/CD8^+$ progenitor cells in the thymus, and $CD4^+$ T cells and B cells in the spleen. Similarly, in transgenic mice that overexpress GHRH and GH, there is an increase in the thymus and spleen weight, and in the B- and T-cell mitogen-induced proliferation in splenocytes (213). Addition of bovine GH stimulates the *in vitro* proliferation of lectin- or anti-CD3-activated T lymphocytes in mice, presumed to be a direct effect of GH on T lymphocytes that is mediated by cytokine release (214). *In vitro* incubation of human peripheral blood mononuclear cells with hGH stimulates the proliferation of IFN-γ-secreting cells and IFN-γ production (215). There is no difference in basal Con A-, phytohaemagglutinin (PHA)-, and pokeweed mitogen-induced lymphocyte proliferation in hGH-deficient children; however, therapy with hGH increases PHA-induced proliferation (205).

GH enhances NK-cell activity, possibly through hGH and IGF-1 receptors on these cells. In patients with GH deficiency, NK-cell activity is reduced, the expression of GH-binding sites is increased on NK cells, and NK-cell numbers remain unchanged (216). A similar reduction in NK-cell activity is found in children with GH deficiency, but administration of GH does not increase cytolytic activity in these children, possibly due to developmental deficits in NK cells. Acute and chronic administration of GH to healthy human subjects significantly enhances NK-cell activity (217). Saxena and colleagues (218) report reduced NK-cell killing of virus-infected targets in hypophysectomized mice. Administration of ovine GH to these animals for 10 days significantly increased the cytolytic activity of NK cells in these mice.

Postoperative infections are common in patients with low levels of IGF-1 and GH. It is speculated that this may be the due to chronic activation of the immune system by LPS, a component of bacterial cell walls, followed by reduced proliferation and migration of peripheral mononuclear cells and monocytes, phagocytic activity and opsonic activity (219, 220). Supplemental GH and IGF-1 therapy in mice and humans prevents septic shock by enhancing the bactericidal functions of macrophages, augmenting IgG production by B lymphocytes, and preventing TNF-α release through a reduction in nuclear translocation of nuclear factor-kappa B (NF-κB) (219, 221). GH also promotes the bactericidal functions of peripheral mononuclear cells through the downregulation of Fas expression. Furthermore, GH inhibits apoptosis in mononuclear cells, prolonging the viability of these cells and inducing reactive oxygen intermediates that are responsible for the killing of ingested bacteria (222). Stimulation of humoral immunity with restoration of GH in hypophysectomized rainbow trout occurs by implantation of GH, a procedure that reverses the reduction in IgM levels (223).

Clinical studies indicate a role for GH in immune regulation. There is an increase in phagocytic activity and CD71 expression of CD4⁺ and CD8⁺ T cells in patients with acromegaly compared to normal individuals, indicating that either GH or IGF-1 may be responsible for the enhancement of T-cell activity (224). This hypothesis is supported by the finding that the age-related decline in Con A-induced T-cell proliferation is linked to a reduction in IGF-1 levels in the elderly population (225). A correlative study between serum GH and IGF-1 levels and stages of lung cancer reveals an increase in GH, and a decrease in IGF-1 levels with advancing stages of cancer (226). In chronically stressed female caregivers, GH mRNA expression is significantly lower in blood mononuclear cells and B cells, resulting in diminished antibody response to influenza virus vaccination (227). Preliminary evidence suggests that IGF-1 levels are lower in patients with the juvenile form of degenerative arthritis than normal, age-matched subjects, suggesting that GH administration to such patients may be helpful in arresting the progression of the disease. In support of this potential therapy, IGF-1 promotes the synthesis of proteoglycan and enhances the formation of extracellular matrix in articular cartilage (228), important for repairing tissue damage to the joints.

In HIV patients treated with rhGH and rhIGF-1, an increase in *in vitro* IL-2 production by peripheral blood mononuclear cells in response to an HIV-1 envelope peptide supports the use of GH and/or IGF-1 as an immunostimulatory agent in HIV, as well as other diseases, including cancer, where augmenting cell-mediated immunity would be beneficial (229). Similarly, in mice, HIV-1-gp120 enhances IL-4 production, indicating a shift towards humoral Th2-type immune responses, which are not as effective in handling the HIV infection (230). Conversely, administration of hGH increases the synthesis of IL-2 and IFN-γ and decreases IL-4 production, attributable to a GH-evoked shift from Th2-lymphocyte activation to Th1-cell activation in these mice (230).

3.2 PROLACTIN

Prolactin (PRL) is critical for the maintenance of immunocompetence, and is produced by both the anterior pituitary and lymphocytes from the human thymus, spleen, tonsil, and mesenteric lymph nodes (MLNs). PRL-producing lymphoid cells are primarily T lymphocytes localized in the subcapsular cortex of thymus, paracortex of tonsil and lymph nodes, and in the PALS of the white pulp and marginal zone of spleen (231). CD4$^-$CD8$^-$ and CD4$^+$ T cells in the human thymus, and B cells, monocytes and T cells in the peripheral blood, express a high density of PRL receptors (232). The two isoforms of the PRL receptor and PRL protein levels are differentially regulated in the thymus and spleen during the various stages of the oestrous cycle, and during pregnancy and lactation in rats, indicating that other hormones such as LH, FSH, progesterone, and oestrogen may be involved in regulating PRL-receptor expression on cells of the immune system (233). It should be noted that besides these hormones, GH can also activate PRL receptors in humans, because PRL receptors belong to the class of haematopoietic receptor superfamily that include erythropoietin, ILs, growth factors, and GH (234). Binding of PRL to PRL receptors results in dimerization or oligomerization of the receptor, followed by activation of PRL-receptor-associated JAK2 kinases. Multiple targets are phosphorylated within the cytoplasm and then translocated to the nucleus to activate interferon regulatory factor-1 (IRF-1) (235).

Grafting of the thymus and pituitary in athymic nude mice increases the CD4/CD8 ratio, similar to that seen in immunocompetent BALB/c mice, and with stimulation of CD4$^+$ T-cell development. This finding suggests that PRL is important for maturation and migration of T cells from the thymus into the periphery (235). Several studies have demonstrated that the effects of PRL on the immune system are dependent upon the circulating levels of this hormone, with physiological plasma concentrations of PRL providing a stimulatory influence, and supra-physiological plasma PRL levels providing an inhibitory effect on immune functions. Hyper- and hypoprolactinaemia cause abnormal B-cell, T-cell, and NK-cell functions, changes that may be responsible for the development and progression of autoimmune disorders such as experimentally induced arthritis and encephalomyelitis. Restoration of PRL in the plasma to physiological levels restores these immune responses to normal ranges (236, 237). PRL is capable of transcriptionally regulating interferon regulatory factor-1 (IRF-1), a factor encoded by the PRL-inducible gene that can regulate gene expression in B and T lymphocytes, myeloid cells, and fibroblasts, as well as NK-cell cytotoxic activity (236, 238). *In vitro* addition of PRL enhances proliferation of Con A-induced splenocytes, peripheral blood cells, and thymocytes, effects mediated through either IRF-1 or an upregulation of receptors for the cytokine, erythropoietin, and for PRL on these cells. The inhibition of glucocorticoid (GC)-induced apoptosis by PRL in T cells and the enhancement of IgG and IgM antibody production by B cells suggests that PRL has multiple functions in the regulation of the immune system (236). Physiological levels of PRL may participate in the differentiation of Th cells to Th1 type, indicated by its ability to induce expression of splenic IL-2 receptors and IFN-γ synthesis (239, 240).

PRL-receptor-bearing macrophages synthesize PRL. In mice, hypoprolactinaemia results in suppression of macrophage functions, including antigen processing and phagocytic activity, while administration of PRL activates these macrophage functions (241). Incubation of murine peritoneal macrophages with PRL enhances NO and IL-1 production through the activation of PKC (242). PRL treatment of mice infected with *Salmonella typhimurium* confers immunoprotection, an effect that is mediated via PRL receptor activation and subsequent production of NO (243). Suppression of both inducible and constitutively expressed IL-1β, IL-6, and TNF-α in peritoneal macrophages from mice with sepsis is reversed by treatment with PRL and a dopamine antagonist (244). High doses of PRL suppress NK-cell activity while there was an enhancement of cytolytic activity in purified NK cells. Inhibition of NK-cell activity in hyperprolactinaemia may be due to interruption of PRL to PRL-receptor signalling due to high amounts of PRL. Besides inducing the differentiation of NK cells, PRL is responsible for promoting lymphokine-activated killer-cell activity by IL-2 (237).

Hyperprolactinaemia is evident in patients with AIDS, rheumatoid and psoriatic arthritis, multiple sclerosis, and systemic lupus erythematosus. Administration of bromocriptine, a dopamine agonist, corrects deficiencies in T-cell and NK-cell functions in patients with hyperprolactinaemia (236, 237). The immunomodulatory role of PRL in breast cancer is yet to be understood, but recent evidence reveals that PRL is produced by the mammary gland in rodents and also by breast tissue in humans. The trophic effects of PRL in other target tissues raises the question as to whether it may have similar effects on mammary tumours.

Recent studies indicate that PRL and PRL-receptor pathways are not essential for immunomodulation. In PRL-deficient mice, myelopoiesis and lymphopoiesis is normal, but defects in the development of the mammary glands are apparent (245). Similarly, there are no alterations in thymic and splenic cellularity, antibody response to T-cell-dependent antigen, production of antibodies, regulation of bacterial infection, or NK-cell cytotoxic activity in PRL-receptor-deficient mice (246). However, these studies are not sufficiently conclusive to discount the role of PRL in immunoregulation, because the existence of yet to be identified subtypes of PRL receptors, interactions with GH and placental lactogen receptors, signalling through other members of cytokine receptor family by PRL, and altered development may contribute to their findings. For the same reasons it is difficult to interpret the immunoregulatory functions of PRL, since most of the data are obtained with Nb2, a T-lymphoma cell line that is different from normal lymphoid cells. However, PRL is clearly important for the development, maturation, and migration of T and B lymphocytes in the thymus and in other peripheral lymphoid organs.

3.3 THE HYPOTHALAMIC–PITUITARY–ADRENAL AXIS

3.3.1 *Corticotrophin-releasing hormone*

Corticotrophin-releasing hormone (CRH) plays a major role in modulating endocrine, autonomic, behavioural, and immune responses to stress. CRH can influence immune responses to stress through a variety of mechanisms. First, CRH secreted from the PVN of the hypothalamus integrates the stress response in the CNS through two different pathways. CRH acts on the pituitary to release proopiomelanocortin (POMC) from the anterior pituitary. POMC is cleaved enzymatically to form ACTH, α-melanocyte-stimulating hormone (α-MSH), and β-endorphin. ACTH releases GC from the zona fasciculata of the adrenal gland. GCs interact with specific receptors inside cells of the immune system to alter immune function. Stress responses are also mediated through the action of CRH on central descending autonomic pathways, which ultimately enhances sympathetic outflow.

CRH also has direct effects on cells of the immune system via binding to receptors on their cell surface. High-affinity binding sites for CRH are present on rat monocyte/macrophages, and on human T-helper and B lymphocytes (247–249). These receptors have structural and pharmacological characteristics similar to those expressed in brain, pituitary, and placental tissue. mRNA and protein for CRH-receptor 1 (CRH-R1) in splenic neutrophils can be induced by acute systemic inflammation induced by i.p. administration of LPS (250).

CRH and its mRNA are also present in lymphoid organs, and are produced by a subset of macrophages, human peripheral blood T and B lymphocytes, neutrophils, and erythrocytes (251–256). Human lymphocytes and Jurkat T lymphoma cells are reported to produce urocortin, a recently identified neuropeptide related to CRH, but not CRH (257). NA sympathetic nerves course adjacent to CRH-producing cells in lymphoid organs, suggesting that NE can modulate CRH production and/or release from these cells, perhaps in a way similar to that seen in the HPA axis (256). Functional studies indicate that CRH is released from these cells in lymphoid organs upon cell activation, which, in turn, modulates immune responses. CRH stimulates activated monocytes to produce IL-1, which then induces B-lymphocyte secretion of POMC-derived peptides (ACTH and β-endorphin) (258, 259). CRH alters the secretion of other cytokines, including IL-2 and IL-6, stimulates mitogen-induced T-lymphocyte proliferation, enhances IL-2 receptor expression, and alters NK-cell activity (260–263).

Regardless of the source of CRH, it is clear that this signalling molecule is important for coordinating immune, endocrine, and CNS responses to stressors imposed by a variety of immunological challenges (bacteria, viruses, or neoplastic cells) and inflammatory responses that result from injury. Intracerebroventricular (i.c.v.) administration of urocortin markedly decreased the proliferative responses of splenocytes to a mitogen, an effect blocked by interfering with sympathetic outflow but not by adrenalectomy (264). These findings are consistent with the literature, indicating that the enhancing effects of CRH appear to be indirect, via IL-1-stimulated release of β-endorphin from B lymphocytes, while the suppressive effects of CRH are thought to be mediated via central release of CRH with consequent sympathetic activation.

α-MSH blocks the effects of CRH on immune cells by interfering with the action IL-1 on target cells. CRH responses that are blockable by α-MSH, as well as ACTH, include IL-1-mediated fever, anorexia, elevation of ACTH and corticosterone, and suppression of NK-cell activity. These studies suggest that ACTH, α-MSH, and possibly GC may serve as negative feedback mechanisms to suppress the excess release of CRH-induced cytokines by lymphoid cells in response to various stressors or pathogenic stimuli (viruses, bacteria, or tumour cells) (265, 266).

Recent studies indicate a role for CRH in inflammation. In animals models of rheumatoid arthritis, CRH is elevated in affected joints and acts as both an autocrine and paracrine mediator at these sites (267, 268). Centrally administered CRH blunts endothelial upregulation of ICAM-1 and attenuates the recruitment of leukocytes during endotoxaemia. Anti-inflammatory effects of CRH are mediated by adrenocortical activation, and possibly other mechanisms that are independent of α-MSH (269).

Cytokines (IL-1, IL-2, and IL-6) modulate release of CRH from neurons in the HPA axis, and from cells of the immune system (270–277). In mice that are CRH-R1 (the receptor type that predominantly mediates CRH-induced

ACTH secretion) deficient, it is still possible to mount a pituitary–adrenal response to turpentine-induced local inflammation via mechanisms that do not depend critically on either CRH or AVP action. Resting levels of ACTH in these mice are attributable, in part, to arginine vasopressin (AVP)-dependent mechanisms. Interpretation of these data is difficult, but suggests multiple mechanisms for the regulation of ACTH release from the pituitary gland.

AVP is also involved in stress-induced suppression of immune function. AVP, as well as oxytocin, is produced and secreted into the posterior pituitary from axons that arise from neurons in the mPVN and the SON. AVP can also be secreted from CRH neurons that regulate ACTH release (278, 279), particularly during increased pituitary–adrenal activity (280). Additionally, AVP and oxytocin from other sources can contribute to the pool of ACTH secretagogues in the hypophyseal portal blood (281–283). AVP, and possibly oxytocin, interact synergistically with CRH to stimulate ACTH secretion (284). The extent to which this occurs varies with the nature of the physiological threat. Suppression of proliferative response of splenic T cells to Con A and NK activity from intermittent electrical footshock for 60 minutes is blocked (partially and completely, respectively) by i.c.v. pre-administration of a V1 receptor antagonist (285). Footshock-induced suppression of the T-cell proliferative response is completely abolished by co-administration of a CRH-receptor antagonist, and the V1-receptor antagonist, but does not involve the adrenal gland. So AVP, in conjunction with CRH, suppresses immune function through V1 receptors in rats, at least under certain types of stressor.

3.3.2   POMC-derived products: ACTH, α-MSH, and endorphins

ACTH, α-MSH, and endorphin modulate immune function. ACTH indirectly modulates immune reactivity through its ability to stimulate the release of glucocorticoids (GCs) from the adrenal gland. ACTH from the anterior pituitary can be released by hormones other than CRH, including AVP, oxytocin, and leukaemia inhibitory factor (LIF). LIF increases ACTH secretion and POMC mRNA level in murine corticotroph tumour cell line (AT-20), and primary cultured normal rat pituitary cells, but does not augment CRH-induced ACTH secretion by these cells.

In addition to its ability to stimulate the release of GCs from the adrenal gland, ACTH also has a direct effect on cells of the immune system by binding to high-affinity and low-affinity receptors on mononuclear leukocytes that are very similar in structure and pharmacology to ACTH receptors present on adrenal cells (286). B cells express approximately three times more ACTH receptors than T cells (287). $ACTH_{1-39}$ added to lymphocyte cultures suppresses *in vitro* antibody production (288) and macrophage-mediated tumoricidal activity (289), alters B-lymphocyte function (290), and decreases IFN-γ production (288).

IgM secretion by a B-cell line is enhanced by exposure of 10^{-12} to 10^{-10} M ACTH *in vitro*, with or without LPS stimulation (291). ACTH may also act to increase B-cell proliferation at later stages of B-cell stimulation, in concert with IL-5 (292). However, *in vivo* treatment of adrenalectomized mice with ACTH has no effect on spleen cell antibody production *in vitro* (293). NK-cell activity is enhanced in pigs treated with ACTH (294), but ACTH has no effect on NK-cell activity when added *in vitro*, suggesting that ACTH acts indirectly to effect NK-cell activity, possibly through reduced CRH production by cells in the culture. Both ACTH and β-endorphin, as well as other opioid peptides, modulate immune responses by altering receptors on lymphocytes, including CD2 expression, expression and conformation of CD3, and the affinity of IL-2 receptors for IL-2 (reviewed in 295). Further research using both *in vitro* and *in vivo* techniques is needed to fully elucidate the role of ACTH as an immunomodulator.

α-MSH (ACTH$_{1-13}$) has similar actions to ACTH. α-MSH is more potent and faster acting than the parent ACTH in inhibiting migration in response to IL-1 and other chemotactic agents (296). A similar ability of α-MSH over ACTH occurs in the prevention of spontaneous neutrophil activation. The ability of α-MSH to block several functions of IL-1 suggests that it may have an important role in downregulating immune responses (266, 296, 297).

The products obtained from β-lipotropin (pituitary-derived opioid peptides) include α-endorphin (31 amino acids) and products derived from its N-terminus, including β-endorphin (16 amino acids), δ-endorphin (27 amino acids), and γ-endorphin (17 amino acids). This family of opioid peptides is also an important group of immunomodulators. β-Endorphin alters the proliferative activity of lymphocytes (298, 299), NK-cell activity (300–302), antibody synthesis by B cells (288, 303), and IFN-γ production by T cells (304, 305). β-Endorphin also inhibits production of a T-lymphocyte chemotactic factor by Con A-stimulated human peripheral blood mononuclear cells (306), and may serve as a chemotactic factor itself since increased migration of human T lymphocytes was demonstrated *in vitro* in the presence of this peptide (307). Enhancement of Con A-stimulated splenocyte proliferation (298, 308, 309), suppression of PHA-stimulated human lymphocyte proliferation (310), and inhibition of prostaglandin E$_1$ (PGE$_1$)-induced suppression (311) by β-endorphin appear to be mediated through a non-opioid receptor-mediated mechanism. Non-opioid-mediated effects of β-endorphin may be due to C-terminal binding to an as yet unidentified receptor. Whether other effects of β-endorphin are mediated through the interaction of β-endorphin with genuine opioid receptors or some form of a non-opioid receptor has yet to be resolved.

3.3.3 Glucocorticoids

Glucocorticoids (GCs) are potent modulators of immune and inflammatory responses. GCs generally, but not always, downregulate the immune and inflammatory responses during stressful conditions, presumably to prevent defence mechanisms from overshooting, and subsequently damaging the organism or inducing autoimmune diseases. GCs are potent inhibitors of inflammation, and synthetic GCs are widely used to treat inflammatory disorders such as rheumatoid arthritis, inflammatory bowel disease, asthma, and autoimmune diseases (312–316). The anti-inflammatory effects of GCs are mediated either by direct binding of the GC–GC-receptor complex to GC-responsive elements in the promoter regions of genes, or by an interaction of this complex with other transcription factors; in particular, activating protein-1 (AP-1) or nuclear factor-kappa B (NF-κB). GCs inhibit many mediators of inflammatory responses. The most striking effect of GCs is the inhibition of expression of multiple inflammatory genes encoding proinflammatory cytokines, chemokines, enzymes for arachidonic acid metabolism, receptors, and adhesion molecules. These effects of GCs cannot be due to direct interaction of GC-bound GC receptors and GC response elements, as these binding sites are not present in the promoter regions of most inflammatory genes. These effects result from an inhibitory action of the GC–GC-receptor complex with activated transcription factors, such as AP-1 and NF-κB, which regulate inflammatory gene expression. In addition, GCs often upregulate anti-inflammatory mediators, such as lipocortin-1, IL-10, IL-1 receptor antagonist and neutral endopeptidase, by direct GC–GC receptor complex interaction with GC response elements present within genes encoding for these proteins. This further increases their effectiveness as anti-inflammatory agents.

The anti-inflammatory properties of GCs are attributed in part to their interference with prostaglandin and leukotriene synthesis. GCs reduce the production of prostaglandins and leukotrienes by inhibiting cellular phospholipases and COX (312–315). These are enzymes that degrade membrane phospholipids to release arachidonic acid, a precursor for prostaglandin and leukotriene synthesis. GC-induced synthesis of phospholipase and COX mRNA occurs around 1 hour after treatment with GCs. Protein synthesis of these enzymes occurs within 5 hours of GC treatment in various tissues and cells. Under normal physiological conditions, GCs do not affect prostaglandin synthesis mediated by constitutively expressed COX-1. In contrast, during an inflammatory response, GC treatment inhibits the increase in production of phospholipase A2 and COX-2 that occur as a result of inflammation.

Immune cell trafficking is crucial to immune surveillance and effector functions. Recent studies suggest that GCs diminish the ability of endothelial cells to direct leukocyte traffic into inflamed tissues by inhibiting adhesion molecule expression. GCs inhibit leukocyte recruitment to inflamed areas (317), and cause retention of lymphocytes in the lymphatic circulation with shrinkage of peripheral lymph nodes (318). Following conditions of acute, mild stress, increases in plasma corticosterone are accompanied by a decline in the numbers and percentages of lymphocytes, and an increase in the numbers and percentages of neutrophils in the blood (319). B-cell, NK-cell, and monocyte numbers decrease to a greater extent than T-lymphocyte numbers. Adrenalectomy reduces these stress-induced changes, and treatment with corticosterone in adrenalectomized animals replicates the stress-induced changes in peripheral blood lymphocytes and neutrophils in unmanipulated animals. This suggests that GCs modulate leukocyte trafficking, and the distribution of leukocytes between the blood and other immune compartments.

The expression of adhesive molecules by both the endothelium and leukocytes plays a critical role in immune responses by directing circulating leukocytes into sites of inflammation and infection. GCs modulate trafficking of leukocytes by regulating the expression of adhesion molecules on endothelial cells and leukocytes. Expression of endothelial–leukocyte adhesion molecule 1 (ELAM-1) and ICAM-1 is inhibited in LPS-stimulated endothelial cells (320). Treatment with GCs reduces the expression of leukocyte function antigen on T lymphocytes in patients with multiple sclerosis (321). Alloreactive lymphocytes and monocytes upregulate the expression of VCAM-1 and ICAM-1 on target cells (322). Treatment with GCs prevents mixed leukocyte reaction-induced upregulation of VCAM-1 and ICAM-1. GCs attenuate platelet-activating factor-induced changes in L-selectin and CD18 expression on human neutrophils at clinically relevant doses (323). These GC effects are inhibited by treatment with a GC receptor antagonist, and by a protein synthesis inhibitor. Similarly, downregulation of L-selectin and CD18 adhesion molecules on bovine neutrophils occurs following treatment with GCs for 3 days in dairy cows (324).

It is well known that GCs suppress production of several cytokines involved in the acute phase of inflammation, and in the balance of the Th1 and Th2 responses (325). GCs can regulate the synthesis of numerous cytokines, including, IL-1, IL-2, IL-6, IL-8, IFN-γ, TNF-α, and macrophage migration inhibitory factor (MIF). Decreased production of the cytokines IL-1, IL-2, IL-6, IFN-γ, and TNF-α, following GC treatment, also results in an increase in their corresponding receptors, IL-1 receptor (IL-1R) type II, IL-2Ra, IL-6Ra, IFN-γ, and TNF-R type I (326). IL-1, IL-6, and TNF-α are multifunctional pro-inflammatory cytokines produced primarily by activated monocytes and macrophages. In addition to their role as immunological mediators, these molecules have CNS effects, such as induction of fever, sickness, and activation of the HPA axis (discussed in greater detail later in this chapter). The effect of GCs on the production of cytokines is not always inhibitory. Exposure of different cell lines to physiological GC concentrations results in an increase of macrophage MIF, a key cytokine in the control of hormone–immune interactions at the inflammatory site.

GCs also regulate Th1 and Th2 subset development by strongly inhibiting production of Th1 cytokines, while having little effect on Th2 cytokine production. This results in suppression of Th1 cell-mediated responses, and enhancement of Th2 humoral immune functions. GCs selectively inhibit Th1 production of IL-2 and IFN-γ. The effects of GCs on cytokine production by lymphocytes has been addressed by analysing the regulation of genes which code for ILs and IFNs (318). Many of these genes are upregulated substantially by the nuclear transcription factors, AP-1, C/EBP, and especially NF-κB (327). Studies examining the mechanisms by which GCs inhibit T-cell proliferation and IL-2 production have focused on the interference of GCs with the transcriptional activation of the IL-2 gene. Although the IL-2 promoter lacks a GC response element, GCs inhibit IL-2 gene transcription following binding of GC to its intracellular receptor. The GC–GR complex then interferes with the activity of AP-1 and NF-κB nuclear proteins that bind to the IL-2 promoter (328). GCs also inhibit the activity of NF-κB by elevating transcription and protein synthesis of its cytoplasmic inhibitor, IκBα (329).

GCs play a crucial role in T-cell development and maturation, both at the thymic level and in secondary lymphoid tissue, where they control the peripheral tolerance of activated T lymphocytes, through the regulation of apoptosis. GCs induce apoptosis of DP thymocytes (330–332), which is inhibited by proper stimulation of DP thymocytes through TCR/CD3 and co-stimulation through the co-receptor, CD4 or CD8, and the integrin, leukocyte function-associated antigen 1 (LFA-1) (333, 334). The anti-apoptotic effects following TCR/CD3 ligation and accessory molecule stimulation induce differentiation and commitment of DP thymocytes to either CD4$^+$ or CD8$^+$ T cells (335–337).

GC-induced apoptosis requires binding of GCs to cytosolic GC hormone receptors (GRs) and protein synthesis. Inhibitors of either mRNA or protein synthesis block GC-induced apoptosis in thymocytes (335). The binding of GCs to GRs stimulates translocation of the ligand–receptor complex from the cytosol to the nucleus. The ligand–receptor complex functions as a translation regulatory factor and induces, enhances, or represses the expression of certain genes. Thus, the principal mechanism whereby they exert their powerful effects is through modulation of the transcription of specific sets of genes. In contrast to mature T cells, GC-induced apoptosis in DP thymocytes is not dependent on p53, Nur77, or Fas/Fas ligand, apoptosis-related gene products.

Although the requirement has been established for functional GR in GC-induced apoptosis sensitivity, certain lymphoid cells resist apoptosis *in vitro* and *in vivo* despite having a GR content equivalent to, or greater than, GC-sensitive T cells, and have similar binding properties to GC-sensitive T cells (338–343). Clearly, other factors control GC-induced apoptosis, such as secretion of protein factors that attenuate the lytic response (344, 345). Immature CD4/CD8 dual-negative cells (precursors of DP thymocytes) or mature T cells are much less sensitive to GCs (343, 346). Although resistant, a significant number of mature splenic T cells do succumb to apoptotic death following treatment with dexamethasone, a synthetic GC, in the same concentration range that induces apoptosis in immature thymocytes (347). However, the mechanism of GC-induced apoptosis in mature T cells differs from that of DP thymocytes. Apoptosis in mature T cells is modulated by T-cell growth factors. IL-4 rescues Th2 cells from GC-induced apoptosis. In contrast to Th2 cells where IL-2 and IL-1 rescues these cells, IL-2 is effective in inhibiting GC-induced apoptosis in Th1 cells.

3.4 THE HYPOTHALAMIC–PITUITARY–THYROID AXIS

Like ACTH, TSH can exert direct effects on the immune system, or act indirectly through TSH-stimulated release of the thyroid hormones T_3 (triiodothyronine) and T_4 (thyroxine) from the thyroid gland. In the presence of physiological (nanomolar) concentrations of highly purified TSH *in vitro*, antibody responses by murine splenocytes to both T-dependent and T-independent antigens are enhanced (348, 349). This TSH-mediated potentiation requires suboptimal culture conditions (no 2-mercaptoethanol and low concentrations of antigen). In a subsequent study, thyroid-releasing hormone (TRH), but not other releasing factors, stimulates TSH mRNA and immunoreactive TSH production by murine lymphocytes (350), as it does in the anterior pituitary. TRH, in picomolar concentrations, also enhances antibody production to a T-independent antigen *in vitro*; an effect blocked by anti-TSH antibody. These results suggest that endogenous production of TSH is regulated in a manner similar to pituitary-derived TSH, and that lymphocyte-derived TSH has immunological activity that enhances murine antibody responses. A human T-lymphoma cell line, MOLT-4b, also produces immunoreactive TSH, similar in subunit structure, molecular weight, and antigenicity to pituitary-derived TSH (351). Regulation of immunoreactive TSH release by MOLT-4b cells is induced by TRH and inhibited by T_3, a regulatory mechanism similar to that of pituitary-derived TSH. TSH receptors are expressed on several B-cell lines and LPS-stimulated B cells (352). TRH receptors are present on human peripheral blood mononuclear cells (PBMCs) and rat splenocytes under basal conditions. A significant increase in TRH DNA synthesis is observed in PHA-stimulated PBMCs and Con A-stimulated splenocytes when TRH (10^{-6} -10^{-12} M) is added to the culture medium. After administration of TRH *in vivo*, a significant increase in rat splenocyte proliferation to Con A results, an effect that is blocked by *in vivo* pretreatment with anti-rat TSH antibody (353). These findings suggest that TRH possesses immunostimulatory functions directly via its receptor, and indirectly via release of other immunostimulatory factors such as TSH .

The effects of T_3 and T_4 on immune functions are apparent following thyroidectomy. Thyroidectomy in neonatal and adult rats, or thiouracil-induced hypothyroidism in chickens, decreases lymphoid organ weight, reduces the numbers of circulating lymphocytes, diminishes antibody responses, and decreases mitogen-induced proliferative responses (354–356). T_3 and T_4 replacement in thyroidectomized animals reverses these effects. In euthyroid animals, T_3 or T_4 administration enhances antibody and mitogen responses (354, 355). Administration of T_4 to aged mice restores NK-cell activity to levels observed in young mice, but has no effect in young mice (357). T_4 has no effect on

NK-cell activity *in vitro*, even in the presence of such NK stimulants as IL-2 or IFN-γ. Thus, restoration of immune activity with T_3 and T_4 may have been achieved indirectly through interaction with non-lymphoid cells.

After immunization of rats with sheep red blood cells (SRBCs), a T-cell-dependent antigen, an increase in hypothalamic TRH mRNA is found 4–24 hours post-immunization (LPS decreases the response) (358). There is also an increase in pituitary TRH receptor mRNA and plasma PRL levels, but no changes in TSH and GH. Activation of the HPA suppressive response appears in a late phase, 5–7 days after immunization (occurs early with LPS). Antibody production and plasma PRL levels are blocked by antisense oligonucleotide complementary to rat TRH mRNA, i.c.v. So, the T-cell-dependent immune response is critically dependent on the early activation of TRH and PRL, and the neuroendocrine changes occurring during this response are profoundly different from those occurring during the T-cell-independent and inflammatory responses (LPS model). Demonstrated more recently, stimulation of TSH receptors on bone marrow cells induces the synthesis of cytokines that are classically used in regulation of inflammatory responses, including IL-6, IFN, TNF-α, TNF-β, TGF-α_2, and lymphotoxin-β within 2–3 hours of stimulation (359). This effect of TSH is mediated by a rapid increase in cAMP levels and an elevation in the phosphorylation of the Jak2 protein kinase.

Studies in athymic mice indicate that the neuroendocrine hormones TRH and TSH can influence the development of lymphoid cells associated with intestinal intraepithelial lymphocytes (IELs) (360). IELs in euthymic mice are unaffected by TRH and TSH treatment; however, T_4 administered to adult euthymic mice at 3 or 6 weeks of age causes a dramatic reduction in the number of TCR alpha beta, CD8 alpha beta IELs, which are upregulated by TRH and TSH in athymic mice. Once TCR alpha beta and CD8 alpha beta subsets reach normal developmental levels (about 8 weeks of age), T_4 has minimal effect on IELs, suggesting an effect on developing, but not mature, IELs. Similarly, Mihara *et al.* (361) have demonstrated that addition of T_3 and T_4, but not TSH or TRH, to cultured T lymphocytes enhances apoptosis (DNA ladder formation), reduces mitochondrial transmembrane potential (delta psi), produces reactive oxygen species, and reduces the anti-apoptotic Bcl-2 protein. These findings suggest a role for thyroid hormone in T-cell survival. This effect is more pronounced in lymphocytes from patients with Grave's disease.

3.5 GONADAL STEROIDS

Several lines of evidence have established a significant difference in the immune responsiveness of male and female mammals (362). Females demonstrate more robust antibody responses and have higher levels of serum IgG, IgG_1, IgM, and IgA than males in several species (363, 364). Immunological functions of T-lymphocyte and antigen-presenting cells from female mice vigorously respond to alloantigens, produce higher levels of IL-2, and generate better secondary responses than lymphocytes from male mice, suggesting that gonadal hormonal levels play a contributing role in immunocompetence (365). This significant difference in immune responsiveness may be responsible for the higher incidence of autoimmune diseases in females, such as systemic lupus erythematosus, rheumatoid arthritis, Hashimoto's thyroiditis, and liver diseases (362).

3.5.1 Oestrogen

Oestrogen receptors have been demonstrated on human and rodent thymocytes, suppressor/cytotoxic T cells, and synovial and peritoneal macrophages. The consequences of oestrogen binding to these receptors on immunological functions depend upon the physiological or pharmacological concentrations of the hormone (366). *In vitro* addition of physiological concentrations of 17β-oestradiol inhibits the chemotaxis of polymorphonuclear leukocytes isolated from male subjects, blockable by addition to the culture medium of oestrogen receptor antagonists (367).

The ability of oestrogen to influence immune cells may be responsible for promoting the migration of a higher percentage of macrophages, granulocytes, and dendritic cells in the uterus during oestrus (368). Treatment of mouse splenic macrophages with 17β-oestradiol suppresses LPS-induced IL-1α, IL-6, and TNF-α production, while leaving IL-10 and macrophage inflammatory protein (MIP) production unchanged. These alterations in cytokine production were accompanied by a reduction in NF-κB-binding activity to DNA, suggesting involvement of this transcription factor in the observed effect (369). Chao *et al.* (370) have shown that treatment of male rat peritoneal macrophages with physiological concentrations of 17β-oestradiol stimulates TNF release, but higher or lower concentrations of oestradiol inhibit TNF release. The effects of oestrogen on the release of pro-inflammatory cytokines may be mediated through an increase in the activity of IFN-γ, and modulation of prostaglandin synthesis.

NO is produced by peripheral mononuclear cells, macrophages, and other phagocytic cells in response to bacteria, endotoxin, and other mediators of inflammation to confer some protective effect on the host. Ovariectomy inhibits spontaneous production of NO by alveolar macrophages, suggesting that physiological concentrations of oestrogen are essential for the induction of NO synthesis by macrophages (371). Oestrogen enhances the gene expression of inducible NOS and promotes TNF-α gene expression by uterine mast cells, but does not have an effect on macrophages (372). Prolonged administration of physiological doses of oestrogen to ovariectomized mice of various strains results in the suppression of NK-cell activity in a dose-dependent manner that may accelerate with the progression of murine lupus (373).

Oestrogen contributes to the pathogenesis of systemic lupus erythematosus (SLE), a disease that is most common in women of childbearing age. SLE is characterized by enhanced humoral immunity and abnormal apoptosis of peripheral blood lymphocytes. Oestrogen increases *in vitro* IgG and IgM production in PBMCs from healthy men and women, an effect that was abrogated by an anti-IL-10-antibody. This finding suggests that the enhancement of humoral immunity by oestrogen is mediated through IL-10 production by monocytes (374). Oestrogen suppresses *in vitro* apoptosis of PBMCs from normal subjects, and also from SLE patients with normal menstrual cycles (375). Oestrogen-stimulated PBMCs from SLE patients produce significantly lower levels of TNF-α. The more vigorous immune response in females compared to males may be due to the anti-apoptotic action of oestrogen on activated monocytes and macrophages. The decline in autoimmune reactivity in SLE patients after menopause may result from clonal deletion of autoimmune cells by apoptosis, and an increase in TNF production from lower oestrogen levels and fewer oestrogen receptors on these cells.

In contrast to SLE, which tends to exacerbate during pregnancy or following high doses of exogenous oestrogen, the disease symptoms of rheumatoid arthritis and multiple sclerosis are suppressed during pregnancy and by treatment with oestrogen. Rheumatoid arthritis is due to predominant production of Th1 cytokines at the site of inflammation and joint destruction. The suppression of IFN-γ and IL-2 production and the enhancement of IL-4 and IL-10 production that occur during pregnancy may explain, at least in part, the amelioration of this disease during pregnancy. Treatment of mice with oestrogen ameliorates the post-partum progression of the collagen-induced arthritis, possibly by suppressing angiogenesis and NO production by the endothelium (376). In mice with experimental autoimmune encephalomyelitis (EAE) (a model for multiple sclerosis), implants of oestriol, a hormone associated with pregnancy, increases IL-10 production and serum IgG$_1$, the isotype that is specific for the autoantigen myelin basic protein (377). Addition of oestrone and oestriol to CD4$^+$ T-cell clones from patients with multiple sclerosis enhance the secretion of antigen- or anti-CD3-stimulated IL-10 and IFN-γ production. Low concentrations of oestrone, oestradiol, and oestriol enhance, while higher concentrations suppress, TGF-β secretion (378). Altogether, these effects of oestrogens in human cell lines, and in mice, suggest that they exert anti-inflammatory effects through production of specific cytokines similar to those elevated during pregnancy.

The development and progression of breast cancer is thought to be determined, in part, by a plethora of immune functions. Lower T-cell functions associated with suppression of cytokine production, and reduction in NK-cell activity, are some of the important prognostic factors in this disease. Phorbol myristate acetate (PMA)-induced IL-1β, TNF, IFN-γ, IL-4, IL-6, and IL-10 production by B cells is enhanced by tamoxifen and toremifene, anti-oestrogens. In contrast, IL-1β, IL-6, and IFN-γ production is enhanced by tamoxifen in a T-cell line, and both tamoxifen and toremifene have no effect on cytokine production in a myeloid cell line (379). The inability of these anti-oestrogens to shift the balance between Th1 and Th2 cytokine production in the T-cell line suggests that anti-oestrogens may also exert their effects independent of the oestrogen receptor-mediated mechanisms. Alternatively, this T-cell line may not express oestrogen receptors, or may respond to oestrogen through mechanisms that are different from oestrogen-mediated responses in normal T cells.

3.5.2 Progesterone

Progesterone receptors are present in the thymic epithelial cells, in the cytoplasm of macrophages in rats (292), and in B lymphocytes from the chicken bursa of fabricius (380). Peripheral blood lymphocytes from healthy pregnant women contain more progesterone receptors than in non-pregnant women (381). During pregnancy, there is marked suppression of mitogen-induced proliferation of T lymphocytes and NK-cell activity. These effects of progesterone are mediated through a 34-kDa protein, progesterone-induced blocking factor, that enhances Con A-induced murine splenic Th2 cytokine (e.g. IL-3, IL-4, and IL-10) production. Treatment of pregnant mice with anti-progesterone-induced blocking factor leads to lower levels of splenic IL-10 production, higher levels of splenic IFN-γ expression, and higher resorption rates. These effects are reversed by administration of anti-NK-cell antibodies to pregnant mice (382). Progesterone increases IL-5 gene expression in T-cell lines, an effect mediated at the transcription stage, and enhances IL-4 production by CD4$^+$ T-cell clones (378, 383).

Oestrogen and progesterone influence immune responses during the oestrous cycle, pregnancy, and implantation by regulating the migration of macrophages and neutrophils into the uterus and vagina. Simultaneous administration of progesterone and oestrogen to ovariectomized mice prevents the oestrogen-induced entry of macrophages and neutrophils into the uterus. Gomez and colleagues (384) have suggested that progesterone and its analogues should be considered for the treatment of immune disorders because of their ability to decrease the cell-surface expression of Fcγ receptors on macrophages, resulting in the amelioration of immune thrombocytopenic purpura and autoimmune haemolytic anaemia. Progesterone inhibits basal and *in vitro* LPS-stimulated NO production by alveolar macrophages in male rats, possibly mediated via an increase in TNF production (370, 371). Some of the effects of progesterone may be mediated through an interaction with GC receptors on the thymocytes, as both receptors for GCs and progesterone bind to the same elements within the DNA (296, 385).

3.5.3 Androgens

The immunomodulatory effects of androgens may be exerted through the androgen receptors on the macrophages (386) and subsets of CD4$^-$CD8$^-$ and

CD4⁻CD8⁺ T lymphocytes (387). These immunocytes are also capable of synthesizing and metabolizing androgens (389). The inactive dehydroepiandrosterone (DHEA) sulfate, precursor to testosterone and oestrogen, produced in the adrenal cortex is converted to DHEA by enzymes in the immune cells.

Several studies have demonstrated the beneficial effects of DHEA and its metabolites in preventing the progression of experimental neoplastic diseases, atherosclerosis, and other age-related diseases. Administration of DHEA and its metabolite, androstenediol, suppresses the mortality rate of bacterially infected mice; this antibacterial action of DHEA is mediated through the inhibition of TNF-α and IL-1 production (389). DHEA sulfate enhances splenic IL-2 and IFN-γ production in LP-BM5 retrovirus-infected mice, whereas the production of IL-6 and IL-10 is suppressed. These findings indicate that the anti-viral functions of DHEA occur through a shift in Th1/Th2 cytokine profile (390). DHEA treatment also reverses trauma- and haemorrhage-induced suppression of proliferation of splenocytes and splenic IL-2, IL-3, and IFN-γ production in mice. This effect of DHEA may be due to direct stimulation of T cells, and an antagonistic effect on GC functions by DHEA (391).

Pretreatment with DHEA results in an 80 per cent survival rate in mice infected with a lethal strain of influenza virus (392). In contrast, administration of DHEA sulfate to elderly populations as an adjuvant therapy to influenza vaccination did not produce an increase in immune response, indicating that supra-physiological doses of this hormone may be necessary to improve immune responses in human subjects (393). Miller and Chrisp (394) find that DHEA sulfate does not have immunostimulatory properties. Instead, chronic treatment with DHEA sulfate has no effect on age-related immunosenescence, or on the lifespan of ageing mice. They also report that exposing these animals to DHEA increases the risk for hormone-dependent cancers.

3.6 MELATONIN

The pineal gland modulates immune response through its circadian synthesis and release of melatonin. Mice raised for 3–4 generations under constant lighting conditions, inhibiting the dark-dependent synthesis of melatonin (286), resulted in cellular depletion of the thymic cortex, atrophy of the splenic red and white pulp, and inability to mount humoral immune responses to T-dependent antigens (395). Pharmacological intervention to block the synthesis of melatonin reduced the antibody response to SRBCs and lowered the autologous mixed-lymphocyte reaction, while leaving transplantation immunity unaffected (395). These effects were reversible by exogenous administration of melatonin. Similar findings were observed in surgically pinealectomized animals (396).

Exogenous administration of melatonin in the evening, but not in the morning, enhanced the primary antibody response to SRBCs as measured in a plaque-forming assay (397, 398), but had no effect on the primary antibody response to T-independent antigens (224). Melatonin treatment in mice at the time of primary antigenic challenge did not alter the cytotoxic T-lymphocyte (CTL) response to vaccinia virus or SRBCs. However, upon re-exposure to the antigen, the secondary response was significantly higher than in saline-treated control mice (499, 400). Exposure of various strains of mice to melatonin at a range of concentrations and for various periods of time had no significant effect on NK-cell activity of natural CTL activity. These findings suggest that the immunoenhancing effect of melatonin in normal mice is dependent on the presence of T-dependent antigens.

Maestroni and Conti (400) have suggested that melatonin plays a role in preparing the animal to better handle environmental stressors. Thymic atrophy and immunosuppression of secondary antibody response to T-dependent antigen induced by administration of GC or acute restraint stress was blocked by administration of melatonin (221, 401). These effects of melatonin appear not to directly antagonize the effects of GC. The mechanisms through which melatonin exerts its effect on immune responses in not entirely clear. Maestroni and co-workers have evidence to suggest that it may involve the stimulated release of opioid peptides by activated immunocompetent cells and/or that melatonin may influence the binding affinity of opioid receptors for their ligand.

Several investigators have reported the presence of opioid receptors on murine- and human-activated lymphocytes, and that these cells are capable of synthesizing opioid peptides (126, 163, 364). Furthermore, Maestroni and Conti (400) have shown that physiological concentrations of melatonin stimulate activated T-helper lymphocytes to synthesize and release opioid peptides, which in turn can enhance the immune response in normal mice, counteract the effects of acute stress, and selectively displace radiolabelled naloxozone from mouse brain membrane preparations.

4   Immune–CNS regulation

4.1   CNS CIRCUITRY INVOLVED IN IMMUNE REGULATION

The PVN of the hypothalamus is a major regulator of both autonomic and neuroendocrine outflow. Caudal cell groups in this nucleus give rise to long descending projections to brain stem autonomic structures (280). These neurons contain CRH, AVP, and oxytocin. Other regions of the nervous system that regulate automonic outflow include the nucleus solitarius, raphe nuclei, tegmental NA nuclei, PVN of the hypothalamus, lateral hypothalamus, posterior hypothalamus, dorsal hypothalamus, central amygdaloid nucleus, and frontal, cingulate, and insular cortex (limbic cortex).

Additionally, indirect regulation of autonomic activity arises from regions such as the parabrachial nuclei, central grey, and reticular formation of the brain stem, numerous hypothalamic nuclei and cell groups, limbic forebrain areas such as the hippocampal formation and septum, and cortical association areas. The central autonomic system has an integrated circuitry with extensive ascending and descending connections among the regions mentioned above, and is intimately involved in visceral, autonomic, and neuroendocrine regulation.

The more medial aspect of the parvocellular PVN (pPVN) is the major source of hypophysiotropic CRH neurons, which release CRH into the hypophyseal portal circulation. As discussed above, under certain situations these neurons can also synthesize and secrete AVP, which acts synergistically with CRH to secrete ACTH. The extreme diversity of stressful stimuli that can activate the HPA axis reflects the diverse inputs to this portion of the PVN. The pPVN receives visceral, somatosensory, auditory, nociceptive, and visual information, input from limbic regions involved in the integration of cognitive and emotional factors. The pPVN receives projections from other hypothalamic nuclei (i.e. medial preoptic area and anterior hypothalamus), from nucleus of the solitary tract and other medullary catecholaminergic cell groups, the organum vascularis of the lamina terminalis (OVLT), and subfornical organ (SFO).

Therefore, for both the ANS and the neuroendocrine system, there are multiple levels through which these systems can be modulated. This is the same circuitry through which signal molecules from the immune system exert their effects on brain function, and through which the brain modulates immune function. Brain-mediated changes in immune responses that result from psychosocial stressors and behavioural conditioning occur via cortical and limbic circuitry. These are sites that respond to the administration of cytokines and to immunization by altered neuronal activity, and changes in neurotransmitter metabolism. These brain regions also possess the highest density of GC receptors and regulate the balance between neuroendocrine and autonomic outflow.

Stereotactically applied electrolytic lesions in the anterior hypothalamus result in decreased nucleated splenocytes, reduced proliferation of T cells in response to the mitogen Con A, thymic involution, decreased NK-cell activity, reduced antibody production, altered tumour cell growth, and inhibited development of lethal anaphylactic response (reviewed in 403). Most of these responses were transient in nature, and some of the responses were reversible with hypophysectomy indicating that the effects are mediated through neuroendocrine mechanisms.

Ablation studies involving other sites in the hypothalamus have produced more variable results (402). Lesions in the medial hypothalamus have been reported to decrease T- and B-cell number and enhance graft rejection, although no alterations in immune functions were detected with lesions in the region of the hypothalamus. Posterior hypothalamic lesions decreased T-helper/T-suppressor cell ratio and enhanced tumour growth, while lesions in the medial or posterior hypothalamus had no effect on the development of lethal anaphylaxis. These findings suggest involvement of the anterior hypothalamus and perhaps other hypothalamic regions in immune modulation; however, problems inherent in the experimental design of these types of studies limit interpretation of the data, such as accurate placement of the lesion in small discrete hypothalamic nuclei, the presence of many subsets of chemically specific neurons that can be compact or scattered in the nucleus, and bundles of fibres arising from other CNS sites that may pass through the hypothalamus.

Electrical recordings of neuronal firing in discrete nuclear regions of rats provide further evidence for hypothalamic involvement in immune modulation (402). An extensive body of literature has documented electrophysiological responses in the hypothalamus, limbic forebrain structures, and midbrain reticular formation in response to antigenic challenge (reviewed in 403). At the peak of an antibody response after immunization, neurons in the ventromedial nucleus of the hypothalamic exhibit an increased activity (402). Antigenic challenge also increased neuronal firing rates in the preoptic/anterior hypothalamic area at peak antibody production (day 5) and suppressed neuronal activity in the PVN of the hypothalamus during the first 3 days after immunization followed by enhancement in neuronal activity by day 6. Secondary immunization produced a similar neuronal firing pattern in the preoptic/anterior hypothalamus, but the response was not as abrupt or as robust as that seen with primary immunization. Changes in neuronal firing patterns in specific regions of the brain are thought to result from immune-derived cytokines that interact either directly or indirectly with neurons in these brain regions. Differences in neuronal firing patterns in response to primary and secondary immunization may result from differences in cytokine secretion that occur under these two conditions.

Discrete lesions in the limbic forebrain structures produce changes in immune reactivity, generally favouring immune enhancement (402). Ablations of the dorsal hippocampus and amygdaloid complex transiently elevated splenocyte and thymocyte number, and mitogen-induced T-cell proliferation. These effects were reversible by HypoX, indicating mediation via neuroendocrine routes. Lesions in these sites do not affect the development and progression of experimental allergic encephalomyelitis (EAE) and graft rejection. After lesioning the lateral septal area and its connections to the hippocampus, Nance *et al.* (404) found chronic alterations in T-cell-mediated responses. Through the extensive connections between limbic structures and the hypothalamus, altered T-cell functions could result from either altered neuroendocrine or autonomic outflow.

Evidence for brain stem involvement of immune modulation is provided from ablation studies showing suppressed DTH responses following lesions in the caudal reticular formation of the medulla and pons (405), and enhancement of DTH by lesions in the rostral medial reticular formation and raphe nuclei (406). Lesions in the reticular formation also result in thymic involution. The reticular formation is a diffuse network of neurons and connections that link together many neuronal systems. This means that identification of the chemically specific neurons involved in modulating immune function is not possible with ablation techniques. Monoaminergic systems in the reticular formation lesions may be involved, since NA and serotonergic cell bodies in the caudal reticular formation and rostral raphe nuclei, respectively, project extensively to the hypothalamus and some limbic structures (402). These two monoaminergic systems regulate numerous visceral and neuroendocrine events, and clearly are involved in both affective and cognitive processes. Because these monoaminergic systems also regulate descending autonomic preganglionic neurons in the brain stem and spinal cord, destruction of these connections would alter autonomic outflow as well.

Central administration of 6-OHDA, a neurotoxin specific for NA nerve fibres, into the cisterna magna enhanced suppressor T-cell activity in immunized rats (407). At the peak of a primary antibody response, NE concentrations in the hypothalamus declined (408). Similarly, 2 hours after administration of supernatants from cultures of Con A-stimulated lymphocytes, hypothalamic NE content decreased, suggesting that cytokine secretion from lymphocytes is responsible for altered monoamine content in the hypothalamus. Turnover studies indicate a reduction in hypothalamic NE content after immunization is accompanied by an increase in NE turnover (409, 410). Neurochemical measurement of monoamines from specifically microdissected regions of hypothalamus and other CNS sites revealed that an altered monoamine content was specific both to certain brain regions and to the time course of the antibody response. NE content in the PVN of the hypothalamus (but not in the SON, the anterior or medial hypothalamus) decreased at the peak of the antibody response (day 4), and at the peak time of secretion of GC (411). Changes in monoamine metabolism and electrophysiological activity in the PVN in response to immunological stimuli provides a potential mechanism for mediating the activity of the CRH–ACTH–GC axis, which is known to modulate immune function. Decreased NA and serotonin (5-HT) content in the dorsal hippocampus and increased 5-HT content in the nucleus solitarius were also found during the rising phase of the immune response. No alterations in monoamine content were found in other discrete brain regions, or during the declining phase of the immune response. These studies support brain modulation by the immune system, through the secretion of one or more cytokines acting on specific hypothalamic, limbic forebrain, and brain stem autonomic nuclei.

Discrete lesions in the ventral and medial aspects of the parabrachial nuclei decreased proliferation of thymocytes (412). These nuclei contribute to the circuitry lining brain stem autonomic nuclei such as the nucleus solitarius with the hypothalamus and the amygdala, a limbic structure. These findings suggest that the parabrachial nuclei process both afferent and efferent information related to autonomic regulation, and influence hypothalamic and limbic modulation of the neuroendocrine system.

Changes in immune parameters resulting from stressors, psychosocial factors, and behavioural conditioning suggest the involvement of the cerebral cortex, particularly the frontal, cingulate, and temporal regions. These cortical regions have direct projections to the limbic forebrain, hypothalamus, brain stem, visceral nuclei, and autonomic preganglionic neurons. A role for the cerebral cortex in immune modulation is indicated by several studies (reviewed in 413), and suggests a lateralization of function by the cortex. Large lesions in the left cerebral hemisphere in mice decreased T-cell numbers, T-cell response, and NK-cell activity. B-cell and macrophage function remained unaffected. Lesions in the right cerebral cortex had the opposite effect, which could result from modulation of efferent signals arising from the left cortex.

Signalling between the nervous and immune systems occurs bidirectionally through short, intermediate, and long communication channels. Signalling occurs via chemical mediators such as hormones, neurotransmitters, and cytokines that bind to receptors present on the cell surface or in the cytosol of target cells located in the nervous system and in the immune system. Binding to specific receptors by these mediators activates common second-messenger systems, changes receptor expression for specific signal molecules on the cell surface, and/or alters membrane permeability.

4.2 CYTOKINE SIGNALLING OF THE HYPOTHALAMIC–PITUITARY–TARGET TISSUE AXIS

In the past 10–15 years, an abundance of articles concerning cytokine activation of the hypothalamic–pituitary–target axis have been published (reviewed in 414). These research efforts reflect the large number of cytokines recently discovered, the complex organization of the HPA, and the importance of the HPA axis in handling stressful stimuli. Circulating GC concentrations rise in response to any stimulus that is perceived to threaten homeostasis. GCs have multiple targets in which they interact to alter a variety of cellular activities aimed at changing metabolic, endocrine, nervous, cardiovascular, and immunological needs that promote survival.

Numerous studies show that a single peripheral treatment of either IL-1α or β to rats or mice stimulates ACTH and GC secretion, as well as AVP, and a hyper-responsiveness of the HPA axis (414). Long-term administration of IL-1β to rats enhances CRH- and ACTH-like immunoreactivities in the hypothalamus and pituitary, respectively, increases adrenal weight, and elevates plasma ACTH concentrations for at least 7 days. Similarly, i.c.v. administration of IL-1, or microinjection into the PVN, median eminence, or hippocampus, in much lower concentrations than given by peripheral routes also elicits pituitary ACTH secretion. Central and peripheral administration of IL-1 also induces cfos mRNA and Fos protein in the pPVN.

In addition to IL-1, other cytokines derived from both myeloid and lymphoid cells influence HPA-axis secretory activity, including IL-2, IL-4,

IL-6, IL-11, IL-12, LIF, oncostatin, cardiotropin-1, ciliary neurotrophic factor (CNTF), TNF-α, IFN-α, activin, epidermal growth factor (EGF), NGF, and colony-stimulating factor (CSF) (reviewed in 414). With the exception of activin, all other cytokines studied are reported to either enhance or have no effect on ACTH secretion. Some cytokines act synergistically to enhance ACTH secretion. All haematopoietic cytokines enhance IL-1-induced ACTH and/or corticosterone secretion to a greater extent than the additive effects when administered alone. TNF-α also augments IL-1-evoked release of ACTH and GC (415).

TNF-α given peripherally generally enhances HPA activity; however, i.c.v. TNF-α administration elevates, or has no effect on, HPA activity (414). These discrepancies are attributed to the use of different sources of TNF-α, with murine TNF-α augmenting and human TNF-α having no effect on HPA activity. This has been a problem for other cytokine effects of HPA activity, such as IL-6. While the majority of cytokines examined in animal studies have been found to exert an enhancing effect on the HPA axis, IL-4 (416) and low concentrations of IFN-γ (418) inhibit HPA-axis activity *in vivo*. At higher concentrations IFN-γ given i.c.v. enhances plasma GC levels (417). Similarly, IL-2, IL-6, TNF-α, and EGF elevate plasma ACTH and/or GC concentrations when administered i.c.v. (414). Interestingly, the pattern of gene expression in the PVN and/or pharmacological profiles differs for IL-1β and TNF-α, depending on the route of administration (peripheral or central), indicating distinct pathways for stimulated HPA activity. With both central and peripheral administration of these cytokines, it is clear that activation at or above the level of the hypothalamus is required for HPA activation.

Clinical trials using a number of human-derived cytokines as anti-cancer therapies have assessed their effects on the human HPA axis. Plasma ACTH and/or cortisol concentrations are rapidly (within 1 hour or 1–4 hours after treatment, respectively) elevated in patients receiving either i.v. or subcutaneous administration of IL-1α, IL-1β, IL-2, IL-6, TNF-α, IFN-α, IFN-β, and IFN-γ (415). AVP is also elevated by many of these cytokines. The rise in neuroendocrine hormones after these anti-cancer therapies contributes to the severe side-effects of these treatment strategies.

Elaboration of cytokines from injury, inflammation, and infectious diseases influences HPA activity (414). Administration of Newcastle disease virus (NDV) to rodents resulted in marked increases in plasma ACTH and GC concentrations within 1–2 hours after injection (418, 419). This rise in ACTH and CG in the blood results from the production of IL-1 that, in turn, activates CRH release from the hypothalamus. Polyinosinic polycytidylic acid (Poly I:C), a synthetic, double-stranded polyribonucleotide commonly used to mimic viral exposure, also induces rapid activation of the HPA axis (420, 421), a response that is not present in IL-6-deficient mice. In mice infected with murine cytomegalovirus, circulating levels of IL-12, IFN-γ, TNF-α, IL-1α, and IL-6, but not IL-1β, are elevated 24–48 hours after infection (421).

During this period plasma concentrations of GC and, to a lesser extent, ACTH rise significantly. This effect on the HPA axis is attributable to the increase in IL-6, since enhanced HPA activity is not seen in IL-6-deficient mice even though IL-1α is elevated (421). Treatment of normal mice with IL-1 receptor antagonist (IL-1Ra) also blunts HPA activation, an effect mediated via IL-1-induced release of IL-6 (421).

Administration of LPS, either i.v. or i.p., produces marked elevations in ACTH and GC secretion; however, the two administration routes may influence the HPA axis via different pathways (422, 423). LPS also produces an increase in cfos mRNA and Fos protein in the pPVN and elevates CRH mRNA (424, 425). These effects are mediated via LPS-induced release of IL-1, IL-6, and TNF-α (426), since they are attenuated by inhibiting IL-1, IL-6, or TNF-α, and destroying macrophages (414). However, the precise role played by these cytokines in HPA activation by LPS is not fully understood.

Turpentine-induced local inflammation produces a biphasic activation of the HPA axis in the rat. The first peak results from activation of nociceptive sensory afferents (427), and the second peak parallels the development of the local inflammatory response (428). This second rise in ACTH is mediated predominantly by a rise in plasma IL-6, although other cytokines are clearly involved in this response.

The effect of cytokines on the release of other pituitary hormones is variable, depending on the route of administration, the dose used, and the *in vivo* or *in vitro* system examined. I.c.v. infusion of IL-1 at low doses stimulates GH release (429). In contrast, IL-1α and IL-1β administered via the same route inhibits GH surges (greater effect with IL-1β), suggesting that GHRH and/or somatostatin may be involved in GH release. Administration of IL-1α and IL-1β (i.v.) has similar effects on GH surges as seen centrally, while IL-2 and IL-6 have no effect on GH release (430). The finding that dose-dependent increases in somatostatin and its mRNA in foetal rat diencephalic cell culture incubated with IL-1β provides evidence for somatostatin involvement in IL-1β-induced inhibition of GH secretion (431). Further support for a role for somatostatin in cytokine-mediated regulation of GH release is obtained from *in vitro* incubation of the anterior pituitary and medial basal hypothalamus, showing that IL-2 suppresses GH and stimulates somatostatin release, respectively (432). Central administration of IL-1β reduces IGF-1 levels in the periphery, including plasma, liver, and gastrocnemius muscle but does not have an effect on soleus muscle, kidney, spleen, intestine, or whole brain, indicating that IGF-1 may control cytokine-induced GH release (433). TNF-α increases GH secretion from ovine and rodent pituitary cells *in vitro* and after intraventricular infusion (434, 435). The inhibitory effect of IFN-γ on GH and PRL release is mediated through increased production of NO (436).

A large number of *in vitro* studies indicate possible direct effects of cytokines on pituitary ACTH secretion and adrenal GC secretion (414). There is evidence for IL-1β and IL-1Ra binding sites in the anterior pituitary of the mouse (437), and in both the anterior and posterior pituitary of the rat (438). IL-1 binding in the mouse anterior pituitary decreases after systemic treatment with LPS (439, 440), and increases after immobilization stress (50, 87), ether-laparotomy stress (441, 442), and long-term treatment with GC (437). Enhanced IL-1 binding in the pituitary after ether-laparotomy stress can be prevented by treatment with a CRH receptor antagonist. IL-1R1 and IL-1R2 are present in the anterior pituitary of the rat (438, 443, 444). In the murine anterior pituitary IL-1R1 and IL-1R2 are co-expressed, and predominantly found on somatrope (GH-producing) cells (445). IL-6 binding sites have been demonstrated in the rodent and human anterior pituitary gland (414). TNF-α binding sites are present in murine and rat anterior pituitary (446).

Rey and Melmed (447) have reviewed the diverse range of cytokines that are present in the pituitary. These include IL-2, IL-10, LIF, and MIF localized to corticotropes. In the pituitary mRNA encoding IL-1α, IL-1β, IL-6, LIF, IFN-γ, and TNF-α is elevated 45 minutes to 6 hours after LPS treatment (447–449). IL-1Ra has been reported to be unchanged (450) or elevated (451–453) after systemic treatment with LPS (454–457). MIF is found in high concentrations in the pituitary, and is released into the systemic circulation within 2 hours after LPS treatment. MIF plays an important role in endotoxaemia, with inhibition promoting protection from endotoxaemia and prevention of death as an end point (454).

Pituitary cells constitutively produce IL-6 (458), and its secretion can be induced within 6 hours of treatment with LPS (414, 459, 460), IL-1α, IL-1β (459, 460), TNF-α (434), IFN, phorbol myristate, and agents that elevate cAMP (414, 461; reviewed in 448). IL-1β-evoked secretion of IL-6 is not, however, mediated by cAMP-dependent pathways (414, 460, 462). GCs inhibit basal (463) and IL-1β-stimulated (460) release of IL-6 from the pituitary. Chronic inflammation elevates IL-6 in the anterior pituitary (464, 465). IL-6 is produced by folliculostellate cells (of monocyte lineage) in the anterior lobe (466–468), and is also found in the intermediate pituitary where IL-1β and LPS are potent secretagogues (459). Release of IL-6 from folliculostellate cells is thought to regulate hormone secretion from the pituitary in a paracrine manner.

Whether IL-1 has direct effects on pituitary cells to secrete ACTH is not clear; some studies have shown a direct effect on pituitary cells in culture, while others have found no effect (reviewed in 414). These discrepancies may result from sex differences or the period of IL-1 incubation. Similarly, data regarding the ability of IL-2, IL-6, IL-8, TNF-α, and EGF to directly stimulate ACTH secretion are contradictory (414). Buckingham et al. (468A) demonstrated that IL-1α, IL-1β, IL-6, IL-8, and TNF-α when administered alone have no effect on ACTH secretion from rat pituitary fragments, but conditioned media from macrophages stimulated with LPS produce a dose-dependent increase in ACTH secretion within just 30 minutes. This finding suggests that another macrophage-derived cytokine stimulates ACTH production and/or there are synergistic effects of macrophage products on ACTH secretion.

There is also evidence that cytokines directly affect GC secretion from the adrenal gland. While IL-1R1 is not expressed in the adrenal gland (444), IL-6Ra mRNA is present in the zona glomerulosa and fasciculata in human adrenals and in the adrenal medulla (469, 470). IL-1α, IL-1β, IL-1 cleaving enzyme (ICE), and IL-1Ra are constitutively expressed in the adrenal gland (471–473). Systemic LPS treatment augments IL-1α, IL-1β, ICE, and IL-1Ra within 90 minutes of treatment (473, 474). The IL-1-related cytokine, IL-18/IL-1γ, is constitutively expressed in the rat adrenal cortex, and is strongly induced by acute cold stress (475). IL-6 is present throughout the human adrenal cortex (469, 476), and in rat adrenal gland extracts (333, 470, 477), and can also be augmented by LPS administration (477). TNF-α mRNA occurs throughout the human cortex, particularly in steroid-producing cells (478), but whether the human cortex has TNF-α protein is inconclusive (476).

In the rat, IL-6 is mainly found in the zona glomerulosa, with small amounts of IL-6 and TNF-α produced in the zona fasciculata/reticulata (414, 479, 480). Both TNF-α and IL-6 secretion is stimulate in a dose-dependent fashion by IL-1α, IL-1β, and LPS (414, 479, 480). IL-1-evoked IL-6 release from the adrenal gland is not potentiated by dexamethasone (481). ACTH also stimulates IL-6 production from zona glomerulosa cells, but not zona fasciculata/reticularis (479). IL-6 secretion from these cells is enhanced by PKC activators, the calcium ionophore, ionomycin, PGE_2, forskolin, and angiotensin II (414). Similarly, TNF-α secretion is stimulated by PKC activators and ionomycin, but in contrast to IL-6, TNF-α is inhibited by ACTH and dibutyryl cAMP (480).

Direct actions of cytokines on GC secretion in rats have been demonstrated, including stimulation with TNF-α, IFN-γ, IL-1α, IL-1β, IL-2, IL-3, and IL-6 (414). Generally, IL-1α, IL-1β, IL-2, IL-3, TNF-α, IFN-γ, and IL-6 augment GC release from various preparations of adrenal cells. IL-6 and TNF-α potentiated and inhibited ACTH-induced GC secretion, respectively. In the majority of these reports, however, it should be noted that lengthy incubation periods (more than 12 hours) were required to observe these effects, suggesting that *in vivo* direct cytokine action on the GC secretion is not likely to account for the rapid effects of administered cytokines on plasma GC concentrations.

Several of the cytokines, including IL-1, IL-2, IL-6, IFN-γ, and TNF-α, exert their effects directly on the pituitary to influence the secretion of pituitary hormones. IL-1 infusion (i.c.v.) stimulates PRL release, but inhibits TSH secretion (429). Addition of IL-2 to anterior pituitary cells *in vitro* elevates basal PRL and TSH release and suppresses basal LH and FSH release (481). Co-incubation of IL-6 with anterior pituitary cells stimulates PRL, GH, and LH release (482); this effect may be due to IL-1β-enhanced spontaneous release of IL-6 (334). Administration of TNF-α (i.v.) significantly suppresses serum TSH, T_4, free T_4, T_3, and hypothalamic TRH in rats, and also induces profound alteration in TSH glycosylation, reduction in pituitary TSH mRNA expression, and thyroid radioiodinated uptake (483).

The cytokines have direct effects on gonadal steroidogenesis. IL-1 suppresses gonadotropin-induced oestradiol production from human granulosa luteal cells in a dose-dependent fashion (484). Similar to IL-1, TNF-α decreases oestrone and oestradiol synthesis in human granulosa cells regardless of the dose of the cytokine (485). IL-1α stimulates gonadotropin-induced release of progesterone synthesis in the rodent thecal cells (486) and human granulosa cells (487). The effects of TNF-α on progesterone secretion from human granulosa cells are dependent upon cytokine dose, with lower doses increasing progesterone secretion and higher doses suppressing hormone secretion (485). *In vitro* incubation of rodent ovarian follicles with TNF-α increases the release of progesterone and other progestins, resulting from enhanced conversion of cholesterol to progestins (488). In contrast, Adashi and colleagues (489) ascribe an inhibitory role for TNF-α on gonadotropin-induced progesterone production by the granulosa and luteal cells that may cause attrition of corpus luteum. *In vivo* administration of IL-1β significantly reduces gonadotropin-induced secretion of testosterone *in vitro*. This effect is mediated through the reduction in steroidogenic acute regulatory protein important for biosynthesis of testosterone (490). *In vitro* addition of IL-1α to rat Leydig cells prevents gonadotropin-induced testosterone synthesis, an effect mediated through the inhibition of cytochrome P450 side-chain cleavage (491).

4.3 CYTOKINES SYNTHESIZED IN THE BRAIN

Cytokines such as IL-1, IL-6, and TNF-α are synthesized by the brain but under normal, healthy, stress-free conditions their expression is low. IL-1β immunoreactivity is expressed in neurons of the hypothalamus (periventricular region, pPVN, and median eminence of the human brain (414, 492, 493). Similarly, IL-1β low-level immunoreactivity occurs in the rat brain; however, more prominent staining is found in extrahypothalamic sites, particularly in the hippocampus and in the cerebrovasculature. mRNA for ICE, the enzyme responsible for cleaving pro-IL-1β to mature, active IL-1β, is expressed in murine microglia, whole brain homogenates, homogenates of hypothalamus, and hippocampus, and blood vessels throughout the brain parenchyma. IL-1Ra mRNA is present in the hypothalamus (particularly the PVN), hippocampus, cerebellum, choroid plexus, and blood vessels throughout the brain.

TNF-α immunoreactivity occurs in the hypothalamus, caudal raphe nuclei, and ventral medulla and pons of the normal murine brain (414, 492, 493). Two TNF-α immunoreactive fibre pathways have been described, one that courses along the ventricular system (periventricular pathway) and one associated with the medial forebrain bundle. The PVN receives terminal fields from fibres in the medial forebrain bundle that originate from neurons in the bed nucleus of the stria terminalis, one of the most intensely stained cell groups. IL-6 mRNA has not been detected in the normal rat brain in one study (494), but in another article IL-6 mRNA was co-localized with IL-6Ra mRNA in the hypothalamus, cerebellum, hippocampus, striatum, neocortex, and pons/medulla (495).

Cytokines, particularly IL-1β, IL-6, and TNF-α, can be induced in the brain with cellular damage that results from CNS bacterial or viral infections, brain trauma, cerebral ischaemia, and convulsions, and in chronic CNS disorders such as multiple sclerosis, Alzheimer's disease, and Down's syndrome (496, 497). Under these conditions, microglia are the major cell type in which IL, chemokines, TNF, and IFN are synthesized, although vascular cells, astrocytes, and neurons contribute to the cytokine production. Peripheral administration of LPS in doses that do not compromise the integrity of the blood–brain barrier can induce cytokine expression in several brain regions, including cortex, cerebellum, thalamus, striatum, hippocampus, brain stem, and hypothalamus (mRNA for IL-1β, IL-6, TNF-α, and IFN-α) (448). Other studies in rodents have demonstrated IL-1β mRNA and protein after systemic i.v. or i.p. LPS in circumventricular organs (OVLT, SFO median eminence, area postrema, and pineal gland), meninges, and choroid plexus, with staining occurring in macrophages, microglia, and perivascular cells (414). Intraperitoneal administration of LPS also augments IL-1β immunoreactivity in the rat hypothalamus (498, 499). Induction of TNF-α and IL-6 mRNAs by LPS treatment occurs in perivascular and neuronal elements in the circumventricular organs (OVLT, area postrema, SFO (IL-6), and median eminence), in the meninges and in choroid plexus within 2 hours after treatment (495, 500). By 9–18 hours after LPS treatment, TNF-α mRNA is induced in the hypothalamus and nucleus tractus solitarius (500).

Enhanced production of cytokines derived from the immune system and from the brain occurs under certain stressful conditions. Psychosocial stressors induce cytokine synthesis in the hypothalamus. Immobilization stress in the rat induces hypothalamic expression of IL-1β mRNA (501, 502), IL-1Ra mRNA (502), and IL-1 bioactivity (503) within 30 minutes of initiation, and IL-6 mRNA is elevated in the midbrain 4–24 hours after restraint stress (504). In mouse brain homogenates from animals exposed to similar restraint paradigms, IFN-γ mRNA was elevated (505).

IL-1, IL-6, and brain-derived neurotrophic factor synthesis and/or secretion are altered during acute physical or psychological stresses, including exposure to a novel environment (506, 507), conditioned aversive stimuli (509), electroshock (508, 509), restraint in rodents (508, 511), treadmill exercise (511), and combat-related stress disorder in humans (512). In the CNS, IL-6 mRNA is elevated in the midbrain and hypothalamus 4–24 hours after restraint stress in rats (504). Similarly, acute and chronic restraint increases hypothalamic IL-1β mRNA (501, 502), IL-1 protein (503), and IL-1Ra mRNA (502). I.c.v. administration of IL-1Ra before inescapable shock blocks the subsequent interference with escape learning and enhancement of fear conditioning normally produced by such a stressor (513).

Collectively, these studies indicate that cytokines mediate some of the behavioural effects of non-inflammatory/infectious stressors, and that they play a role in homeostasis unrelated to immune function. Psychological/physical stressors produce many aspects of the acute phase response to sickness, and psychological/physical stress commonly precedes inflammatory/infectious stress in animals in the wild. These findings and observations suggest common mechanisms through which the body copes with infectious/inflammatory stressors, and physical/psychological stressors.

4.4   CYTOKINE RECEPTORS ARE EXPRESSED IN THE BRAIN

Cytokine effects in the CNS are mediated via interaction with specific receptors. Cytokine receptors for most of the ILs, IFNs, TNF, MIF, MIP, growth factors (CNTF, IGF-1 and 2, EGF, basic fibroblast growth factor, TGF, CSF), and neurotrophins have been reported in the brain (414). IL-1, IL-6, and TNF-α receptors have been investigated most extensively, and are most relevant for HPA activation. IL-1 receptors have a widespread distribution in the rat brain, including choroid plexus, cerebellum, cerebral cortex, and olfactory bulb, with low levels in the hypothalamus and median eminence (514, 515). Differences exist in the distribution of IL-1 receptors in brains from rats and mice. Overall, the murine brain exhibits consistently high levels of IL-1 receptors in the hippocampus (dentate gyrus, but not CA1 to CA4), choroid plexus, and meninges (414). IL-1 receptor mRNA is expressed predominantly in the dentate gyrus (granule cell layer), the entire midline raphe system, the choroid plexus, and endothelial cells. Very little IL-1 receptor or IL-1 receptor mRNA expression is present in the hypothalamus. IL-1 receptors are present on neurons (in mouse, and to a much lesser extent in rats), astrocytes, cerebrovascular endothelia, neuroblastoma cells, and glioblastoma cells, but not microglia (414). Moderate levels of IL-1 receptor-expressing neurons in the rat are found in the basolateral nucleus of the amygdala, the arcuate nucleus of the hypothalamus, the trigeminal and hypoglossal motor nuclei, and the area postrema (516). IL-2R2 mRNA is undetectable in both the rat and murine brain by *in situ* hybridization histochemistry, but can be induced by systemic treatment with kainic acid (517). Systemic LPS reduces IL-1 binding in rat and mouse brain, while RT–PCR (reverse transcription polymerase chain reaction) and RPA (ribonuclease protection assay) have demonstrated that either IL-1β or LPS increases the expression of IL-1R1 and IL-1R2, suggesting either increased receptor occupancy after immune activation or decreased translation of IL-1 receptor mRNA into protein (492, 496, 518).

IL-6 binding sites are expressed in extracts of bovine hypothalamus (519), and mRNA encoding the α subunit of the IL-6 receptor is present in neurons, microglia, and astrocytes from either normal brain tissue, primary cell cultures, or tumour cell lines (492, 498, 518). In the rat brain, IL-6Ra is most abundant in pyramidal cells of the hippocampus (CA1 and CA4) and in the dentate gyrus (granule cell layer) and has been detected in the hypothalamus, cerebellum, hippocampus, striatum, neocortex, and pons/medulla. IL-6Ra mRNA hybridization signals are also found in glial cells of the lateral olfactory tract, in ependymal cells of the olfactory and anterior lateral ventricle, and in neurons of the piriform cortex, medial habenular nucleus, neocortex, hippocampus, and hypothalamus (ventromedial and dorsomedial regions, including periventricular region and medial preoptic nucleus, but not the anterior hypothalamus and PVN) (496). Treatment with LPS markedly elevates IL-6Ra mRNA levels in the area postrema, bed nucleus of the stria terminalis, amygdala, cerebral cortex, claustrum, hippocampus, median eminence, piriform cortex, septohippocampal nucleus, PVN, SFO, OVLT, and in blood vessels throughout the rat brain (414).

Few studies have investigated the distribution or physiological role of TNF receptors in the brain. Binding studies in tissue homogenates of the murine brain reveal TNF-binding sites in the brain stem, cortex, thalamus, basal ganglia, and cerebellum (520). *In vitro* studies demonstrate TNF-R1 and TNF-R2 mRNA in murine cerebrovascular endothelium (521), and in human microglia, astrocytes, and oligodendrocytes (522, 523). TNF receptors have also been demonstrated in human neurons of the substantia nigra (TNF-R1), and hippocampal and striatal neurons (TNF-R1 and TNF-R2) (524), but there is no evidence for either TNF-α receptor subtype in the hypothalamus.

4.5 MECHANISMS OF CYTOKINE ENTRY INTO THE BRAIN

There are many proposed mechanisms through which cytokines such as IL-1 influence the HPA axis, these include: (a) direct actions on the pituitary and adrenal gland; (b) transport of cytokines across the blood–brain barrier either by diffusion through the disrupted blood–brain barrier or by transport mechanisms; (c) cytokine-induced prostaglandin-mediated mechanisms; (d) induction of intermediates at the blood–brain barrier, including prostaglandins and NO; (e) cytokine interaction at sites devoid of a blood–brain barrier (e.g. circumventricular organs); (f) cytokine activation of medullary catecholaminergic pathways; (g) cytokine stimulation of the vagus nerve; and (h) synthesis of cytokines within the CNS (414). A large body of evidence indicates that IL-1, regardless of the route of administration, acts at the hypothalamus, although the mechanisms are not entirely clear. Increased permeability of the blood–brain barrier during infection, inflammation, and administration of high doses of TNF-α or LPS has been demonstrated, indicating that this is a possible mechanism through which cytokine can enter the brain under certain conditions, but is does not explain the initial neuroendocrine effects of peripherally administered cytokines or LPS which occurs more quickly, and at lower doses of LPS and cytokines, does not compromise the integrity of the blood–brain barrier (414).

Carrier-facilitated transport of cytokines that are saturable has also been demonstrated (525–529). What has been questioned is whether the small amount of cytokine that enters the brain by this mechanism is physiologically significant. It seems likely that under conditions where peripheral blood levels remain elevated for a long period of time, this mechanism may provide cytokine–brain signalling of physiological relevance, but it seems unlikely that this route of communication accounts for the effects of peripherally administered cytokines on the HPA axis.

The relative lack of IL-1R on neurons in the pPVN and the limited entry of IL-1 into the brain have led to the hypothesis that IL-1 interacts with receptors at specific sites in the brain or cerebrovasculature, that in turn generate secondary molecules capable of diffusing into and then signalling the brain. Examples of secondary signalling molecules that have been investigated include CAs, 5-HT, histamine, lipid autocoids, eicosanoids, and NO. In the rat, PGE_2 concentrations in the OVLT, the posterior anterior hypothalamus, PVN, hippocampus, and cerebrospinal fluid of the lateral ventricle increase within 20 minutes of i.v. IL-1β injection (530, 531). Similarly, systemic LPS administration increases hypothalamic PGE_2 production (504). Peripheral administration of indomethacin attenuates the rise in plasma ACTH levels that result from i.v. administration of IL-1α, IL-1β, or TNF-α, but the inhibition is not always complete, and is short in duration even with multiple treatments of indomethacin or ibuprofen (414). A similar response to indomethacin occurs after i.c.v. injection of IL-1β, but the results from i.p. administration have been inconsistent (532, 533). Pretreatment systemically with indomethacin also blocks cfos expression in the pPVN of rats injected i.v., i.p., or i.c.v. with IL-1β or LPS, or continuously infused with IL-6, i.v. (423, 534–537). These effects are not explained by a direct action of indomethacin on enhanced feedback by elevated GC secretion from the adrenal gland. Interestingly, ACTH secretion caused by a variety of other stimuli is not affected by COX inhibition, including i.v. CRH (538, 539), electrofootshock (539), immobilization (505), or insulin-induced hypoglycaemia (538).

In vitro studies support a role for prostaglandins as an intermediary for cytokine actions on the HPA axis. Indomethacin prevents IL-1α-, IL-1β-, or IL-6-evoked CRH release from hypothalamic explants (540–543). Lastly, antibodies directed against PGE_1, PGE_2, or PGF_{2a} injected i.c.v. significantly reduce IL-1-stimulated ACTH secretion (544). Collectively, these studies support a direct role for prostaglandins in the mediation of IL-1 effects on the HPA axis. The anatomical sites and the cell types involved in prostaglandin synthesis are less clear; two sites have received much attention, the cerebrovasculature and the circumventricular organs.

NO, synthesized from the enzyme NOS is another possible mediator of IL-1 effects on the brain (414). NO is present in the PVN and SON of the hypothalamus (545, 546) and appears to have a restraining effect on IL-1-induced HPA activation (426, 547). Immobilization stress (545), i.c.v. CRH injection

(414), i.c.v. IL-1β (414), or systemic LPS (546) augment NOS expression in the PVN, indicating a role for NO in the regulation of the HPA axis. NOS is also expressed in cerebrovasculature (548) and hypophyseal portal blood vessels (549), as well as in the posterior (550) and anterior (551) pituitary. Pretreatment with the NOS substrate L-arginine (i.v.) blunts the rise in plasma ACTH induced by IL-1 (552), while NOS inhibitors administered i.v. exaggerate and prolong the ACTH and GC responses to IL-1β (414, 553). NOS inhibitors do not markedly influence ACTH secretion stimulated by treatment with CRH, but do potentiate the ACTH response to AVP and oxytocin, perhaps by increasing the sensitivity of corticotropes to AVP and/ or oxytocin (552). NO released from endothelial cells of the cerebrovasculature may mediate IL-1β-stimulated HPA activation, or alternatively NO may act indirectly by augmenting the suppressive effects of catecholaminergic pathways (414, 547).

Studies over the past several years indicate that cytokine may influence the CNS via interaction with receptors on peripheral nerves. Subdiaphragmatic transection of the vagus nerve (SDVX) several days before i.p. injection of LPS or IL-1β prevents the induction of Fos protein in the PVN and SON of the hypothalamus, and ACTH secretion (423). SDVX also reduces sickness behaviour (fever, sleep, loss of appetite), NE turnover, elevation of hypothalamic IL-1β mRNA, and hyperalgesia after i.p. LPS (553–556). Similarly, hyperalgesia and conditioned taste aversion induced by i.p. TNF-α are also inhibited by SDVX (557). While IL-1 receptors have not been found on vagal nerve fibres, they are expressed in abdominal paraganglia, which closely appose vagal fibres, and bind biotinylated IL-1Ra specifically (558). These findings suggest that the vagus provides an afferent route by which inflammation in the peritoneal cavity can influence the brain; sensory afferents in other sites of the body are likely to play a similar role in mediating inflammatory signals to the CNS (427, 559).

5 Discussion and concluding remarks

This chapter describes the anatomical associations between nerves and immunocytes in lymphoid tissue, with the assumption that they form an anatomical substrate for direct neural modulation of the immune system. The presence of receptors on cells of the immune system for all neurotransmitter-defined nerve fibres thus far described and the functional consequences of receptor activation on these cells support this route of neural–immune communication. Conversely, it is likely that immune cell products, upon release, can modulate nerve terminal activity, viability, and neurotransmitter release. We have also described hormonal effects on immune functions, and some of the mechanisms that mediate this interaction. Finally, we have discussed briefly some of the feedback mechanisms through which immune cell products regulate CNS activity. From this discussion it is clear that the distinction of what is a neurotransmitter/hormone vs. a cytokine has become less clear, since neurons, glia, and endocrine cells can synthesize and release cytokines, and cells of the immune system can synthesize and secrete neurotransmitters or neurohormones in some cases. These signalling molecules have been found to have a minimal effect on a particular immune parameter alone, but when administered with another signalling molecule they have a dramatic effect on the immune response. Thus, synergistic, as well as countersynergistic, modulation is likely to occur between signalling molecules.

The neurotransmitters thus far described in nerves in lymphoid tissues all have vasoactive capability to some extent, and can modulate blood flow, perfusion pressure, blood volume, and cell trafficking. Changes in vasculature alone can influence cell traffic to and from the lymphoid organ. Additionally, specific neurotransmitters could directly interact with lymphoid cells to direct trafficking, as is the case for VIP in the GALT. Additionally, dynamic changes can occur in innervation in lymphoid compartments, cellular components of the immune system, and in neuroendocrine regulation over the life span of an individual, and under a variety of physiological conditions. These changes clearly are important to immunocompetences and in determining whether the immune system can successful eliminate pathogens, suppress autoimmunity, and prevent tumour development. Aberrant neural–immune interactions that result from age-related changes of life insults also influence neurogenic inflammation and chronic inflammatory diseases.

The age-associated development of mammary and pituitary tumours and the inhibition of reproductive functions in old rats are due to a decline in the secretion of hormones by the neuroendocrine system, and by hypothalamic catecholaminergic activity. Pituitary PRL, considered as the major hormone regulating the tumour growth in rats, is inhibited by dopamine release from the hypothalamic tuberoinfundibular system. The ovarian steroids, oestrogen and progesterone, also directly and/or indirectly control mammary tumour development. Recent studies have demonstrated that PRL plays a critical role in the progression of breast cancer in women. Treatments that enhance or suppress CAs in the hypothalamus inhibit and promote, respectively, the development and growth of mammary tumours in rodents. A number of other hormones (thyroid hormones, insulin, corticosteroids, GH, melatonin), neurotransmitters (histamine, acetylcholine, 5-HT), and neuropeptides (VIP, opioids, LH-releasing hormone) are also involved in the onset and progression of mammary tumours (560).

Paralleling these changes in the neuroendocrine system, there is a profound decline in immune system functions, especially T-cell-mediated immunity, characterized by suppression of T-cell proliferation and IL-2 production in response to mitogens and antigens (561, 562). As described earlier, the functions of the immune system are influenced by NE released from NA nerve fibres that distribute to lymphoid organs and reside in close proximity to immunocytes. The age-related decline in the sympathetic NA innervation in spleens from F344 rats is accompanied by a decrease in NE content, lower total-uptake of NE, and increased β-adrenergic receptor density on splenocytes. Recently, ThyagaRajan and colleagues have demonstrated that deprenyl, a monoamine oxidase inhibitor, enhances sympathetic NA neuronal activity in spleen of old rats, an effect that is accompanied by an increase in mitogen-stimulated IL-2 production and NK-cell activity (563).

Immunosuppression in tumour-bearing rats is associated with lower dopaminergic activity in the hypothalamus and sympathetic NA activity in the spleen (ThyagaRajan, unpublished data). Treatment with deprenyl increases splenic NK-cell activity, mitogen-induced IL-2 and IFN-γ production, hypothalamic dopaminergic activity, and splenic NE concentration, suggesting that bidirectional communication between the neuroendocrine system and the immune system is critical in the treatment of breast cancer. Similar effects, such as enhanced splenic IFN-γ production, CD8$^+$ T cells, NE concentration, and hypothalamic dopamine concentration are found in deprenyl-treated rats with spontaneously occurring mammary tumours (564). Deprenyl treatment of rats with carcinogen-induced and spontaneously developing mammary tumours inhibits PRL secretion, which is associated with reduced monoamine metabolism in the medial basal hypothalamus (565–567). Although the mechanisms of action are not clear, deprenyl may be mediating its effects either directly on T and B lymphocytes to influence cytokine and growth factor production, or indirectly through the regulation of splenic sympathetic NA activity and secretion of hormones, such as PRL and GH, by the anterior pituitary, thymus, and spleen.

Studies examining the mechanisms of action, routes of communication, and the neural and immune mediators involved in disease processes are currently under way in many laboratories. The development of new technologies has contributed significantly to our current understanding of neural–immune interactions, and will continue to advance this multidisciplinary field. Future studies will provide critical information for understanding of CNS–immune mechanisms *in vivo*, and ultimately stimulate advances in novel interventions that work through neural–immune circuits.

Summary

This chapter summarizes the vast literature supporting bidirectional communication between the nervous system and the immune system. In recent years, research efforts have begun to identify neurotransmitter-, hormonal-, and cytokine-specific pathways through which these two systems interact. The central nervous system (CNS) influences the immune system via neuroendocrine outflow, and autonomic and sensory nerves that innervate lymphoid tissue. Neurotransmitter-specific nerves distribute to specific lymphoid compartments in lymphoid organs. Pharmacological studies have indicated that cells of the immune system possess receptors for these neurotransmitters, whereas functional studies have shown neurotransmitters to be capable of altering immune function. The neuroendocrine system also regulates the immune system through the release of a variety of hormones released by the pituitary gland, under the regulation of the hypothalamus. Conversely, immune-derived mediators called cytokines regulate neuroendocrine and autonomic outflow from the brain. Autonomic and neuroendocrine regulation of immune functions are discussed in this chapter. How cytokines modulate the CNS, pituitary, and endocrine target tissues is also presented. There is considerable complexity in neural–immune interactions. Future research needs to continue to focus on the mechanisms through which these two systems communicate under normal physiological conditions across the life span, during stressful life events, and in disease states. Additionally, research efforts should be concentrated on delineating neural–immune and/or immune–neural signalling involved in the etiology of specific disease states, and contributing factors that are important in increasing and decreasing susceptibility of the host to these diseases. Clearly of importance is the fact that stressful life events alter immunological function, with important consequences to health. These questions will only be answered through integrative approaches involving behavioural, pharmacological, neurological, and immunological hypothesis testing. We anticipate that a multidisciplinary approach to understanding neural–immune interaction will lead to the novel multifaceted and individualized therapies involving prophylactic measures, psychosocial interventions (behaviour modification, support groups, and relaxation therapies), and drug treatments that direct immunity (either cellular or humoral) towards the arm that most efficiently deals with infectious agents, autoimmunity, and cancer.

References

1. DePace, D. M. and Webber, R. H. (1975). Electrostimulation and morphologic study of the nerves to the bone marrow of the albino rat. *Acta Anat.*, **93**, 1–18.
2. Kawahara, G. and Osada, N. (1962). Studies on the innervation of bone marrow with special reference to the intramedullary fibres in the dog and goat. *Arch. Histol. Jpn*, **24**, 471–487.
3. Takase, B. and Nomura, S. (1957). Studies on the innervation of the bone marrow. *J. Comp. Neurol.*, **108**, 421–443.
4. Felten, D. L., Felten, S. Y., Carlson, S. L., Olschowka, J. A., and Livnat, S. (1985). Noradrenergic and peptidergic innervation of lymphoid tissue. *J. Immunol.*, **135**, 755s–765s.
5. Felten, S. Y. and Felten, D. L. (1991). The innervation of lymphoid tissue. In *Psychoneuroimmunology* (2nd edn), (eds R. Ader, D. L. Felten, and N. Cohen), pp. 27–69. Academic Press, New York.
6. Tabarowski, Z., Gibson-Berry, K., and Felten, S. Y. (1996). Noradrenergic and peptidergic innervation of the mouse femur. *Acta Histochem.*, **98**, 453–457.

7. Maestroni, G. J. and Conti, A. (1994). Modulation of hematopoiesis via alpha 1-adrenergic receptors on bone marrow cells. *Exp. Hematol.*, **22**, 313–320.
8. Setchenska, M. S., Bonanou-Tzedaki, S. A., and Arnstein, H. R. (1986). Classification of beta-adrenergic subtypes in immature rabbit bone marrow erythroblasts. *Biochem. Pharmacol.*, **35**, 3679–3684.
9. Maestroni, G. J. M., Cosentino, M., Marino, F., Togni, M., Conti, A., Lecchini, S. *et al.* (1998). Neural and endogenous catecholamines in the bone marrow. Circadian association of norepinephrine with hematopoiesis. *Exp. Hematol.*, **26**, 1172–1177.
10. Besedovsky, H. O., del Rey, A., Sorkin, E., Da Prada, M., and Keller, H. H. (1979). Immunoregulation mediated by the sympathetic nervous system. *Cell. Immunol.*, **48**, 346–355.
11. Madden, K. S., Sanders, V. M., and Felten, D. L. (1995). Catecholamine influences and sympathetic neural modulation of immune responsiveness. *Annu. Rev. Pharmacol. Toxicol.*, **35**, 417–448.
12. Yamazaki, K. and Allen, T. D. (1990). Ultrastructural morphometric study of efferent nerve terminals on murine bone marrow stromal cells, and the recognition of a novel anatomical unit: the 'neuro-reticular complex'. *Am. J. Anat.*, **187**, 261–276.
13. Afan, A. M., Broome, C. S., Nicholls, S. E., Whetton, A. D., and Miyan, J. A. (1997). Bone marrow innervation regulates cellular retention in the murine haemopoietic system. *Br. J. Haematol.*, **98**, 569–577.
14. Garcia, J. F. and van Dyke, D. C. (1961). Response of rats of various ages to erythropoietin. *Proc. Soc. Exp. Biol. Med.*, **106**, 585–588.
15. Calvo, W. and Forteza-Vila, J. (1969). On the development of bone marrow innervation in new-born rats as studied with silver impregnation and electron microscopy. *Am. J. Anat.*, **126**, 355–359.
16. Cosentino, M., Marino, F., Bombelli, R., Ferrari, M., Maestroni, G. J., Conti, A. *et al.* (1998). Association between the circadian course of endogenous noradrenaline and the hematopoietic cell cycle in mouse bone marrow. *J. Chemother.*, **10**, 179–181.
17. Maestroni, G. J. M., Conti, A., and Pedrinis, E. (1992). Effect of adrenergic agents on hematopoiesis after syngeneic bone marrow transplantation in mice. *Blood*, **80**, 1178.
18. Felten, D. L., Gibson-Berry, K., and Wu, J. H. D. (1996). Innervation of bone marrow by tyrosine hydroxylase-immunoreactive nerve fibres and hemopoiesis-modulating activity of a β-adrenergic agonist in mouse. *Mol. Biol. Hematopoiesis*, **5**, 627–636.
19. Benestad, H. B., Strom-Gundersen, I., Ole Iversen, P., Haug, E., and Nja, A. (1998). No neuronal regulation of murine bone marrow function. *Blood*, **91**, 1280–1287.
20. Tran, M. A., Dang, T. L., Lafontan, M. S., and Montastruc, P. (1985). Adrenergic neurohumoral influences of FFA release from bone marrow adipose tissue. *J. Pharmacol.*, **16**, 171–179.
21. Feldman, S., Rachmilewitz, E. A., and Izak, G. (1966). The effect of central nervous system stimulation on erythropoiesis in rat with chronically implanted electrodes. *J. Lab. Clin. Med.*, **67**, 713–725.
22. Müller, S. and Weihe, E. (1991). Interrelation of peptidergic innervation with mast cells and ED1-positive cells in rat thymus. *Brain Behav. Immun.*, **5**, 55–72.
23. Bellinger, D. L., Lorton, D., Romano, T., Olschowka, J. A., Felten, S. Y., and Felten, D. L. (1990). Neuropeptide innervation of lymphoid organs. *Ann. N. Y. Acad. Sci.*, **594**, 17–33.

24. Al Shawaf, A. A., Kendall, M. D., and Cowen, T. (1991). Identification of neural profiles containing vasoactive intestinal polypeptide, acetylcholinesterase and catecholamines in the rat thymus. *J. Anat.*, **174**, 131–143.
25. Thompson, R. J., Doran, J. F., Jackson, P., Dhillon, A. P., and Rode, J. (1983). PGP 9.5: a new marker for vertebrate neurons and neuroendocrine cells. *Brain Res.*, **278**, 224–228.
26. Kurz, B., Feindt, J., von Gaudecker, B., Kranz, A., Loppnow, H., and Mentlein, R. (1997). Beta-adrenoceptor-mediated effects in rat cultured thymic epithelial cells. *Br. J. Pharmacol.*, **120**, 1401–1408.
27. Chan, A. S. (1992). Association of nerve fibres with myoid cells in the chick thymus. *J. Anat.*, **181**, 509–512.
28. Singh, U. (1979). Effect of catecholamines on lymphopoiesis in fetal mouse thymic explants. *J. Anat.*, **129**, 279–292.
29. Singh, U. (1979). Effect of catecholamines on lymphopoiesis in fetal mouse thymic explants. *Eur. J. Immunol.*, **14**, 757–759.
30. Singh, U. (1985). Effect of sympathectomy on the maturation of fetal thymocytes grown within the anterior eye chambers in mice. *Adv. Exp. Biol. Med.*, **186**, 349–356.
31. Singh, U. (1985). Lymphopoiesis in the nude fetal mouse thymus following sympathectomy. *Cell. Immunol.*, **93**, 222–228.
32. Singh, U. and Owen, J. J. T. (1975). Studies on the effect of various agents on the maturation of thymus stem cells. *Eur. J. Immunol.*, **5**, 286–288.
33. Singh, U. and Owen, J. J. T. (1976). Studies on the maturation of thymus stem cells. The effects of catecholamines, histamine, and peptide hormones on the expression of T alloantigens. *Eur. J. Immunol.*, **6**, 59–62.
34. Felten, D. L., Felten, S. Y., Bellinger, D. L., Carlson, S. L., Ackerman, K. D., Madden, K. S. *et al.* (1987). Noradrenergic sympathetic neural interactions with the immune system: structure and function. *Immunol. Rev.*, **100**, 225–260.
35. Livnat, S., Felten, S. Y., Carlson, S. L., Bellinger, D. L., and Felten, D. L. (1985). Involvement of peripheral and central catecholamine systems in neural–immune interactions. *J. Neuroimmunol.*, **10**, 5–30.
36. Carlson, S. L., Albers, K. M., Beiting, D. J., Parish, M., Conner, J. M., and Davis, B. M. (1995). NGF modulates sympathetic innervation of lymphoid tissues. *J. Neurosci.*, **15**, 5892.
37. Felten, S. Y. and Olschowka, J. A. (1987). Noradrenergic sympathetic innervation of the spleen: II. Tyrosine hydroxylase (TH)-positive nerve terminals form synaptic-like contacts on lymphocytes in the splenic white pulp. *J. Neurosci. Res.*, **18**, 37–48.
38. Kelley, S. P., Grota, L. J., Felten, S. Y., Madden, K. S., and Felten, D. L. (1996). Norepinephrine in mouse spleen shows minor strain differences and no diurnal variation. *Pharmacol. Biochem. Behav.*, **53**, 141–146.
39. Ackerman, K. D., Felten, S. Y., Bellinger, D. L., and Felten, D. L. (1987). Noradrenergic sympathetic innervation of the spleen: III. Development of innervation in the rat spleen. *J. Neurosci. Res.*, **18**, 49–54.
40. Ackerman, K. D., Felten, S. Y., Bellinger, D. L., Livnat, S., and Felten, D. L. (1987). Noradrenergic sympathetic innervation of spleen and lymph nodes in relation to specific cellular compartments. *Prog. Immunol.*, **6**, 588–600.
41. Bellinger, D. L., Ackerman, K. D., Felten, S. Y., Lorton, D., and Felten, D. L. (1989). Noradrenergic sympathetic innervation of thymus, spleen and lymph

nodes: aspects of development, aging and plasticity in neural–immune interactions. In *Proceedings of a Symposium on Interactions Between the Neuroendocrine and Immune Systems* (ed. G. Nistico), pp. 35–66. Pythogora Press, Rome.

42. Bellinger, D. L., Felten, S. Y., Ackerman, K. D., Lorton, D., Madden, K. S., and Felten, D. L. (1992). Noradrenergic sympathetic innervation of lymphoid organs during development, aging, and autoimmune disease. In *Aging of the Autonomic Nervous System* (ed. F. Amenta), pp. 243–284. CRC Press, Boca Raton, FL.

43. Felten, D. L., Livnat, S., Felten, S. Y., Carlson, S. L., Bellinger, D. L., and Yeh, P. (1984). Sympathetic innervation of lymph nodes in mice. *Brain Res. Bull.*, **13**, 693–699.

44. Fink, T. and Weihe, E. (1988). Multiple neuropeptides in nerves supplying mammalian lymph nodes: messenger candidates for sensory and autonomic neuroimmunomodulation? *Neurosci. Lett.*, **90**, 39–44.

45. Ernström, U. and Sandberg, G. (1974). Stimulation of lymphocyte release from the spleen by theophylline and isoproterenol. *Acta Physiol. Scand.*, **90**, 202–209.

46. Ernström, U. and Söder, O. (1975). Influence of adrenaline on the dissemination of antibody-producing cells from the spleen. *Clin. Exp. Immunol.*, **21**, 131–140.

47. Kostrzewa, R. M. and Jacobwitz, D. M. (1974). Pharmacological actions of 6-hydroxydopamine. *Pharmacol. Rev.*, **26**, 199–288.

48. Madden, K. S., Felten, S. Y., Felten, D. L., Moynihan, J., Hardy, C. A., and Livnat, S. (1994). Sympathetic nervous modulation of the immune system. II. Induction of lymphocyte proliferation and migration *in vivo* by chemical sympathectomy. *J. Neuroimmunol.*, **49**, 67–75.

49. Madden, K. S. and Livnat, S. (1991). Catecholaminergic action on immunologic reactivity. In *Psychoneuroimmunology* (2nd edn), (eds R. Ader, D. L. Felten, and N. Cohen), pp. 283–310. Academic Press, New York.

50. Kruszewska, B., Felten, S. Y., and Moynihan, J. A. (1995). Alterations in cytokine and antibody production following chemical sympathectomy in two strains of mice. *J. Immunol.*, **155**, 4613–4620.

51. Kruszewska, B., Felten, D. L., Stevens, S. Y., and Moynihan, J. A. (1998). Sympathectomy-induced immune changes are not abrogated by the glucocorticoid receptor blocker RU-486. *Brain Behav. Immun.*, **12**, 181–200.

52. Madden, K. S., Felten, S. Y., Felten, D. L., Sundaresan, P. R., and Livnat, S. (1989). Sympathetic neural modulation of the immune system. I. Depression of T cell immunity *in vivo* and *in vitro* following chemical sympathectomy. *Brain Behav. Immun.*, **3**, 72–89.

53. Benschop, R. J., Rodriquez-Feuerhahn, M., and Schedlowski, M. (1996). Catecholamine-induced leukocytosis. Early observations, current research, and future directions. *Brain Behav. Immun.*, **10**, 77–91.

54. Carlson, S. L., Beiting, D. J., Kiani, C. A., Abell, K. M., and McGillis, J. P. (1996). Catecholamines decrease lymphocyte adhesion to cytokine-activated endothelial cells. *Brain Behav. Immun.*, **10**, 55–67.

55. Benschop, R. J., Schedlowski, M., Wienecke, H., Jacobs, R., and Schmidt, R. E. (1997). Adrenergic control of natural killer cell circulation and adhesion. *Brain Behav. Immun.*, **11**, 321–332.

56. Li, Y. S., Kouassi, E., and Revillard, J. P. (1990). Differential regulation of mouse B-cell activation of β-adrenoceptor stimulation depending on type of mitogens. *Immunology*, **69**, 367–372.

57. Sanders, V. M. and Powell-Oliver, F. E. (1992). b2-adrenoceptor stimulation increases the number of antigen specific precursor B lymphocytes that differentiate into IgM-secreting cells without affecting burst size. *J. Immunol.*, **148**, 1822–1828.

58. Bartik, M. M., Brooks, W. H., and Roszman, T. L. (1993). Modulation of T cell proliferation by stimulation of the β-adrenergic receptor: lack of correlation between inhibition of T cell proliferation and cAMP accumulation. *Cell. Immunol.*, **148**, 408–421.

59. Hatfield, S. M., Petersen, B. H., and DiMicco, J. A. (1986). Beta adrenoceptor modulation of the generation of murine cytotoxic T lymphocytes *in vitro*. *J. Pharmacol. Exp. Ther.*, **239**, 460–466.

60. Ramer-Quinn, D. S., Baker, R. A., and Sanders, V. M. (1997). Activated T helper 1 and T helper 2 cells differentially express the β-2-adrenergic receptor A mechanism for selective modulation of T helper 1 cell cytokine production. *J. Immunol.*, **159**, 4857–4867.

61. Landmann, R. (1992). Beta-adrenergic receptors in human leukocyte subpopulations. *Eur. J. Clin. Invest.*, **22**(Suppl. 1), 30–36.

62. Shakhar, G. and Ben-Eliyahu, S. (1998). *In vivo* β-adrenergic stimulation suppresses natural killer activity and compromises resistance to tumour metastasis in rats. *J. Immunol.*, **160**, 3251–3258.

63. Brenner, G. J., Felten, S. Y., Felten, D. L., and Moynihan, J. A. (1992). Sympathetic nervous system modulation of tumour metastases and host defense mechanisms. *J. Neuroimmunol.*, **37**, 191–202.

64. Bellinger, D. L., Felten, S. Y., and Felten, D. L. (1988). Maintenance of noradrenergic sympathetic innervation in the involuted thymus of the aged Fischer 344 rat. *Brain Behav. Immun.*, **2**, 133–150.

65. Madden, K. S., Bellinger, D. L., Felten, S. Y., Synder, E., Maida, M. E., and Felten, D. L. (1997). Alterations in sympathetic innervation of thymus and spleen in aged mice. *Mech. Ageing Dev.*, **94**, 165–175.

66. Josefsson, E., Bergquist, J., Ekman, R., and Tarkowski, A. (1996). Catecholamines are synthesized by mouse lymphocytes and regulate function of these cells by induction of apoptosis. *Immunology*, **88**, 140–146.

67. Berquist, J., Josefsson, E., Tarkowski, A., Ekman, R., and Ewing, A. (1997). Measurements of catecholamine-mediated apoptosis of immunocompetent cells by capillary electrophoresis. *Electrophoresis*, **18**, 1760–1766.

68. Bellinger, D. L., Felten, S. Y., Collier, T. J., and Felten, D. L. (1987). Noradrenergic sympathetic innervation of the spleen: IV. Morphometric analysis in adult and aged F344 rats. *J. Neurosci. Res.*, **18**, 55–63.

69. Felten, S. Y., Bellinger, D. L., Collier, T. J., Coleman, P. D., and Felten, D. L. (1987). Decreased sympathetic innervation of spleen in aged Fischer 344 rats. *Neurobiol. Aging*, **8**, 159–165.

70. Bellinger, D. L., Ackerman, K. D., Felten, S. Y., and Felten, D. L. (1992). A longitudinal study of age-related loss of noradrenergic nerves and lymphoid cells in the aged rat spleen. *Exp. Neurol.*, **116**, 295–311.

71. Carlson, S. L., Felten, D. L., Livnat, S., and Felten, S. Y. (1987). Noradrenergic sympathetic innervation of the spleen: V. Acute drug-induced depletion of lymphocytes in the target fields of innervation results in redistribution of noradrenergic fibres but maintenance of compartmentation. *J. Neurosci. Res.*, **18**, 64–69.

72. Ackerman, K. D., Bellinger, D. L., Felten, S. Y., and Felten, D. L. (1991). Ontogeny and senescence of noradrenergic innervation of the rodent thymus and spleen. In *Psychoneuroimmunology* (2nd edn), (eds R. Ader, D. L. Felten, and N. Cohen), pp. 72–125. Academic Press, New York.

73. Madden, K. S., Felten, S. Y., Felten, D. L., and Bellinger, D. L. (1995). Sympathetic nervous system–immune system interactions in young and old Fischer 344 (F344) rats. *Ann. N. Y. Acad. Sci.*, **771**, 523–534.

74. Bjurholm, A., Kreicbergs, A., Broden, E., and Schultzberg, M. (1989). Substance P- and CGRP-immunoreactive nerves in bone. *Peptides*, **9**, 165–171.

75. Iwasaki, A., Inoue, K., and Hukuda, S. (1995). Distribution of neuropeptide-containing nerve fibres in the synovium and adjacent bone of the rat knee joint. *Clin. Exp. Rheumatol.*, **13**, 173–178.

76. Imai, S., Tokunaga, Y., Maeda, T., Kikkawa, M., and Hukuda, S. (1997). Calcitonin gene-related peptide, substance P, and tyrosine hydroxylase-immunoreactive innervation of the rat bone marrow: an immunohistochemical and ultrastructural investigation on possible efferent and afferent mechanisms. *J. Orthop. Res.*, **15**, 133–140.

77. Ahmed, M., Srinivasan, G. R., Theodorsson, E., Bjurholm, A., and Kreicbergs, A. (1994). Extraction and quantitation of neuropeptides in bone by radioimmunoassay. *Regul. Pept.*, **51**, 179–188.

78. Maestroni, G. J. (1998). Is hematopoiesis under the influence of neural and neuroendocrine mechanisms? *Histol. Histopathol.*, **13**, 271–274.

79. Rameshwar, P., Ganea, D., and Gascon, P. (1993). In vitro stimulatory effect of substance P on hematopoiesis. *Blood*, **81**, 391–398.

80. Rameshwar, P., Ganea, D., and Gascon, P. (1994). Induction of IL-3 and granulocyte-macrophage colony-stimulating factor by substance P in bone marrow cells is partially mediated through the release of IL-1 and IL-6. *J. Immunol.*, **152**, 4044–4054.

81. Rameshwar, P., Poddar, A., and Gascon, P. (1997). Hematopoietic regulation mediated by interactions among the neurokinins and cytokines. *Leuk. Lymphoma*, **28**, 1–10.

82. Rameshwar, P. and Gascon, P. (1996). Induction of negative hematopoietic regulators by neurokinin-A in bone marrow stroma. *Blood*, **88**, 98–106.

83. Rameshwar, P. and Gascon, P. (1997). Hematopoietic modulation by the tachykinins. *Acta Haematol.*, **98**, 59–64.

84. Manske, J. M., Sullivan, E. L., and Andersen, S. M. (1995). Substance P mediated stimulation of cytokine levels in cultured murine bone marrow stromal cells. *Adv. Exp. Med. Biol.*, **383**, 53–64.

85. McGillis, J. P., Rangnekar, V., and Ciallella, J. R. (1995). A role for calcitonin gene-related peptide (CGRP) in the regulation of early B lymphocyte differentiation. *Can. J. Physiol. Pharmacol.*, **73**, 1057–1064.

86. Elhassan, A. M., Adem, A., Hultenby, K., and Lindgren, J. U. (1998). Somatostatin immunoreactivity in bone and joint tissues. *NeuroReport*, **9**, 2573–2575.

87. Weihe, E., Müller, S., Fink, T., and Zentel, H. J. (1989). Tachykinins, calcitonin gene-related peptide and neuropeptide Y in nerves of the mammalian thymus: interactions with mast cells in autonomic and sensory neuroimmunomodulation. *Neurosci. Lett.*, **100**, 77–82.

88. Kendall, M. D. and Al-Shawaf, A. A. (1991). Innervation of the rat thymus gland. *Brain Behav. Immun.*, 5, 9–28.

89. Kranz, A., Kendall, M. D., and von Gaudecker, B. (1997). Studies on rat and human thymus to demonstrate immunoreactivity of calcitonin gene-related peptide, tyrosine hydroxylase and neuropeptide Y. *J. Anat.*, 191, 441–450.

90. Gulati, P., Tay, S. S., and Leong, S. K. (1997). Nitrergic, peptidergic and substance P innervation of the chick thymus. *J. Hirnforsch.*, 38, 553–564.

91. Bellinger, D. L., Felten, S. Y., and Felten, D. L. (1992). Neural–immune interactions: neurotransmitter signaling of cells of the immune system. *Annu. Rev. Psychiatry*, 11, 127–144.

92. Bulloch, K., Hausman, J., Radojcic, T., and Short, S. (1991). Calcitonin gene-related peptide in the developing and aging thymus. An immunocytochemical study. *Ann. N. Y. Acad. Sci.*, 621, 218–228.

93. Bulloch, K., Radojcic, T., Yu, R., Hausman, J., Lenhard, L., and Baird, S. (1991). The distribution and function of calcitonin gene-related peptide in the mouse thymus and spleen. *Prog. NeuroEndocrinImmunol.*, 4, 186–194.

94. Lorton, D., Bellinger, D. L., Felten, S. Y., and Felten, D. L. (1990). Substance P innervation of the rat thymus. *Peptides*, 11, 1269–1275.

95. Jurjus, A. R., More, N., and Walsh, R. J. (1998). Distribution of substance P positive cells and nerve fibres in the rat thymus. *J. Neuroimmunol.*, 90, 143–148.

96. Geppetti, P., Maggi, C. A., Zecchi-Orlandini, S., Santicioli, P., Meli, A., Frilli, S. *et al.* (1987). Substance P-like immunoreactivity in capsaicin-sensitive structures of the rat thymus. *Regul. Pept.*, 18, 321–329.

97. Geppetti, P., Frilli, S., Renzi, D., Santicioli, P., Maggi, C. A., Theodorsson, E. *et al.* (1988). Distribution of calcitonin gene-related peptide-like immunoreactivity in various rat tissues: correlation with substance P and other tachykinins and sensitivity to capsaicin. *Regul. Pept.*, 23, 289–298.

98. Elfvin, L. G., Aldskogius, H., and Johansson, J. (1993). Primary sensory afferents in the thymus of the guinea pig demonstrated with anterogradely transported horseradish peroxidase conjugates. *Neurosci. Lett.*, 150, 35–38.

99. Bellinger, D. L., Lorton, D., Brouxhon, S., Felten, S. Y., and Felten, D. L. (1996). The significance of vasoactive intestinal polypeptide (VIP) in immunomodulation. *Adv. Neuroimmunol.*, 6, 5–27.

100. Bellinger, D. L., Lorton, D., Horn, L., Felten, S. Y., and Felten, D. L. (1997). Vasoactive intestinal polypeptide (VIP) innervation of rat spleen, thymus, and lymph nodes. *Peptides*, 18, 1139–1149.

101. Stead, R. H., Tomioka, M., Quinonez, G., Simon, G., Felten, S. Y., and Bienenstock, J. (1987). Intestinal mucosal mast cells in normal and nematode-infected rat intestines are in intimate contact with peptidergic nerves. *Proc. Natl. Acad. Sci. USA*, 84, 2975–2979.

102. Aguila, M. C., Dees, W. L., Haensely, W. E., and McCann, S. M. (1991). Evidence that somatostatin is localized and synthesized in lymphoid organs. *Proc. Natl. Acad. Sci. USA*, 88, 11485–11489.

103. Clements, J. A. and Funder, J. W. (1986). Arginine vasopressin (AVP) and AVP-like immunoreactivity in peripheral tissues. *Endocr. Rev.*, 7, 449–460.

104. Geenen, V., Legros, J.-J., Franchimont, P., Baudrihaye, M., Defresne, M. P., and Boniver, J. (1986). The neuroendocrine thymus: coexistence of oxytocin and neurophysin in the human thymus. *Science*, 232, 508–510.

105. Geenen, V., Legros, J.-J., Franchimont, P., Defresne, M. P., Boniver, J., Ivell, R. *et al.* (1987). The thymus as a neuroendocrine organ: synthesis of vasopressin and oxytocin in human thymic epithelium. *Ann. N. Y. Acad. Sci.*, **496**, 56–66.
106. Markwick, A. J., Lolait, S. J., and Funder, J. W. (1986). Immunoreactive arginine vasopressin in the rat thymus. *Endocrinology*, **119**, 1690–1696.
107. Gulati, P., Leong, S., and Chan, A. S. (1998). Ontogeny of NADPH-d expression in the thymic microenvironment of the chick embryo. *Cell Tissue Res.*, **294**, 335–343.
108. Romano, T. A., Felten, S. Y., Felten, D. L., and Olschowka, J. A. (1991). Neuropeptide-Y innervation of the rat spleen: another potential immunomodulatory neuropeptide. *Brain Behav. Immun.*, **5**, 116–131.
109. Romano, T., Felten, S. Y., Olschowka, J. A., and Felten, D. L. (1994). Noradrenergic and peptidergic innervation of lymphoid organs in the beluga, *Delphinapterus leucas*: an anatomical link between the nervous and immune systems. *J. Morphol.*, **221**, 243–259.
110. Olschowka, J. A., Felten, S. Y., Bellinger, D. L., Lorton, D., and Felten, D. L. (1988). NPY-positive nerve terminals contact lymphocytes in the periarteriolar lymphatic sheath of the rat splenic white pulp. *Soc. Neurosci. Abstr.*, **14**, 1280.
111. Meltzer, J. C., Grimm, P. C., Greenberg, A. H., and Nance, D. M. (1997). Enhanced immunohistochemical detection of autonomic nerve fibres, cytokines and inducible nitric oxide synthase by light and fluorescent microscopy in rat spleen. *J. Histochem. Cytochem.*, **45**, 599–610.
112. Fried, G., Terenius, L., Brodin, E., Efendic, S., Dockray, G., Fahrenkrug, J. *et al.* (1986). Neuropeptide Y, enkephalin and noradrenaline coexist in sympathetic neurons innervating the bovine spleen. Biochemical and immunohistochemical evidence. *Cell Tissue Res.*, **243**, 495–508.
113. Rosenstein, J. M. and Brightman, M. W. (1983). Circumventing the blood–brain barrier with autonomic ganglion transplants. *Science*, **221**, 879–881.
114. Lundberg, J. M., Änggård, A., Pernow, J., and Hökfelt, T. (1985). Neuropeptide Y-, substance P- and VIP-immunoreactive nerves in cat spleen in relation to autonomic vascular and volume control. *Cell Tissue Res.*, **239**, 9–18.
115. Lundberg, J. M., Rudehill, A., Sollevi, A., Theodorsson-Norhein, E., and Hamberger, B. (1986). Frequency- and reserpine-dependent chemical coding of sympathetic transmission: differential release of noradrenaline and neuropeptide Y from pig spleen. *Neurosci. Lett.*, **63**, 96–100.
116. Lorton, D., Bellinger, D. L., Felten, S. Y., and Felten, D. L. (1991). Substance P innervation of spleen in rats: nerve fibres associate with lymphocytes and macrophages in specific compartments of the spleen. *Brain Behav. Immun.*, **5**, 29–40.
117. Baron, R. and Jänig, W. (1988). Sympathetic and afferent neurons projecting in the splenic nerve of the cat. *Neurosci. Lett.*, **94**, 109–113.
118. Fillenz, M. (1970). The innervation of the cat spleen. *Proc. R. Soc. London*, **174**, 459–468.
119. Bellinger, D. L., Felten, S. Y., Lorton, D., and Felten, D. L. (1989). Origin of noradrenergic innervation of the spleen in rats. *Brain Behav. Immun.*, **3**, 291–311.
120. Nance, D. M. and Burns, J. (1989). Innervation of the spleen in the rat: evidence for absence of afferent innervation. *Brain Behav. Immun.*, **3**, 281–290.
121. Elfvin, L.-G., Aldskogius, H., and Johansson, J. (1992). Splenic primary sensory afferents in the guinea pig demonstrated with anterogradely transported

wheat-germ agglutinin conjugated to horseradish peroxidase. *Cell Tissue Res.*, **269**, 229–234.

122. Bellinger, D. L., Earnest, D. J., Gallagher, M., and Felten, D. L. (1992). Presence and availability of VIP in primary and secondary lymphoid organs. *Soc. Neurosci. Abstr.*, **18**, 1009.

123. Chevendra, V. and Weaver, L. C. (1992). Distribution of neuropeptide Y, vasoactive intestinal peptide and somatostatin in populations of postganglionic neurons innervating the rat kidney, spleen and intestine. *Neuroscience*, **50**, 727–743.

124. Schultzberg, M., Svenson, S. B., Unden, A., and Bartfai, T. (1987). Interleukin-1-like immunoreactivity in peripheral tissues. *J. Neurosci. Res.*, **18**, 184–189.

125. Nohr, D., Michel, S., Fink, T., and Weihe, E. (1995). Pro-enkephalin opioid peptides are abundant in porcine and bovine splenic nerves, but absent from nerves of rat, mouse, hamster, and guinea-pig spleen. *Cell Tissue Res.*, **281**, 215–219.

126. Romeo, H. E., Fink, T., Yanaihara, N., and Weihe, E. (1994). Distribution and relative proportions of neuropeptide Y- and proenkephalin-containing noradrenergic neurones in rat superior cervical ganglion: separate projections to submaxillary lymph nodes. *Peptides*, **15**, 1479–1487.

127. Enzmann, V. and Drossler, K. (1994). Immunohistochemical detection of substance P and vasoactive intestinal peptide fibres in the auricular lymph nodes of sensitized guinea-pigs and mice. *Acta Histochem. Jena*, **96**, 15–18.

128. Popper, P., Mantyh, C. R., Vigna, S. R., Magioos, J. E., and Mantyh, P. W. (1988). The localization of sensory nerve fibres and receptor binding sites for sensory neuropeptides in canine mesenteric lymph nodes. *Peptides*, **9**, 257–267.

129. Kurkowski, R., Kummer, W., and Heym, C. (1990). Substance P-immunoreactive nerve fibres in tracheobronchial lymph nodes of the guinea pig: origin, ultrastructure and coexistence with other peptides. *Peptides*, **11**, 13–20.

130. Reubi, J. C., Horisberger, U., Dappeler, A., and Laissue, J. A. (1998). Localization of receptors for vasoactive intestinal peptide, somatostatin, and substance P in distinct compartments of human lymphoid organs. *Blood*, **92**, 191–197.

131. Dureus, P., Louis, D., Grant, A. V., Bilfinger, T. V., and Stefano, G. B. (1993). Neuropeptide Y inhibits human and invertebrate immunocyte chemotaxis, chemokinesis, and spontaneous activation. *Cell. Mol. Neurobiol.*, **13**, 541–546.

132. Nair, M. P., Schwartz, S. A., Wu, K., and Kronfol, Z. (1993). Effect of neuropeptide Y on natural killer activity of normal human lymphocytes. *Brain Behav. Immun.*, **7**, 70–78.

133. De La Fuente, M., Bernaez, I., Del Rio, M., and Hernanz, A. (1993). Stimulation of murine peritoneal macrophage functions by neuropeptide Y and peptide YY. Involvement of protein kinase C. *Immunology*, **80**, 259–265.

134. Sung, C. P., Arleth, A. J., and Feuerstein, G. Z. (1991). Neuropeptide Y upregulates the adhesiveness of human endothelial cells for leukocytes. *Circ. Res.*, **68**, 314–318.

135. Hafstrom, I., Ringertz, B., Lundeberg, T., and Palmblad, J. (1993). The effect of endothelin, neuropeptide Y, calcitonin gene-related peptide and substance P. *Acta Physiol. Scand.*, **148**, 341–346.

136. Foreman, J. C. and Jordan, C. C. (1983). Histamine release and vascular changes induced by neuropeptides. *Agents Actions*, **13**, 105–111.

137. Payan, D. G., McGillis, J. P., Renold, F. K., Mitsuhashi, M., and Goetzl, E. J. (1987). The immunomodulating properties of neuropeptides. In *Hormones and Immunity* (eds I. Berczi and K. Kovacs), pp. 203–214. MTP, Norwell, MA.

138. Lofstrom, B., Pernow, B., and Wahren, J. (1985). Vasodilating action of substance P in human forearm. *Acta Physiol. Scand.*, **63**, 311–315.

139. Lundbert, J. M., Saria, A., Brodin, E., Rosell, S., and Folkars, K. (1983). A substance P antagonist inhibits vagally-induced increase in vascular permeability and bronchial smooth muscle contraction in the guinea pig. *Proc. Natl. Acad. Sci. USA*, **80**, 1120–1124.

140. Ruff, M. R., Wahl, S. M., and Pert, C. B. (1985). Substance P receptor-mediated chemotaxis of human monocytes. *Peptides*, **6**, 107–111.

141. Hartung, H. P. and Toyka, K. V. (1983). Activation of macrophages by substance P: induction of oxidative burst and thromboxane release. *Eur. J. Pharmacol.*, **89**, 301–305.

142. Hartung, H.-P., Wolters, K., and Toyka, K. V. (1986). Substance P: binding properties and studies on cellular responses in guinea pig macrophages. *J. Immunol.*, **136**, 3856–3863.

143. Lotz, M., Vaughan, J. H., and Carson, D. A. (1988). Effect of neuropeptides on production of inflammatory cytokines by human monocytes. *Science*, **241**, 1218–1221.

144. Braun, A., Wiebe, P., Pfeufer, A., Gessner, R., and Renz, H. (1999). Differential modulation of human immunoglobulin isotype production by the neuropeptides, substance P, NKA and NKB. *J. Neuroimmunol.*, **97**, 43–50.

145. Payan, D. G., Brewster, D. R., and Goetzl, E. J. (1983). Specific stimulation of human T lymphocytes by substance P. *J. Immunol.*, **131**, 1613–1615.

146. Stanisz, A. M., Befus, D., and Bienenstock, J. (1986). Differential effects of vasoactive intestinal peptide, substance P, and somatostatin on immunoglobulin synthesis and proliferations by lymphocytes from Peyer's patches, mesenteric lymph nodes, and spleen. *J. Immunol.*, **136**, 152–156.

147. Payan, D. G., Brewster, D. R., Missirian-Bastian, A., and Goetzl, E. J. (1984). Substance P recognition by a subset of human T lymphocytes. *J. Clin. Invest.*, **74**, 1532–1539.

148. Stanisz, A. M., Scicchitano, R., Dazin, P., Bienenstock, J., and Payan, D. G. (1987). Distribution of substance P receptors on murine spleen and Peyer's patch T and B cells. *J. Immunol.*, **139**, 749–754.

149. Weinstock, J. V., Blum, A., and Khetarpal, S. (1988). Eosinophils from granulomas in murine *Schistosomiasis mansoni* produce substance P. *Immunology*, **71**, 52–56.

150. Nilsson, J., von Euler, A. M., and Dalsgaard, C.-J. (1985). Stimulation of connective tissue cell growth by substance P and substance K. *Nature*, **315**, 61–63.

151. Payan, D. G. (1985). Receptor-mediated mitogenic effects of substance P on cultured smooth muscle cells. *Biochem. Biophys. Res. Commun.*, **130**, 104–109.

152. McGillis, J. P., Organist, M. L., and Payan, D. G. (1987). Substance P and immunoregulation. *Fed. Proc.*, **46**, 196–199.

153. Okiji, T., Jontell, M., Belichenko, P., Dahlgren, U., Bergenholtz, G., and Dahlstrom, A. (1997). Structural and functional association between substance P- and calcitonin gene-related peptide-immunoreactive nerves and accessory cells in the rat dental pulp. *J. Dent. Res.*, **76**, 1818–1824.

154. Bulloch, K., McEwen, B. S., Diwa, A., Radojcic, T., Hausman, J., and Baird, S. (1994). The role of calcitonin gene-related peptide in the mouse thymus revisited. *Ann. N. Y. Acad. Sci.*, **741**, 129–136.

155. Wang, X., Fiscus, R. R., Tang, Z., Yany, L., Wu, J., Fan, S. *et al.* (1994). CGRP in the serum of endotoxin-treated rats suppresses lymphoproliferation. *Brain Behav. Immun.*, **8**, 282–292.

156. Bulloch, K., McEwen, B. S., Diwa, A., and Baird, S. (1995). Relationship between dehydroepiandrosterone and calcitonin gene-related peptide in the mouse thymus. *Am. J. Physiol.*, **2689**, E168–E173.

157. Umeda, Y. and Arisawa, M. (1990). Characterization of the calcitonin gene-related peptide receptor in mouse T lymphocytes. *Neuropeptides*, **14**, 237–242.

158. Asahina, A., Hosoi, J., Beissert, S., Stratigos, A., and Granstein, R. D. (1995). Inhibition of the induction of delayed-type and contact hypersensitivity by calcitonin gene-related peptide. *J. Immunol.*, **154**, 3056–3061.

159. Torii, H., Hosoi, J., Beissert, S., Xu, S., Fox, F. E., Asahina, A. *et al.* (1997). Regulation of cytokine expression in macrophages and the Langerhans cell-like XS-52 by calcitonin gene-related peptide. *J. Leukocyte Biol.*, **61**, 216–223.

160. Fox, R. E., Kubin, M., Cassin, M., Niu, Z., Hosoi, J., Torii, H. *et al.* (1997). Calcitonin gene-related peptide inhibits proliferation and antigen presentation by human peripheral blood mononuclear cells: effects on B7, interleukin 10 and interleukin 12. *J. Invest. Dermatol.*, **108**, 43–48.

161. Gespach, C., Chedeville, A., Hurbain-Kosmath, I., Housset, B., Derenne, J.-P., and Abita, J.-P. (1989). Adenylate cyclase activation by VIP-helodermin and histamine H_2 receptors in human THP-1 monocytes/macrophages: a possible role in the regulation of superoxide anion production. *Regul. Pept.*, **26**, 158.

162. Abello, J., Damien, C., De Neef, P., Tastenoy, M., Googhe, R., Robberecht, P. *et al.* (1989). Properties of vasoactive-intestinal-peptide receptors and β-adrenoceptors in the murine radiation leukemia virus-induced lymphoma cell line BL/VL₃. *Eur. J. Biochem.*, **183**, 263–267.

163. Calvo, J. R., Montilla, M. L., Guerrero, J. M., and Segura, J. J. (1994). Expression of VIP receptors in mouse peritoneal macrophages: functional and molecular characterization. *J. Neuroimmunol.*, **50**, 85–93.

164. Segura, J. J., Guerrero, J. M., Goberna, R., and Calvo, J. R. (1991). Characterization of functional receptors for vasoactive intestinal peptide (VIP) in rat peritoneal macrophages. *Regul. Pept.*, **35**, 133–143.

165. Bondesson, L., Norolind, K., Liden, S., Gafvelin, G., Theodorsson, E., and Mutt, V. (1991). Dual effects of vasoactive intestinal peptide (VIP) on leucocyte migration. *Acta Physiol. Scand.*, **141**, 477–481.

166. Ottaway, C. A. (1984). *In vitro* alteration of receptors for vasoactive intestinal peptide changes the *in vivo* localization of mouse T cells. *J. Exp. Med.*, **160**, 1054–1069.

167. Moore, T. C., Spruck, C. H., and Said, S. I. (1988). *In vivo* depression of lymphocyte traffic in sheep by VIP and HIV (AIDS)-related peptides. *Immunopharmacology*, **16**, 181–189.

168. Ohkubo, N., Miura, S., Serizawa, H., Yan, H. J., Kimura, H., Imaeda, H. *et al.* (1994). *In vivo* effect of chronic administration of vasoactive intestinal peptide on gut-associated lymphoid tissues in rats. *Regul. Pept.*, **50**, 127–135.

169. Ottaway, C. A., Lewis, D. L., and Asa, S. L. (1987). Vasoactive intestinal peptide-containing nerves in Peyer's patches. *Brain Behav. Immun.*, 1, 148–158.
170. Johnston, J. A., Taub, D. D., Lloyd, A. R., Conlon, K., Oppenheim, J. J., and Kevlin, D. J. (1994). Human T lymphocyte chemotaxis and adhesion induced by vasoactive intestinal peptide. *J. Immunol.*, 153, 1762–1768.
171. Robichon, A., Sreedharan, S. P., Yang, J., Shames, R. S., Gronroos, E. C., Cheng, P. P.-J. *et al.* (1993). Induction of aggregation of Raji human B-lymphoblastic cells by vasoactive intestinal peptide. *Immunology*, 79, 574–579.
172. Peuriere, S., Susini, C., Alvinerie, M., Vaysse, N., and Escoula, L. (1991). Interactions between neuropeptides and dexamethasone on the mitogenic response of rabbit spleen lymphocytes. *Peptides*, 12, 645–651.
173. Stanisz, A. M., Scicchitano, R., and Bienenstock, J. (1988). The role of vasoactive intestinal peptide and other neuropeptides in the regulation of the immune response *in vitro* and *in vivo*. *Ann. N. Y. Acad. Sci.*, 527, 478–485.
174. Neil, G. A., Blum, A., and Weinstock, J. V. (1991). Substance P but not vasoactive intestinal peptide modulates immunoglobulin secretion in murine schistosomiasis. *Cell. Immunol.*, 135, 394–401.
175. Kimata, H., Yoshida, A., Ishioka, C., and Mikawa, H. (1992). Differential effect of vasoactive intestinal peptide, somatostatin, and substance P on human IgE and IgG subclass production. *Cell. Immunol.*, 144, 429–442.
176. Kimata, H., Yoshida, A., Fujimoto, M., and Mikawa, H. (1993). Effect of vasoactive intestinal peptide, somatostatin, and substance P on spontaneous IgE and IgG4 production in atopic patients. *J. Immunol.*, 150, 4630–4640.
177. Kimata, H. and Fujimoto, M. (1995). Induction of IgA1 and IgA2 production in immature human fetal B cells and pre-B cells by vasoactive intestinal peptide. *Blood*, 85, 2098–2104.
178. Drew, P. and Shearman, D. (1985). Vasoactive intestinal peptide: a neurotransmitter which reduces human NK cell activity and increases Ig synthesis. *Aust. J. Exp. Biol. Med. Sci.*, 63, 313–318.
179. Rola-Pleszczynski, M., Bulduc, D., and St Pierre, A. (1985). The effects of VIP on human NK cell function. *J. Immunol.*, 135, 2659–2673.
180. Sirianni, M. C., Annibale, B., Tagliaferri, F., Fais, S., De Luca, S., Pallone, F. *et al.* (1992). Modulation of human natural killer activity by vasoactive intestinal peptide (VIP) family. VIP, glucagon, and GHRF specifically inhibit NK activity. *Regul. Pept.*, 38, 79–87.
181. van Tol, E. A. F., Verspaget, H. W., Pena, A. S., Jansen, J. B. M. J., Aparicio-Pages, N., and Lamers, C. B. H. W. (1991). Modulatory effects of VIP and related peptides from the gastrointestinal tract on cell mediated cytotoxicity against tumour cells *in vitro*. *Immunol. Invest.*, 20, 257–267.
182. van Tol, E. A. F., Verspaget, H. W., Hansen, B. E., and Lamers, C. B. H. W. (1993). Neuroenteric peptides affect natural killer activity by intestinal lamina propria mononuclear cells. *J. Neuroimmunol.*, 42, 139–146.
183. Ginsburg, C. H., Dambrauskas, J. T., Ault, K. A., and Falchuk, Z. M. (1983). Impaired natural killer cell activity in patients with inflammatory bowel disease: evidence for a qualitative defect. *Gastroenterology*, 85, 846–851.
184. Koch, T. R., Carney, J. A., and Go, V. L. W. (1987). Distribution and quantitation of gut neuropeptides in normal intestine and inflammatory bowel disease. *Dig. Dis. Sci.*, 32, 369–376.

185. Koch, T. R., Carney, J. A., Go, V. L. W., and Szurszewski, J. H. (1990). Altered inhibitory innervation of circular smooth muscle in Crohn's colitis: association with decreased vasoactive intestinal polypeptide levels. *Gastroenterology*, **98**, 1437–1444.

186. Foda, H. D., Iwanaga, T., Liu, L. W., and Said, S. I. (1988). Vasoactive intestinal peptide protects against HCl-induced pulmonary edema in rats. *Ann. N. Y. Acad. Sci.*, **527**, 633–636.

187. Berisha, H., Foda, H. D., Sakakibara, H., Trotz, M., Pakbaz, H., and Said, S. I. (1990). Vasoactive intestinal peptide prevents lung injury due to xanthine/xanthine oxidase. *Am. J. Physiol.*, **259**, L151–L155.

188. Kurosawa, M. and Ishizuka, T. (1993). Inhibitory effects of vasoactive intestinal peptide on superoxide anion formation by N-formyl-methionyl-leucyl-phenylalanine-activated inflammatory cells *in vitro*. *Int. Arch. Allergy Appl. Immunol.*, **100**, 28–34.

189. Said, S. I. (1988). Vasoactive intestinal peptide in the lung. *Ann. N. Y. Acad. Sci.*, **527**, 450–464.

190. Wiik, P. (1989). Vasoactive intestinal peptide inhibits the respiratory burst in human monocytes by a cyclic AMP-mediated mechanism. *Regul. Pept.*, **25**, 187–197.

191. Undem, B. J., Dick, E. C., and Buckner, C. K. (1983). Inhibition by vasoactive intestinal peptide of antigen-induced histamine release from guinea-pig minced lung. *Eur. J. Pharmacol.*, **88**, 247–249.

192. Di Marzo, V., Tippins, J. R., and Morris, H. R. (1986). The effect of vasoactive intestinal peptide and calcitonin gene-related peptide on peptidoleukotriene release from platelet activating factor stimulated rat lungs and ionophore stimulated guinea pig lungs. *Biochem. Int.*, **13**, 933–942.

193. Fjellner, B. and Hagermark, O. (1981). Studies on pruritogenic and histamine-releasing effects of some putative peptide neurotransmitters. *Acta Derm. (Stockholm)*, **61**, 245–250.

194. Church, M. K., El-Lati, S., and Caulfield, J. P. (1991). Neuropeptide-induced secretion from human skin mast cells. *Int. Arch. Allergy Appl. Immunol.*, **94**, 310–318.

195. Shanahan, F., Denburg, J. A., Fox, J., Bienenstock, J., and Befus, D. (1985). Mast cell heterogeneity: effects of neuroenteric peptides on histamine release. *J. Immunol.*, **135**, 1331–1337.

196. Pawlikowski, M., Stepien, H., Kunert-Radek, J., and Schally, A. V. (1985). Effect of somatostatin on the proliferation of mouse spleen lymphocytes *in vitro*. *Biochem. Biophys. Res. Commun.*, **129**, 52–55.

197. Stanisz, A. M., Scicchitano, R., Payan, D. G., and Bienenstock, J. (1987). *In vitro* studies of immunoregulation of substance P and somatostatin. *Ann. N. Y. Acad. Sci.*, **496**, 217–225.

198. Payan, D. G., Hess, C. A., and Goetzl, E. J. (1984). Inhibition by somatostatin of the proliferation of T-lymphocytes and Molt-4 lymphoblasts. *Cell. Immunol.*, **84**, 433–438.

199. Theoharides, T. C. and Douglas, W. W. (1981). Mast cell histamine secretion in response to somatostatin analogues: structural considerations. *Eur. J. Pharmacol.*, **73**, 131–136.

200. Bar-Shavit, Z., Goldman, R., Stabinsky, Y., Gottleib, F., Fridkin, M., Teichberg, V. *et al.* (1980). Enhancement of phagocytosis—a newly found activity of

substance P residing in its N-terminal tetrapeptide sequence. *Biochem. Biophys. Res. Commun.*, **94**, 1445–1451.

201. Goetzl, E. J. and Payan, D. G. (1984). Inhibition by somatostatin of the release of mediators from human basophils and rat leukemic basophils. *J. Immunol.*, **133**, 3255–3259.

202. Payan, D. G., McGillis, J. P., and Goetzl, E. J. (1986). Neuroimmunology. In *Advances in Immunology* (eds F. J. Dixon, K. F. Austen, L. Hood, and J. W. Uhr), pp. 299–323. Academic Press, New York.

203. Blum, A. M., Metwall, A., Mathew, R. C., Elliot, D., and Weinstock, J. V. (1993). Substance P and somatostatin can modulate the amount of IgG_{2a} secreted in response to schistosome egg antigens in murine *Schistosomiasis mansoni. J. Immunol.*, **151**, 6694–7004.

204. Elliott, D. E., Blum, A. M., Li, J., Metwali, A., and Weinstock, J. V. (1998). Pre-prosomatostatin messenger RNA is expressed by inflammatory cells and induced by inflammatory mediators and cytokines. *J. Immunol.*, **160**, 3997–4003.

205. Auernhammer, C. J. and Strasburger, C. J. (1995). Effects of growth hormone and insulin-like growth factor I on the immune system. *Eur. J. Endocrinol.*, **133**, 635–645.

206. Gagnerault, M. C., Postel-Vinay, M. C., and Dardenne, M. (1996). Expression of growth hormone receptors in murine lymphoid cells analyzed by flow cytofluorimetry. *Endocrinology*, **137**, 1719–1726.

207. Badamchian, M., Spangelo, B. L., Damavandy, T., MacLeod, R. M., and Goldstein, A. L. (1991). Complete amino acid sequence analysis of a peptide isolated from the thymus that enhances release of growth hormone and prolactin. *Endocrinology*, **128**, 1580–1588.

208. Goya, R. G., Sosa, Y. E., Brown, O. A., and Dardenne, M. (1994). *In vitro* studies on the thymus–pituitary axis in young and old rats. *Ann. N. Y. Acad. Sci.*, **741**, 108–114.

209. Binder, G., Revskoy, S., and Gupta, D. (1994). *In vivo* growth hormone gene expression in neonatal rat thymus and bone marrow. *J. Endocrinol.*, **140**, 137–143.

210. Chen, H. T., Schuler, L. A., and Schultz, R. D. (1999). Growth hormone receptor and regulation of gene expression in fetal lymphoid cells. *Mol. Cell. Endocrinol.*, **137**, 21–29.

211. Yang, Y., Guo, L., Ma, L., and Liu, X. (1999). Expression of growth hormone and insulin-like growth factor in the immune system of children. *Horm. Metab. Res.*, **31**, 380–384.

212. Johnson, R. W., Arkins, S., Dantzer, R., and Kelley, K. W. (1997). Hormones, lymphohemopoietic cytokines and the neuroimmune axis. *Comp. Biochem. Physiol. A. Physiol.*, **116**, 183–201.

213. Dialynas, E., Brown-Borg, H., and Bartke, A. (1999). Immune function in transgenic mice overexpressing growth hormone (GH) releasing hormone, GH or GH antagonist. *Proc. Soc. Exp. Biol. Med.*, **221**, 178–183.

214. Postel-Vinay, M. C., de Mello Coelho, V., Gagnerault, M. C., and Dardenne, M. (1997). Growth hormone stimulates the proliferation of activated mouse T lymphocytes. *Endocrinology*, **138**, 1816–1820.

215. Mustafa, A., Nyberg, F., Mustafa, M., Bakhiet, M., Mustafa, E., Winblad, B. *et al.* (1997). Growth hormone stimulates production of interferon-gamma by human peripheral mononuclear cells. *Horm. Res.*, **48**, 11–15.

216. Bidlingmaier, M., Auernhammer, C. J., Feldmeier, H., and Strasburger, C. J. (1997). Effects of growth hormone and insulin-like growth factor I binding to natural killer cells. *Acta Paediatr. Suppl.*, **423**, 80–81.

217. Crist, D. M. and Kraner, J. C. (1990). Supplemental growth hormone increases the tumour cytotoxic activity of natural killer cells in healthy adults with normal growth hormone secretion. *Metabolism*, **39**, 1320–1324.

218. Saxena, Q. B., Saxena, R. K., and Adler, W. H. (1982). Regulation of natural killer activity *in vivo*. III. Effect of hypophysectomy and growth hormone treatment on the natural killer activity of the mouse spleen cell population. *Int. Arch. Allergy Appl. Immunol.*, **67**, 169–174.

219. Saito, H., Inoue, T., Fukatsu, K., Ming-Tsan, L., Inaba, T., Fukushima, R. *et al.* (1996). Growth hormone and the immune response to bacterial infection. *Horm. Res.*, **45**, 50–54.

220. Soto, L., Martin, A. I., Millan, S., Vara, E., and Lopez-Calderon, A. (1998). Effects of endotoxin lipopolysaccharide administration on the somatotropic axis. *J. Endocrinol.*, **159**, 239–246.

221. Haeffner, A., Thieblemont, N., Deas, O., Marelli, O., Charpentier, B., Senik, A. *et al.* (1997). Inhibitory effect of growth hormone on TNF-alpha secretion and nuclear factor-kappaB translocation in lipopolysaccharide-stimulated human monocytes. *J. Immunol.*, **158**, 1310–1314.

222. Matsuda, T., Saito, H., Inoue, T., Fukatsu, K., Han, I., Furukawa, S. *et al.* (1998). Growth hormone inhibits apoptosis and upregulates reactive oxygen intermediates production by human polymorphonuclear neutrophils. *J. Parenter. Enteral Nutr.*, **22**, 368–374.

223. Yada, T., Nagae, M., Moriyama, S., and Azuma, T. (1999). Effects of prolactin and growth hormone on plasma immunoglobulin M levels of hypophysectomized rainbow trout, *Oncorhynchus mykiss*. *Gen. Comp. Endocrinol.*, **115**, 46–52.

224. Kotzmann, H., Koller, M., Czernin, S., Clodi, M., Svoboda, T., Riedl, M. *et al.* (1994). Effect of elevated growth hormone concentrations on the phenotype and functions of human lymphocytes and natural killer cells. *Neuroendocrinology*, **60**, 618–625.

225. Krishnaraj, R., Zaks, A., and Unterman, T. (1998). Relationship between plasma IGF-I levels, *in vitro* correlates of immunity, and human senescence. *Clin. Immunol. Immunopathol.*, **88**, 264–270.

226. Mazzoccoli, G., Giuliani, A., Bianco, G., De Cata, A., Balzanelli, M., Carella, A. M. *et al.* (1999). Decreased serum levels of insulin-like growth factor (IGF)-I in patients with lung cancer: temporal relationship with growth hormone (GH) levels. *Anticancer Res.*, **19**, 1397–1399.

227. Wu, H., Wang, J., Cacioppo, J. T., Glaser, R., Kiecolt-Glaser, J. K., and Malarkey, W. B. (1999). Chronic stress associated with spousal caregiving of patients with Alzheimer's dementia is associated with downregulation of B-lymphocyte GH mRNA. *J. Gerontol. A. Biol. Sci. Med. Sci.*, **54**, M212–M215.

228. Heemskerk, V. H., Daemen, M. A., and Buurman, W. A. (1999). Insulin-like growth factor-1 (IGF-1) and growth hormone (GH) in immunity and inflammation. *Cytokine Growth Factor Rev.*, **10**, 5–14.

229. Nguyen, B. Y., Clerici, M., Venzon, D. J., Bauza, S., Murphy, W. J., Longo, D. L. *et al.* (1998). Pilot study of the immunologic effects of recombinant human

growth hormone and recombinant insulin-like growth factor in HIV-infected patients. *AIDS*, **12**, 895–904.

230. Mellado, M., Llorente, M., Rodriguez-Frade, J. M., Lucas, P., Martinez, C., and del Real, G. (1998). HIV-1 envelope protein gp120 triggers a Th2 response in mice that shifts to Th1 in the presence of human growth hormone. *Vaccine*, **16**, 1111–1115.

231. Wu, H., Devi, R., and Malarkey, W. B. (1996). Expression and localization of prolactin messenger ribonucleic acid in the human immune system. *Endocrinology*, **137**, 349–353.

232. Dardenne, M., Leite-de-Moraes, M. C., Kelly, P. A., and Gagnerault, M. C. (1994). Prolactin receptor expression in human hematopoietic tissues analyzed by flow cytofluorometry. *Endocrinology*, **134**, 2108–2114.

233. Gunes, H. and Mastro, A. M. (1997). Prolactin receptor gene expression in rat splenocytes and thymocytes during oestrous cycle, pregnancy and lactation. *Cell Prolif.*, **30**, 213–219.

234. Ferrag, F., Goffin, V., Buteau, H., and Kelly, P. A. (1997). Immune function of prolactin (PRL) and signal transduction by PRL/GH/cytokine receptors: specificity, redundancy and lessons from chimaeras. *Cytokines Cell. Mol. Ther.*, **3**, 197–213.

235. Bole-Feysot, C., Goffin, V. M., Goffin, V., Edery, M., Binart, N., and Kelly, P. A. (1998). Prolactin (PRL) and its receptor: actions, signal transduction pathways and phenotypes observed in PRL receptor knockout mice. *Endocr. Rev.*, **19**, 225–268.

236. Yu-Lee, L. Y. (1997). Molecular actions of prolactin in the immune system. *Proc. Soc. Exp. Biol. Med.*, **215**, 35–52.

237. Matera, L. (1997). Action of pituitary and lymphocyte prolactin. *Neuroimmunomodulation*, **4**, 171–180.

238. Duncan, G. S., Mittrucker, H. W., Kagi, D., Matsuyama, T., and Mak, T. W. (1996). The transcription factor interferon regulatory factor-1 is essential for natural killer cell function *in vivo*. *J. Exp. Med.*, **184**, 2043–2048.

239. Mukherjee, P., Mastro, A. M., and Hymer, W. C. (1990). Prolactin induction of interleukin-2 receptors on rat splenic lymphocytes. *Endocrinology*, **126**, 88–94.

240. Cesario, T. C., Yousefi, S., Carandang, G., Sadati, N., Le, J., and Vaziri, N. (1994). Enhanced yields of gamma interferon in prolactin treated human peripheral blood mononuclear cells. *Proc. Soc. Exp. Biol. Med.*, **205**, 89–95.

241. Murphy, W. J., Rui, H., and Longo, D. L. (1995). Effects of growth hormone and prolactin immune development and function. *Life Sci.*, **57**, 1–14.

242. Kumar, A., Singh, S. M., and Sodhi, A. (1997). Effect of prolactin on nitric oxide and interleukin-1 production of murine peritoneal macrophages: role of Ca^{2+} and protein kinase C. *Int. J. Immunopharmacol.*, **19**, 129–133.

243. Meli, R., Raso, G. M., Bentivoglio, C., Nuzzo, I., Galdiero, M., and Di Carlo, R. (1996). Recombinant human prolactin induces protection against *Salmonella typhimurium* infection in the mouse: role of nitric oxide. *Immunopharmacology*, **34**, 1–7.

244. Zhu, X. H., Zellweger, R., Wichmann, M. W., Ayala, A., and Chaudry, I. H. (1997). Effects of prolactin and metoclopramide on macrophage cytokine gene expression in late sepsis. *Cytokine*, **9**, 437–446.

245. Horseman, N. D., Zhao, W., Montecino-Rodriguez, E., Tanaka, M., Nakashima, K., Engle, S. J. *et al.* (1997). Defective mammopoiesis, but normal

hematopoiesis, in mice with a targeted disruption of the prolactin gene. *EMBO J.*, **16**, 6926–6935.

246. Bouchard, B., Ormandy, C. J., Di Santo, J. P., and Kelly, P. A. (1999). Immune system development and function in prolactin receptor-deficient mice. *J. Immunol.*, **163**, 576–582.

247. Webster, E. L. and De Souza, E. B. (1988). Corticotrophin-releasing factor receptors in mouse spleen: identification, autoradiographic localization, and regulation by divalent cations and guanine nucleotides. *Endocrinology*, **122**, 609–617.

248. Audya, T., Jain, R., and Hollander, C. S. (1991). Receptor mediated immunomodulation by corticotropin-releasing factor. *Cell. Immunol.*, **134**, 77.

249. McGillis, J. P., Park, A., Rubin-Fletter, P., Turck, C., Dallman, M. F., and Payan, D. G. (1989). Stimulation of rat B-lymphocyte proliferation by corticotropin-releasing factor. *J. Neurosci.*, **23**, 346–352.

250. Radulovic, M., Dautzenberg, F. M., Sydow, S., Radulovic, J., and Spiess, J. (1999). Corticotropin-releasing factor receptor 1 in mouse spleen: expression after immune stimulation and identification of receptor-bearing cells. *J. Immunol.*, **162**, 3013–3021.

251. Dave, J. R. and Eskay, R. L. (1986). Demonstration of corticotropin-releasing factor binding sites on human and rat erythrocyte membranes and their modulation by chronic ethanol treatment in rats. *Biochem. Biophys. Res. Commun.*, **136**, 137–144.

252. Ritchie, J. C., Owens, M. J., O'Connor, L., Kegelmeyer, L. W., Walker, J. T., Stanley, M. *et al.* (1986). Measurement of ACTH and CRF immunoreactivity in adrenal gland and lymphocytes. *Soc. Neurosci. Abstr.*, **12**, 1041.

253. Stephanou, A., Jessop, D. S., Knight, R. A., and Lightman, S. L. (1990). Corticotropin-releasing factor-like immunoreactivity and mRNA in human leukocytes. *Brain Behav. Immun.*, **4**, 67–73.

254. Aird, F., Clevenger, C. V., Prystowsky, M. B., and Redei, E. (1993). Corticotropin-releasing factor mRNA in rat thymus and spleen. *Proc. Natl. Acad. Sci. USA*, **90**, 7104.

255. Redei, E. (1992). Immuno-reactive and bioactive corticotrophic-releasing factor in rat thymus. *Neuroendocrinology*, **55**, 115–118.

256. Brouxhon, S. M., Prasad, A. V., Joseph, S. A., Felten, D. L., and Bellinger, D. L. (1998). Localization of corticotropin-releasing factor in primary and secondary lymphoid organs of the rat. *Brain Behav. Immun.*, **12**, 107–122.

257. Bamberger, C. M., Wald, M., Bamberger, A. M., Ergun, S., Beil, F. U., and Schulte, H. M. (1998). Human lymphocytes produce urocortin, but not corticotropin-releasing hormone. *J. Clin. Endocrinol. Metab.*, **83**, 708–711.

258. Smith, E. M., Morrill, A. C., Meyer, W. J. III, and Blalock, J. E. (1986). Corticotropin releasing factor induction of leukocyte-derived immunoreactive ACTH and endorphins. *Nature*, **321**, 881–882.

259. Kavelaars, A., Ballieux, R. E., and Heijnen, C. J. (1990). β-endorphin secretion by human peripheral blood mononuclear cells: regulation by glucocorticoids. *Life Sci.*, **46**, 1233–1240.

260. Irwin, M., Vale, W., and Britton, K. T. (1987). Central corticotropin-releasing factor suppresses natural killer cytotoxicity. *Brain Behav. Immun.*, **1**, 81–87.

261. Carr, D. J. J., De Costa, B. R., Jacobson, A. E., Rice, K. C., and Blalock, J. E. (1990). Corticotropin-releasing hormone augments natural killer cell activity through a nalozone-sensitive pathway. *J. Neuroimmunol.*, **28**, 53.

262. Singh, V. K., Warren, R. P., White, E. D., and Leu, S. J. C. (1990). Corticotropin-releasing factor induced stimulation of immune function. *Ann. N. Y. Acad. Sci.*, **594**, 416–419.

263. Montamant, S. C. and Davies, A. O. (1989). Physiological response to isoproterenol and coupling of beta-adrenergic receptors in young and elderly human subjects. *J. Gerontol.*, **44**, M100–M105.

264. Okamoto, S., Ishikawa, I., Kimura, K., and Saito, M. (1998). Potent suppressive effects of urocortin on splenic lymphocyte activity in rats. *NeuroReport*, **21**, 4035–4039.

265. McCann, S. M., Lyson, K., Karanth, S., Gimeno, M., Belova, N., Kamat, A. *et al.* (1994). Role of cytokines in the endocrine system. *Ann. N. Y. Acad. Sci.*, **741**, 50–63.

266. Smith, E. M., Hughes, T. K. Jr, Hashemi, F., and Stefano, G. B. (1992). Immunosuppressive effects of corticotropin and melanotropin and their possible significance in human immunodeficiency virus infection. *Proc. Natl. Acad. Sci. USA*, **89**, 782–786.

267. Karalis, K., Sano, H., Redwine, J., Listwak, S., Wilder, R. L., and Chrousos, G. P. (1991). Autocrine or paracrine inflammatory actions of corticotropin releasing hormone *in vivo*. *Science*, **254**, 421–423.

268. Crofford, L. J., Sano, H., Karalis, K., Webster, E. L., Goldmuntz, E. A., and Chrousos, G. P. (1992). Local secretion of corticotropin-releasing hormone in the joints of Lewis rats with inflammatory arthritis. *J. Clin. Invest.*, **90**, 2555–2564.

269. Casadevall, M., Saperas, E., Panes, J., Salas, A., Anderson, D. C., Malagelada, J. R. *et al.* (1999). Mechanisms underlying the anti-inflammatory actions of central corticotropin-releasing factor. *Am. J. Physiol.*, **276**, G1016–1026.

270. Berkenbosch, J., van Oers, J., del Rey, A., Tilders, F., and Besedovsky, H. (1987). Corticotropin-releasing factor-producing neurons in the rat activated by interleukin-1. *Science*, **238**, 524–526.

271. Sapolsky, R., Rivier, C., Yamamoto, G., Plotsky, P., and Vale, W. (1987). Interleukin-1 stimulates the secretion of hypothalamic corticotropin-releasing factor. *Science*, **238**, 522–524.

272. Uehara, A., Goltschal, P. E., Dahl, R. R., and Arimura, A. (1987). Interleukin-1 stimulates ACTH release by an indirect action which requires endogenous corticotropin releasing factor. *Endocrinology*, **121**, 1580–1582.

273. Tsagarakis, S., Gillies, G., Rees, L., Besser, M., and Grossman, A. (1989). Interleukin-1 directly stimulates the release of corticotropin-releasing factor from rat hypothalamus. *Neuroendocrinology*, **49**, 98–101.

274. Suda, T., Tozawa, R., Ushiyama, T., Sumitomo, T., Yamada, M., and Demura, H. (1990). Interleukin-1 stimulates corticotropin-releasing factor gene expression in rat hypothalamus. *Endocrinology*, **126**, 1223–1228.

275. Farrar, W. L. (1984). *Opioid Peptides in the Periphery*, pp. 159–165. Elsevier, New York.

276. Milenkovic, L., Rettori, V., Snyder, G. D., Beutler, B., and McCann, S. M. (1989). Cachectin alters anterior pituitary hormone release by a direct action *in vitro*. *Proc. Natl. Acad. Sci. USA*, **86**, 2418–2422.

277. Fukata, J., Usui, T., Naito, Y., Nakai, Y., and Imura, H. (1989). Effects of recombinant human interleukin-1α, 1β, 2 and 6 on ACTH synthesis and release in the mouse pituitary tumour cell line AtT20. *J. Endocrinol.*, **122**, 33–39.

278. Sawchenko, P. E., Swanson, L. W., and Vale, W. W. (1984). Co-expression of CRF- and vasopressin-immunoreactivity in parvocellular neurosecretory neurons in the adrenalectomized rat. *Proc. Natl. Acad. Sci. USA*, **81**, 1883–1887.

279. Tilders, F. J. H., Schmidt, E. D., and De Goeij, D. C. E. (1993). Phenotypic plasticity of CRF neurons during stress. *Ann. N. Y. Acad. Sci.*, **697**, 39–52.

280. Sawchenko, P. E., Brown, E. R., Chan, R. K. W., Ericsson, A., Li, H.-Y., Roland, B. I. *et al.* (1996). The paraventricular nucleus of the hypothalamus and functional neuroanatomy of visceromotor responses to stress. *Prog. Brain Res.*, **107**, 201–222.

281. Antoni, F. A., Fink, G., and Sherwood, W. J. (1990). Corticotropin-releasing peptides in rat hypophysial portal blood after paraventricular nucleus lesions: a marked reduction in the concentration of corticotropin-releasing factor-41, but no change in vasopressin. *J. Endocrinol.*, **125**, 175–183.

282. Plotsky, P. M. (1991). Pathways to the secretion of adrenocorticotropin: a view from the portal. *J. Neuroendocrinol.*, **3**, 1–9.

283. Plotsky, P. M. and Sawchenko, P. E. (1987). Hypophysial portal plasma levels, median eminence content and immunohistochemical staining of corticotropin-releasing factor, arginine vasopressin and oxytocin following pharmacological adrenalectomy. *Endocrinology*, **120**, 1361–1369.

284. Rivier, C. and Vale, W. W. (1983). Interaction of corticotropin-releasing factor (CRF) and arginine vasopressin (AVP) on ACTH secretion *in vivo*. *Endocrinology*, **113**, 939–942.

285. Shibasaki, T., Hotta, M., Sugihara, H., and Wakabayashi, I. (1998). Brain vasopressin is involved in stress-induced suppression of immune function in the rat. *Brain Res.*, **808**, 84–92.

286. Ebadi, M. (1984). Regulation of the synthesis of melatonin and its significance to neuroendocrinology. In *The Pineal Gland* (ed. R. J. Reiter), pp. 1–39. Raven Press, New York.

287. Naray, A. (1981). Progesterone receptor in chick thymus. *Biochem. Biophys. Res. Commun.*, **98**, 866–874.

288. Johnson, H. M., Smith, E. M., Torres, B. A., and Blalock, J. E. (1982). Regulation of the *in vitro* antibody response by neuroendocrine hormones. *Proc. Natl. Acad. Sci. USA*, **79**, 4171–4174.

289. Koff, W. C. and Dunegan, M. A. (1985). Modulation of macrophage-mediated tumouricidal activity by neuropeptides and neurohormones. *J. Immunol.*, **135**, 350–354.

290. Alvarez-Mon, M., Kehrl, J. H., and Fauci, A. S. (1985). A potential role for adrenocorticotropin in regulating human B lymphocyte functions. *J. Immunol.*, **135**, 3823–3826.

291. Ylikomi, T., Gasc, J. M., Tuohimaa, P., and Baulieu, E. E. (1987). Ontogeny of oestrogen-sensitive mesenchymal cells in the bursa of Fabricius of the chick embryo. An immunohistochemical study on progesterone receptor. *Development*, **101**, 61–66.

292. Sakabe, K., Seiki, K., and Fujii, H. (1986). Histochemical localisation of progestin receptor in the rat thymus. *Thymus*, **8**, 97–107.

293. Gisler, R. H. and Schenkel-Hulliger, L. (1971). Hormonal regulation of the immune response. II. Influence of pituitary and adrenal activity on immune responsiveness *in vitro*. *Cell. Immunol.*, **2**, 646–657.
294. Pearce, P. T., Khalid, P. A. K., and Funder, J. W. (1983). Progesterone receptors in rat thymus. *Endocrinology*, **13**, 1287–1291.
295. Heijnen, C. J., Kavelaars, A., and Ballieux, R. E. (1991). CRH and POMC-derived peptides in the modulation of immune function. In *Psychoneuroimmunology* (2nd edn), (eds R. Ader, N. Cohen, and D. L. Felten), pp. 429–446. Academic Press, New York.
296. Strahle, U., Boshart, M., Klock, G., Stewart, F., and Schutz, G. (1989). Glucocorticoid and progesterone specific effects are determined by differential expression of the respective hormone receptors. *Nature*, **339**, 629–632.
297. Sundar, S. K., Cierpial, M. A., Kamaraju, L. S., Long, S., Hsieh, S., Lorenz, C. *et al.* (1991). Human immunodeficiency virus glycoprotein (gp120) infused into rat brain induces interleukin 1 to elevate pituitary–adrenal activity and decrease peripheral cellular immune responses. *Proc. Natl. Acad. Sci. USA*, **88**, 11246–11250.
298. Gilman, S. C., Schwartz, J. M., Milner, R. J., Bloom, F. E., and Feldman, J. D. (1982). β-Endorphin enhances lymphocyte proliferative responses. *Proc. Natl. Acad. Sci. USA*, **79**, 4226–4230.
299. Fontana, L., Fattorossi, A., D'Amelio, R., Migliorati, A., and Perricone, R. (1987). Modulation of human concanavalin A-induced lymphocyte proliferative response by physiological concentrations of β-endorphin. *Immunopharmacology*, **13**, 111–115.
300. Kay, N., Allen, J., and Morley, J. E. (1984). Endorphins stimulate normal human peripheral blood lymphocyte natural killer activity. *Life Sci.*, **35**, 53–59.
301. Mathews, P. M., Froelich, C. J., Sibbitt, W. L. Jr, and Bankhurst, A. D. (1983). Enhancement of natural cytotoxicity by β-endorphin. *J. Immunol.*, **130**, 1658–1662.
302. Froehich, C. J. and Bankhurst, A. D. (1984). The effect of β-endorphin on natural cytotoxicity and antibody dependent cellular cytotoxicity. *Life Sci.*, **35**, 261–265.
303. Heijnen, C. J., Bevers, C., Kavelaars, A., and Ballieux, R. E. (1986). Effect of alpha-endorphin on the antigen-induced primary antibody response of human blood B cells *in vitro*. *J. Immunol.*, **136**, 213–216.
304. Brown, S. L. and Van Epps, D. E. (1986). Opioid peptides modulate production of interferon gamma by human mononuclear cells. *Cell. Immunol.*, **103**, 19–26.
305. Van Epps, D. E. and Saland, L. (1984). Beta endorphin and met-enkephalin stimulate human peripheral blood mononuclear cell chemotaxis. *J. Immunol.*, **132**, 3046–3053.
306. Brown, S. L. and Van Epps, D. E. (1985). Suppression of T lymphocyte chemotactic factor production by the opioid peptides β-endorphin and met-enkephalin. *J. Immunol.*, **134**, 3384–3390.
307. Heagy, W., Laurance, M., Cohen, E., and Finberg, R. (1990). Neurohormones regulate T cell function. *J. Exp. Med.*, **171**, 1625–1633.
308. Gilmore, W. and Weiner, L. P. (1989). The opioid specificity of beta-endorphin enhancement of murine lymphocyte proliferation. *Immunopharmacology*, **17**, 19–30.
309. Van Den Bergh, P., Rozing, J., and Nagelkerken, L. (1991). Two opposing modes of action of β-endorphin on lymphocyte function. *Immunology*, **72**, 537–543.

310. McCain, H. W., Lamster, I. B., Bozzone, J. M., and Grbic, J. T. (1982). β-endorphin modulates human immune activity via non-opiate receptor mechanisms. *Life Sci.*, **31**, 1619–1624.
311. Bidlack, J. M. and Hemmick, L. M. (1990). Morphine enhancement of mitogen-induced T-cell proliferation. In *The International Narcotics Research Conference (INRC)'89* (eds F. Guirion, K. Jhamandas, and C. Gianoulakis), pp. 405–408. Alan R. Liss, New York.
312. Hirata, F., Stracke, M. L., and Schiffmann, E. (1987). Regulation of prostaglandin formation by glucocorticoids and their second messenger, lipocortins. *J. Steroid Biochem.*, **27**, 1053–1056.
313. Goppelt-Struebe, M. (1997). Molecular mechanisms involved in the regulation of prostaglandin biosynthesis by glucocorticoids. *Biochem. Pharmacol.*, **53**, 1389–1395.
314. van der Velden, V. H. (1998). Glucocorticoids: mechanisms of action and anti-inflammatory potential in asthma. *Mediators Inflamm.*, **7**, 229–237.
315. Masferrer, J. L. and Seibert, K. (1994). Regulation of prostaglandin synthesis by glucocorticoids. *Receptor*, **4**, 25–30.
316. Barnes, P. J. (1999). Anti-inflammatory actions of glucocorticoids: molecular mechanisms. *Clin. Sci. (Colch.)*, **94**, 557–562.
317. Zweiman, B., Slott, R. I., and Atkins, P. C. (1976). Histologic studies of human skin test responses to ragweed and compound 48/80. III. Effects of alternate-day steroid therapy. *J. Allergy Clin. Immunol.*, **58**, 657–663.
318. Parrillo, J. E. and Fauci, A. S. (1979). Mechanisms of glucocorticoid action on immune processes. *Annu. Rev. Pharmacol. Toxicol.*, **19**, 179–201.
319. Dhabhar, F. S., Miller, A. H., McEwen, B. S., and Spencer, R. L. (1995). Effects of stress on immune cell distribution. Dynamics and hormonal mechanisms. *J. Immunol.*, **154**, 5511–5527.
320. Cronstein, B. N., Kimmel, S. C., Levin, R. I., Martiniuk, F., and Weissmann, G. (1992). A mechanism for the antiinflammatory effects of corticosteroids: the glucocorticoid receptor regulates leukocyte adhesion to endothelial cells and expression of endothelial-leukocyte adhesion molecule 1 and intercellular adhesion molecule 1. *Proc. Natl. Acad. Sci. USA*, **89**, 9991–9995.
321. Pitzalis, C., Sharrack, B., Gray, I. A., Lee, A., and Hughes, R. A. (1997). Comparison of the effects of oral versus intravenous methylprednisolone regimens on peripheral blood T lymphocyte adhesion molecule expression, T cell subsets distribution and TNF alpha concentrations in multiple sclerosis. *J. Neuroimmunol.*, **74**, 62–68.
322. Ihm, C. G., Hong, S. P., Park, J. K., Lee, T. W., Cho, B. S., Yang, M. H. *et al.* (1996). Effects of mixed leukocyte reaction, hydrocortisone and cyclosporine on expression of leukocyte adhesion molecules by endothelial and mesangial cells. *J. Korean Med. Sci.*, **11**, 495–500.
323. Filep, J. G., Delalandre, A., Payette, Y., and Foldes-Filep, E. (1997). Glucocorticoid receptor regulates expression of L-selectin and CD11/CD18 on human neutrophils. *Circulation*, **96**, 295–301.
324. Burton, J. L., Kehrli, M. E. Jr, Kapil, S., and Horst, R. L. (1995). Regulation of L-selectin and CD18 on bovine neutrophils by glucocorticoids: effects of cortisol and dexamethasone. *J. Leukocyte Biol.*, **57**, 317–325.

325. Powrie, F. and Coffman, R. L. (1993). Cytokine regulation of T-cell function: potential for therapeutic intervention. *Immunol. Today*, 14, 270–274.
326. Wiegers, G. J. and Reul, J. M. (1998). Induction of cytokine receptors by gluco-corticoids: functional and pathological significance. *Trends Pharmacol. Sci.*, 19, 317–321.
327. Cato, A. C. and Wade, E. (1996). Molecular mechanisms of anti-inflammatory action of glucocorticoids. *BioEssays*, 18, 371–378.
328. Paliogianni, F., Raptis, A., Ahuja, S. S., Najjar, S. M., and Boumpas, D. T. (1993). Negative transcriptional regulation of human interleukin 2 (IL-2) gene by glucocorticoids through interference with nuclear transcription factors AP-1 and NF-AT. *J. Clin. Invest.*, 91, 1481–1489.
329. Auphan, N., DiDonato, J. A., Rosette, C., Helmberg, A., and Karin, M. (1995). Immunosuppression by glucocorticoids: inhibition of NF-kappa B activity through induction of I kappa B synthesis. *Science*, 270, 286–290.
330. Iwata, M., Hanaoka, S., and Sato, K. (1991). Rescue of thymocytes and T cell hybridomas from glucocorticoid-induced apoptosis by stimulation via the T cell receptor/CD3 complex: a possible *in vitro* model for positive selection of the T cell repertoire. *Eur. J. Immunol.*, 21, 643–648.
331. Claman, H. N. (1972). Corticosteroids and lymphoid cells. *N. Engl. J. Med.*, 287, 388–397.
332. Cohen, J. J. and Duke, R. C. (1984). Glucocorticoid activation of a calcium-dependent endonuclease in thymocyte nuclei leads to cell death. *J. Immunol.*, 132, 38–42.
333. Schobitz, B., Van Den Dobbelsteen, M., Holsboer, F., Sutanto, W., and De Kloet, E. R. (1993). Regulation of interleukin 6 gene expression in rat. *Endocrinology*, 132, 1569–1576.
334. Yamaguchi, M., Matsuzaki, N., Hirota, K., Miyake, A., and Tanizawa, O. (1990). Interleukin 6 possibly induced by interleukin 1 beta in the pituitary gland stimulates the release of gonadotropins and prolactin. *Acta Endocrinol. (Copenhagen)*, 122, 201–205.
335. Iwata, M., Iseki, R., Sato, K., Tozawa, Y., and Ohoka, Y. (1994). Involvement of protein kinase C-epsilon in glucocorticoid-induced apoptosis in thymocytes. *Int. Immunol.*, 6, 431–438.
336. Ohoka, Y., Kuwata, T., Tozawa, Y., Zhao, Y., Mukai, M., Motegi, Y. *et al.* (1996). *In vitro* differentiation and commitment of CD4+ CD8+ thymocytes to the CD4 lineage, without TCR engagement. *Int. Immunol.*, 8, 297–306.
337. Iwata, M., Kuwata, T., Mukai, M., Tozawa, Y., and Yokoyama, M. (1996). Differential induction of helper and killer T cells from isolated CD4+ CD8+ thymocytes in suspension culture. *Eur. J. Immunol.*, 26, 2081–2086.
338. Kaspers, G. J., Pieters, R., Klumper, E., De Waal, F. C., and Veerman, A. J. (1994). Glucocorticoid resistance in childhood leukemia. *Leuk. Lymphoma*, 13, 187–201.
339. Daaka, Y., Luttrell, L. M., and Lefkowitz, R. J. (1997). Switching of the coupling of the beta2-adrenergic receptor to different G proteins by protein kinase A. *Nature*, 390, 88–91.
340. Bourgeois, S., Newby, R. F., and Huet, M. (1978). Glucocorticoid resistance in murine lymphoma and thymoma lines. *Cancer Res.*, 38, 4279–4284.

341. Thompson, E. B. and Harmon, J. M. (1986). Glucocorticoid receptors and gluco-corticoid resistance in human leukemia *in vivo* and *in vitro*. *Adv. Exp. Biol. Med.*, **196**, 111–127.

342. Soufi, M., Kaiser, U., Schneider, A., Beato, M., and Westphal, H. M. (1995). The DNA and steroid binding domains of the glucocorticoid receptor are not altered in mononuclear cells of treated CLL patients. *Exp. Clin. Endocrinol. Diabetes*, **103**, 175–183.

343. Homo, F., Duval, D., Hatzfeld, J., and Evrard, C. (1980). Glucocorticoid sensi-tive and resistant cell populations in the mouse thymus. *J. Steroid Biochem.*, **13**, 135–143.

344. Thompson, E. A. (1991). Glucocorticoid insensitivity of P1798 lymphoma cells is associated with production of a factor that attenuates the lytic response. *Cancer Res.*, **51**, 5551–5556.

345. Sakaue, M., Bowtell, D., and Kasuga, M. (1995). A dominant-negative mutant of mSOS1 inhibits insulin-induced Ras activation and reveals Ras-dependent and independent insulin signaling pathways. *Mol. Cell. Biol.*, **15**, 379–388.

346. Hugo, P., Boyd, R. L., Waanders, G. A., and Scollay, R. (1991). CD4$^+$ CD8$^+$ CD3 high thymocytes appear transiently during ontogeny: evidence from pheno-typic and functional studies. *Eur. J. Immunol.*, **21**, 2655–2660.

347. Ito, A., Satoh, T., Kaziro, Y., and Itoh, H. (1995). G protein beta gamma sub-unit activates Ras, Raf, and MAP kinase in HEK 293 cells. *FEBS Lett.*, **368**, 183–187.

348. Blalock, J. E., Johnson, H. M., Smith, E. M., and Torres, B. A. (1984). Enhance-ment of the *in vitro* antibody response by thyrotropin. *Biochem. Biophys. Res. Commun.*, **125**, 30–34.

349. Kruger, T. E. and Blalock, J. E. (1986). Cellular requirements for thyrotropin enhancement of *in vitro* antibody production. *J. Immunol.*, **137**, 197–200.

350. Kruger, T. E., Smith, L. R., Harbour, D. V., and Blalock, J. E. (1989). Thyrotro-pin: an endogenous regulator of the *in vitro* immune response. *J. Immunol.*, **142**, 744–747.

351. Harbour, D. V., Kruger, T. E., Coppenhaver, D., Smith, E. M., and Meyer, W. J. III (1989). Differential expression and regulation of thyrotropin (TSH) in T cell lines. *Mol. Cell. Endocrinol.*, **64**, 229–241.

352. Harbour, D. V., Leon, S., Keating, C., and Hughes, T. K. (1990). Thyrotropin modulates B-cell function through specific bioactive receptors. *Prog. Neuro-EndocrinImmunol.*, **3**, 266–276.

353. Raiden, S., Polack, E., Nahmod, V., Labeur, M., Holsboer, F., and Arzt, E. (1995). TRH receptor on immune cells: *in vitro* and *in vivo* stimulation of human lymphocyte and rat splenocyte DNA synthesis by TRH. *J. Clin. Immu-nol.*, **15**, 242–249.

354. Fabris, N. (1973). Immunodepression in thyroid-deprived animals. *Clin. Exp. Immunol.*, **15**, 601–611.

355. Chatterjee, S. and Chandel, A. S. (1983). Immunomodulatory role of thyroid hormones: *in vivo* effect of thyroid hormones on the blastogenic response of lymphoid tissues. *Acta Endocrinol.*, **103**, 95–100.

356. Scott, T. and Glick, B. (1987). Organ weights, T-cell proliferation, and graft vs host capabilities of hypothyroidic chickens. *Gen. Comp. Endocrinol.*, **67**, 270–276.

357. Provinciali, M., Muzzioli, M., DiStefano, G., and Fabris, N. (1991). Recovery of spleen cell natural killer activity by thyroid hormone treatment in old mice. *Nat. Immun. Cell. Growth Regul.*, **10**, 226–236.

358. Perez Castro, C., Penalva, R., Paez Pereda, M., Renner, U., Reul, J. M., Stalla, G. K. *et al.* (1999). Early activation of thyrotropin-releasing-hormone and prolactin plays a critical role during a T cell-dependent immune response. *Endocrinology*, **140**, 690–697.

359. Whetsell, M., Bagriacik, E. U., Seetharamaiah, G. S., Prabhakar, B. S., and Klein, J. R. (1999). Neuroendocrine-induced synthesis of bone marrow-derived cytokines with inflammatory immunomodulating properties. *Cell. Immunol.*, **15**, 159–166.

360. Wang, J. and Klein, J. R. (1996). Hormone regulation of murine T cells: potent tissue-specific immunosuppressive effects of thyroxine targeted to gut T cells. *Int. Immunol.*, **8**, 231–235.

361. Mihara, S., Suzuki, N., Wakisaka, S., Suzuki, S., Sekita, N., Yamamoto, S. *et al.* (1999). Effects of thyroid hormones on apoptotic cell death of human lymphocytes. *J. Clin. Endocrinol. Metab.*, **84**, 1378–1385.

362. Olsen, N. J. and Kovacs, W. J. (1996). Gonadal steroids and immunity. *Endocr. Rev.*, **17**, 369–384.

363. Butterworth, M., McClellan, B., and Allansmith, M. (1967). Influence of sex on immunoglobulin levels. *Nature*, **214**, 1224–1225.

364. Eidinger, D. and Garrett, T. J. (1972). Studies of the regulatory effects of the sex hormones on antibody formation and stem cell differentiation. *J. Exp. Med.*, **136**, 1098–1116.

365. Weinstein, Y., Ran, S., and Segal, S. (1984). Sex-associated differences in the regulation of immune responses controlled by the MHC of the mouse. *J. Immunol.*, **132**, 656–661.

366. Cutolo, M., Sulli, A., Seriolo, B., Accardo, S., and Masi, A. T. (1995). Oestrogens, the immune response and autoimmunity. *Clin. Exp. Rheumatol.*, **13**, 217–226.

367. Ito, I., Hayashi, T., Yamada, K., Kuzuya, M., Naito, M., and Iguchi, A. (1995). Physiological concentration of estradiol inhibits polymorphonuclear leukocyte chemotaxis via a receptor mediated system. *Life Sci.*, **56**, 2247–2253.

368. Kaushic, C., Frauendorf, E., Rossoll, R. M., Richardson, J. M., and Wira, C. R. (1998). Influence of the estrous cycle on the presence and distribution of immune cells in the rat reproductive tract. *Am. J. Reprod. Immunol.*, **39**, 209–216.

369. Deshpande, R., Khalili, H., Pergolizzi, R. G., Michael, S. D., and Chang, M. D. (1997). Estradiol downregulates LPS-induced cytokine production and NFκB activation in murine macrophages. *Am. J. Reprod. Immunol.*, **38**, 46–54.

370. Chao, T. C., Van Alten, P. J., Greager, J. A., and Walter, R. J. (1995). Steroid sex hormones regulate the release of tumour necrosis factor by macrophages. *Cell. Immunol.*, **160**, 43–49.

371. Robert, R. and Spitzer, J. A. (1997). Effects of female hormones (17beta-estradiol and progesterone) on nitric oxide production by alveolar macrophages in rats. *Nitric Oxide*, **1**, 453–462.

372. Hunt, J. S., Miller, L., Roby, K. F., Huang, J., Platt, J. S., and DeBrot, B. L. (1997). Female steroid hormones regulate production of pro-inflammatory molecules in uterine leukocytes. *J. Reprod. Immunol.*, **35**, 87–99.

373. Nilsson, N. and Carlsten, H. (1994). Oestrogen induces suppression of natural killer cell cytotoxicity and augmentation of polyclonal B cell activation. *Cell. Immunol.*, **158**, 131–139.

374. Kanda, N. and Tamaki, K. (1999). Oestrogen enhances immunoglobulin production by human PBMCs. *J. Allergy Clin. Immunol.*, **103**, 282–288.

375. Evans, M. J., MacLaughlin, S., Marvin, R. D., and Abdou, N. I. (1997). Oestrogen decreases *in vitro* apoptosis of peripheral blood mononuclear cells from women with normal menstrual cycles and decreases TNF-alpha production in SLE but not in normal cultures. *Clin. Immunol. Immunopathol.*, **82**, 258–262.

376. Ostensen, M. (1999). Sex hormones and pregnancy in rheumatoid arthritis and systemic lupus erythematosus. *Ann. N. Y. Acad. Sci.*, **876**, 131–143.

377. Kim, S., Liva, S. M., Dalal, M. A., Verity, M. A., and Voskuhl, R. R. (1999). Estriol ameliorates autoimmune demyelinating disease: implications for multiple sclerosis. *Neurology*, **52**, 1230–1238.

378. Correale, J., Arias, M., and Gilmore, W. (1998). Steroid hormone regulation of cytokine secretion by proteolipid protein-specific CD4$^+$ T cell clones isolated from multiple sclerosis patients and normal control subjects. *J. Immunol.*, **161**, 3365–3374.

379. Jarvinen, L. S., Pyrhonen, S., Kairemo, K. J., and Paavonen, T. (1996). The effect of anti-oestrogens on cytokine production *in vitro*. *Scand. J. Immunol.*, **44**, 15–20.

380. Pasanen, S., Ylikomi, T., Palojoki, E., Syvala, H., Pelto-Huikko, M., and Tuohimaa, P. (1998). Progesterone receptor in chicken bursa of Fabricius and thymus: evidence for expression in B-lymphocytes. *Mol. Cell. Endocrinol.*, **141**, 119–128.

381. Szekeres-Bartho, J., Reznikoff-Etievant, M. F., Varga, P., Pichon, M. F., Varga, Z., and Chaouat, G. (1989). Lymphocytic progesterone receptors in normal and pathological human pregnancy. *J. Reprod. Immunol.*, **16**, 239–247.

382. Szekeres-Bartho, J., Par, G., Szereday, L., Smart, C. Y., and Achatz, I. (1997). Progesterone and non-specific immunologic mechanisms in pregnancy. *Am. J. Reprod. Immunol.*, **38**, 176–182.

383. Wang, Y., Campbell, H. D., and Young, I. G. (1993). Sex hormones and dexamethasone modulate interleukin-5 gene expression in T lymphocytes. *J. Steroid Biochem. Mol. Biol.*, **44**, 203–210.

384. Gomez, F., Ruiz, P., Briceno, F., Lopez, R., and Michan, A. (1998). Treatment with progesterone analogues decreases macrophage Fcg receptors expression. *Clin. Immunol. Immunopathol.*, **89**, 231–239.

385. Kaiser, N., Mayer, M., Milholland, R. J., and Rosen, F. (1979). Studies of the antiglucocorticoid action of progesterone in rat thymocytes: early *in vitro* effects. *J. Steroid Biochem.*, **10**, 379–386.

386. Cutolo, M., Accardo, S., Villaggio, B., Barone, A., Sulli, A., Coviello, D. A. *et al.* (1996). Androgen and oestrogen receptors are present in primary cultures of human synovial macrophages. *J. Clin. Endocrinol. Metab.*, **81**, 820–827.

387. Viselli, S. M., Olsen, N. J., Shults, K., Steizer, G., and Kovacs, W. J. (1995). Immunochemical and flow cytometric analysis of androgen receptor expression in thymocytes. *Mol. Cell. Endocrinol.*, **109**, 19–26.

388. Zhou, Z., Shackleton, C. H., Pahwa, S., White, P. C., and Speiser, P. W. (1998). Prominent sex steroid metabolism in human lymphocytes. *Mol. Cell. Endocrinol.*, **138**, 61–69.

389. Ben-Nathan, D., Padgett, D. A., and Loria, R. M. (1999). Androstenediol and dehydroepiandrosterone protect mice against lethal bacterial infections and lipopolysaccharide toxicity. *J. Med. Microbiol.*, **48**, 425–431.

390. Araghi-Niknam, M., Liang, B., Zhang, Z., Ardestani, S. K., and Watson, R. R. (1997). Modulation of immune dysfunction during murine leukaemia retrovirus infection of old mice by dehydroepiandrosterone sulphate (DHEAS). *Immunology*, **90**, 344–349.

391. Catania, R. A., Angele, M. K., Ayala, A., Cioffi, W. G., Bland, K. I., and Chaudry, I. H. (1999). Dehydroepiandrosterone restores immune function following trauma-haemorrhage by a direct effect on T lymphocytes. *Cytokine*, **11**, 443–450.

392. Padgett, D. A., Loria, R. M., and Sheridan, J. F. (1997). Endocrine regulation of the immune response to influenza virus infection with a metabolite of DHEA-androstenediol. *J. Neuroimmunol.*, **78**, 203–211.

393. Ben-Yehuda, A., Danenberg, H. D., Zakay-Rones, Z., Gross, D. J., and Friedman, G. (1998). The influence of sequential annual vaccination and of DHEA administration on the efficacy of the immune response to influenza vaccine in the elderly. *Mech. Ageing Dev.*, **102**, 299–306.

394. Miller, R. A. and Chrisp, C. (1999). Lifelong treatment with oral DHEA sulfate does not preserve immune function, prevent disease, or improve survival in genetically heterogeneous mice. *J. Am. Geriatr. Soc.*, **47**, 960–966.

395. Maestroni, G. J. M. and Pierpaoli, W. (1981). Pharmacologic control of the hormonally mediated immune response. In *Psychoneuroimmunology* (ed. R. Ader), pp. 405–425. Academic Press, New York.

396. 396. Becker, J., Veit, G., Handgretinger, R., Attanasio, A., Bruchett, G., Trenner, I. *et al.* (1988). Circadian variations in the immunomodulatory role of the pineal gland. *Neuroendocrinol. Lett.*, **10**, 65–80.

397. Maestroni, G. J. M., Conti, A., and Pierpaoli, W. (1986). Role of the pineal in immunity. Circadian synthesis and release of melatonin modulates the antibody response and antagonizes the immunosuppressive effect of corticosterone. *J. Neuroimmunol.*, **13**, 19–30.

398. Maestroni, G. J. M., Conti, A., and Pierpaoli, W. (1987). The pineal gland and the circadian, opiatergic, immunoregulatory role of melatonin. *Ann. N. Y. Acad. Sci.*, **496**, 67–77.

399. Maestroni, G. J. M., Conti, A., and Pierpaoli, W. (1988). Pineal melatonin, its fundamental immunoregulatory role in aging and cancer. *Ann. N. Y. Acad. Sci.*, **521**, 140–148.

400. Maestroni, G. J. M. and Conti, A. (1991). Role of the pineal neurohormone melatonin in the psycho-neuroendocrine–immune network. In *Psychoneuroimmunology* (2nd edn), (eds R. Ader, N. Cohen, and D. L. Felten), pp. 465–513. Academic Press, New York.

401. Maestroni, G. J. M., Conti, A., and Pierpaoli, W. (1988). Role of the pineal gland in immunity: III. Melatonin antagonizes the immunosuppressive effect of acute stress via an opiatergic mechanism. *Immunology*, **63**, 465–469.

402. Felten, D. L., Cohen, N., Ader, R., Felten, S. Y., Carlson, S. L., and Roszman, T. L. (1991). Central neural circuits involved in neural–immune interactions. In *Psychoneuroimmunology* (2nd edn), (eds R. Ader, D. L. Felten, and N. Cohen), pp. 1–26. Academic Press, New York.

403. Korneva, E. A., Klimenko, V. M., and Shkhinek, E. K. (1985). *Neurohumoral Maintenance of Immune Homeostasis*. University of Chicago Press, Chicago.
404. Nance, D. M., Rayson, D., and Carr, R. I. (1987). The effects of lesions in the lateral septal and hippocampal areas on the humoral immune response of adult female rats. *Brain Behav. Immun.*, 1, 292–305.
405. Masek, K., Kadlecova, O., and Petrovicky, P. (1983). The effect of brain stem lesions on the immune response. In *Advances in Immunopharmacology* (eds J. W. Hadden, L. Chedid, P. Dukor, F. Spreafico, and D. Willoughby), pp. 443–450. Pergamon Press, New York.
406. Isakovic, K. and Jankovic, B. D. (1973). Neuro-endocrine correlates of immune response. II. Changes in the lymphatic organs of brain-lesioned rats. *Int. Arch. Allergy*, 45, 373–384.
407. Cross, R. J., Brooks, W. H., and Roszman, T. L. (1987). Modulation of T-suppressor cell activity by central nervous system catecholamine depletion. *J. Neurosci. Res.*, 18, 75–81.
408. Besedovsky, H. O., del Rey, A., Sorkin, E., Da Prada, M., Burri, R., and Honegger, C. (1983). The immune response evokes changes in brain noradrenergic neurons. *Science*, 221, 564–565.
409. Dunn, A. J. (1988). Systemic interleukin-1 administration stimulates hypothalamic norepinephrine metabolism paralleling the increased plasma corticosterone. *Life Sci.*, 43, 429–435.
410. Kahiersh, A., del Rey, A., Honegger, G., and Besedovsky, H. D. (1988). Interleukin-1 induces changes in norepinephrine metabolism in the rat brain. *Brain Behav. Immun.*, 2, 267–274.
411. Besedovsky, H. O., Sorkin, E., Keller, M., and Müller, J. (1975). Changes in blood hormone levels during the immune response. *Proc. Soc. Exp. Biol. Med.*, 150, 466–470.
412. Kadlecova, O., Masek, K., Seifert, J., and Petrovicky, P. (1987). The involvement of some brain structures in the effects of immunomodulators. *Ann. N. Y. Acad. Sci.*, 496, 394–398.
413. Renoux, G. and Biziere, K. (1991). Neocortex lateralization of immune function and of the activities of imuthiol, a T-cell specific immunopotentiator. In *Psychoneuroimmunology* (2nd edn), (eds R. Ader, D. L. Felten, and N. Cohen), pp. 127–147. Academic Press, New York.
414. Turnbull, A. V. and Rivier, C. L. (1999). Regulation of the hypothalamic–pituitary–adrenal axis by cytokines: actions and mechanisms of action. *Physiol. Rev.*, 79, 1–71.
415. van der Meer, M. J., Sweep, C. G., Pesman, G. J., Borm, G. F., and Hermus, A. R. (1995). Synergism between IL-1 beta and TNF-alpha on the activity of the pituitary–adrenal axis and on food intake of rats. *Am. J. Physiol.*, 268, E551–557.
416. Harbuz, M. S., Stephanou, A., Knight, R. A., Chover-Gonzalez, A. J., and Lightman, S. L. (1992). Action of interleukin-2 and interleukin-4 on CRF mRNA in the hypothalamus and POMC mRNA in the anterior pituitary. *Brain Behav. Immun.*, 6, 214–222.
417. Saphier, D. (1995). Neuroendocrine effects of interferon-alpha in the rat. *Adv. Exp. Med. Biol.*, 373, 209–218.
418. Dunn, A. J. and Vickers, S. L. (1994). Neurochemical and neuroendocrine responses to Newcastle disease virus administration in mice. *Brain Res.*, 645, 103–112.

419. Olsen, N. J., Nicholson, W. E., DeBold, C. R., and Orth, D. N. (1992). Lymphocyte-derived adrenocorticotropin is insufficient to stimulate adrenal steroidogenesis in hypophysectomized rats. *Endocrinology*, 130, 2113–2119.

420. Milton, N. G., Hillhouse, E. W., and Milton, A. S. (1992). Activation of the hypothalamo–pituitary–adrenocortical axis in the conscious rabbit by the pyrogen polyinosinic:polycytidylic acid is dependent on corticotrophin-releasing factor-41. *J. Endocrinol.*, 135, 69–75.

421. Ruzek, M. C., Miller, A. H., Opal, S. M., Pearce, B. D., and Biron, C. A. (1997). Characterization of early cytokine responses and an interleukin (IL)-6-dependent pathway of endogenous glucocorticoid induction during murine cytomegalovirus infection. *J. Exp. Med.*, 185, 1185–1192.

422. Carlson, D. E. (1997). Adrenocorticotropin correlates strongly with endotoxemia after intravenous but not after intraperitoneal inoculations of *E. coli*. *Shock*, 7, 65–69.

423. Wan, W., Wetmore, L., Sorensen, C. M., Greenberg, A. H., and Nance, D. M. (1994). Neural and biochemical mediators of endotoxin and stress-induced cfos expression in the rat brain. *Brain Res. Bull.*, 34, 7–14.

424. Elmquist, J. K., Ackermann, M. R., Register, K. B., Rimler, R. B., Ross, L. R., and Jacobson, C. D. (1993). Induction of Fos-like immunoreactivity in the rat brain following *Pasteurella multocida* endotoxin administration. *Endocrinology*, 133, 3054–3057.

425. Wan, W., Janz, L., Vriend, C. Y., Sorensen, C. M., Greenberg, A. H., and Nance, D. M. (1993). Differential induction of c-Fos immunoreactivity in hypothalamus and brain stem nuclei following central and peripheral administration of endotoxin. *Brain Res. Bull.*, 32, 581–587.

426. Tilders, F. J., DeRijk, R. H., Van Dam, A. M., Vincent, V. A., Schotanus, K., and Persoons, J. H. (1994). Activation of the hypothalamus–pituitary–adrenal axis by bacterial endotoxins: routes and intermediate signals. *Psychoneuroendocrinology*, 19, 209–232.

427. Turnbull, A. V., Dow, R. C., Hopkins, S. J., White, A., Fink, G., and Rothwell, N. J. (1994). Mechanisms of activation of the pituitary–adrenal axis by tissue injury in the rat. *Psychoneuroendocrinology*, 19, 165–178.

428. Turnbull, A. V. and Rivier, C. (1996). Corticotropin-releasing factor, vasopressin, and prostaglandins mediate, and nitric oxide restrains, the hypothalamic–pituitary–adrenal response to acute local inflammation in the rat. *Endocrinology*, 137, 455–463.

429. Rettori, V., Jurcovicova, J., and McCann, S. M. (1987). Control action of interleukin-1 in altering the release of TSH, growth hormone, and prolactin in the male rat. *J. Neurosci. Res.*, 18, 179–183.

430. Wada, Y., Sato, M., Niimi, M., Tamaki, M., Ishida, T., and Takahara, J. (1995). Inhibitory effects of interleukin-1 on growth hormone secretion in conscious male rats. *Endocrinology*, 136, 3936–3941.

431. Scarborough, D. E., Lee, S. L., Dinarello, C. A., and Reichlin, S. (1989). Interleukin-1β stimulates somatostatin biosynthesis in primary cultures of fetal rat brain. *Endocrinology*, 124, 549–551.

432. Karanth, S., Aguila, M. C., and McCann, S. M. (1993). The influence of interleukin-2 on the release of somatostatin and growth hormone-releasing hormone by mediobasal hypothalamus. *Neuroendocrinology*, 58, 185–190.

433. Lang, C. H., Fan, J., Wojnar, M. M., Vary, T. C., and Cooney, R. (1998). Role of central IL-1 in regulating peripheral IGF-I during endotoxemia and sepsis. *Am. J. Physiol.*, **274**, R956–962.

434. Nash, A. D., Brandon, M. R., and Bello, P. A. (1992). Effects of tumour necrosis factor-alpha on growth hormone and interleukin 6 mRNA in ovine pituitary cells. *Mol. Cell. Endocrinol.*, **84**, R31–37.

435. Rettori, V., Milenkovic, L., Beutler, B. A., and McCann, S. M. (1989). Hypothalamic action of cachectin to alter pituitary hormone release. *Brain Res. Bull.*, **23**, 471–475.

436. Vankelecom, H., Matthys, P., and Denef, C. (1997). Involvement of nitric oxide in the interferon-gamma-induced inhibition of growth hormone and prolactin secretion in anterior pituitary cell cultures. *Mol. Cell. Endocrinol.*, **129**, 157–167.

437. Ban, E., Marquette, C., Sarrieau, A., Fitzpatrick, F., Fillion, G., Milon, G. *et al.* (1993). Regulation of interleukin-1 receptor expression in mouse brain and pituitary by lipopolysaccharide and glucocorticoids. *Neuroendocrinology*, **58**, 581–587.

438. Marquette, C., Van Dam, A. M., Ban, E., Laniece, P., Crumeyrolle-Arias, M., Fillion, G. *et al.* (1995). Rat interleukin-1 beta binding sites in rat hypothalamus and pituitary gland. *Neuroendocrinology*, **62**, 362–369.

439. Takao, T., Culp, S. G., and De Souza, E. B. (1993). Reciprocal modulation of interleukin-1 beta (IL-1 beta) and IL-1 receptors by lipopolysaccharide (endotoxin) treatment in the mouse brain–endocrine–immune axis. *Endocrinology*, **132**, 4197–1504.

440. Takao, T., Nakata, H., Tojo, C., Kurokawa, H., Nishioka, T., Hashimoto, K. *et al.* (1994). Regulation of interleukin-1 receptors and hypothalamic–pituitary–adrenal axis by lipopolysaccharide treatment in the mouse. *Brain Res.*, **649**, 265–270.

441. Takao, T., Tojo, C., Nishioka, T., Kurokawa, H., Takemura, T., Hashimoto, K. *et al.* (1994). Reciprocal modulation of corticotropin-releasing factor and interleukin-1 receptors following ether-laparotomy stress in the mouse. *Brain Res.*, **660**, 170–174.

442. Takao, T., Tracey, D. E., Mitchell, W. M., and De Souza, E. B. (1990). Interleukin-1 receptors in mouse brain: characterization and neuronal localization. *Endocrinology*, **127**, 3070–3078.

443. Parnet, P., Brunke, D. L., Goujon, E., Mainard, J. D., Biragyn, A., Arkins, S. *et al.* (1993). Molecular identification of two types of interleukin-1 receptors in the murine pituitary gland. *J. Neuroendocrinol.*, **5**, 213–219.

444. Cunningham, E. T. Jr, Wada, E., Carter, D. B., Tracey, D. E., Battey, J. F., and De Souza, E. B. (1992). *In situ* histochemical localization of type I interleukin-1 receptor messenger RNA in the central nervous system, pituitary, and adrenal gland of the mouse. *J. Neurosci.*, **12**, 1101–1114.

445. French, R. A., Zachary, J. F., Dantzer, R., Frawley, L. S., Chizzonite, R., Parnet, P. *et al.* (1996). Dual expression of p80 type I and p68 type II interleukin-I receptors on anterior pituitary cells synthesizing growth hormone. *Endocrinology*, **137**, 4027–4036.

446. Wolvers, D. A., Marquette, C., Berkenbosch, F., and Haour, F. (1993). Tumour necrosis factor-alpha: specific binding sites in rodent brain and pituitary gland. *Eur. Cytokine Netw.*, **4**, 377–381.

447. Ray, D. and Melmed, S. (1997). Pituitary cytokine and growth factor expression and action. *Endocr. Rev.*, **18**, 206–228.

448. Pitossi, F., del Rey, A., Kabiersch, A., and Besedovsky, H. (1997). Induction of cytokine transcripts in the central nervous system and pituitary following peripheral administration of endotoxin to mice. *J. Neurosci. Res.*, **48**, 287–298.

449. Wang, Z., Ren, S. G., and Melmed, S. (1996). Hypothalamic and pituitary leukemia inhibitory factor gene expression *in vivo*: a novel endotoxin-inducible neuro-endocrine interface. *Endocrinology*, **137**, 2947–2953.

450. Gatti, S. and Bartfai, T. (1993). Induction of tumour necrosis factor-alpha mRNA in the brain after peripheral endotoxin treatment: comparison with interleukin-1 family and interleukin-6. *Brain Res.*, **624**, 291–294.

451. Gabellec, M. M., Griffais, R., Fillion, G., and Haour, F. (1995). Expression of interleukin 1 alpha, interleukin 1 beta and interleukin 1 receptor antagonist mRNA in mouse brain: regulation by bacterial lipopolysaccharide (LPS) treatment. *Brain Res. Mol. Brain Res.*, **31**, 122–130.

452. Licinio, J. and Wong, M. L. (1997). Interleukin 1 receptor antagonist gene expression in rat pituitary in the systemic inflammatory response syndrome: pathophysiological implications. *Mol. Psychiatry*, **2**, 99–103.

453. Wong, M. L., Bongiorno, P. B., Rettori, V., McCann, S. M., and Licinio, J. (1997). Interleukin (IL) 1beta, IL-1 receptor antagonist, IL-10, and IL-13 gene expression in the central nervous system and anterior pituitary during systemic inflammation: pathophysiological implications. *Proc. Natl. Acad. Sci. USA*, **94**, 227–232.

454. Bernhagen, J., Calandra, T., Mitchell, R. A., Martin, S. B., Tracey, K. J., Voelter, W. *et al.* (1995). MIF is a pituitary-derived cytokine that potentiates lethal endotoxaemia. *Nature*, **365**, 756–759.

455. Bernhagen, J., Mitchell, R. A., Calandra, T., Voelter, W., Cerami, A., and Bucala, R. (1994). Purification, bioactivity, and secondary structure analysis of mouse and human macrophage migration inhibitory factor (MIF). *Biochemistry*, **33**, 14144–14155.

456. Bucala, R. (1994). Identification of MIF as a new pituitary hormone and macrophage cytokine and its role in endotoxic shock. *Immunol. Lett.*, **43**, 23–26.

457. Bucala, R. (1994). MIF, a previously unrecognized pituitary hormone and macrophage cytokine, is a pivotal mediator in endotoxic shock. *Circ. Shock*, **44**, 35–39.

458. Spangelo, B. L., MacLeod, R. M., and Isakson, P. C. (1990). Production of interleukin-6 by anterior pituitary cells *in vitro*. *Endocrinology*, **126**, 582–586.

459. Spangelo, B. L., deHoll, P. D., Kalabay, L., Bond, B. R., and Arnaud, P. (1994). Neurointermediate pituitary lobe cells synthesize and release interleukin-6 *in vitro*: effects of lipopolysaccharide and interleukin-1 beta. *Endocrinology*, **135**, 556–563.

460. Spangelo, B. L., Judd, A. M., Isakson, P. C., and MacLeod, R. M. (1991). Interleukin-1 stimulates interleukin-6 release from rat anterior pituitary cells *in vitro*. *Endocrinology*, **128**, 2685–2692.

461. Spangelo, B. L., Isakson, P. C., and MacLeod, R. M. (1990). Production of interleukin-6 by anterior pituitary cells is stimulated by increased intracellular adenosine 3′,5′-monophosphate and vasoactive intestinal peptide. *Endocrinology*, **127**, 403–409.

462.   Spangelo, B. L. and Gorospe, W. C. (1995). Role of the cytokines in the neuroendocrine–immune system axis. *Front. Neuroendocrinol.*, **16**, 1–22.
463.   Carmeliet, P., Vankelecom, H., Van Damme, J., Billiau, A., and Denef, C. (1991). Release of interleukin-6 from anterior pituitary cell aggregates: developmental pattern and modulation by glucocorticoids and forskolin. *Neuroendocrinology*, **53**, 29–34.
464.   Sarlis, N. J., Stephanou, A., Knight, R. A., Lightman, S. L., and Chowdrey, H. S. (1993). Effects of glucocorticoids and chronic inflammatory stress upon anterior pituitary interleukin-6 mRNA expression in the rat. *Br. J. Rheumatol.*, **32**, 653–657.
465.   Stephanou, A., Sarlis, N. J., Knight, R. A., Lightman, S. L., and Chowdrey, H. S. (1992). Effects of cyclosporine A on the hypothalamic–pituitary–adrenal axis and anterior pituitary interleukin-6 mRNA expression during chronic inflammatory stress in the rat. *J. Neuroimmunol.*, **41**, 215–222.
466.   Abraham, E. J. and Minton, J. E. (1997). Cytokines in the hypophysis: a comparative look at interleukin-6 in the porcine anterior pituitary gland. *Comp. Biochem. Physiol. A. Physiol.*, **116**, 203–207.
467.   Vankelecom, H., Carmeliet, P., Van Damme, J., Billiau, A., and Denef, C. (1989). Production of interleukin-6 by folliculo-stellate cells of the anterior pituitary gland in a histiotypic cell aggregate culture system. *Neuroendocrinology*, **49**, 102–106.
468.   Vankelecom, H., Matthys, P., Van Damme, J., Heremans, H., Billiau, A., and Denef, C. (1993). Immunocytochemical evidence that S-100-positive cells of the mouse anterior pituitary contain interleukin-6 immunoreactivity. *J. Histochem. Cytochem.*, **41**, 151–156.
468A.   Buckingham, J.C., Loxley, H.D., Taylor, A.D., and Flowers, R.J. (1994). Cytokines, glucocorticoids and neuroendocrine function. *Pharmacological Rev.* **30**, 35–42.
469.   Path, G., Bornstein, S. R., Ehrhart-Bornstein, M., and Scherbaum, W. A. (1997). Interleukin-6 and the interleukin-6 receptor in the human adrenal gland: expression and effects on steroidogenesis. *J. Clin. Endocrinol. Metab.*, **82**, 2343–2349.
470.   Gadient, R. A., Lachmund, A., Unsicker, K., and Otten, U. (1995). Expression of interleukin-6 (IL-6) and IL-6 receptor mRNAs in rat adrenal medulla. *Neurosci. Lett.*, **194**, 17–20.
471.   Bartfai, T., Andersson, C., Bristulf, J., Schultzberg, M., and Svenson, S. (1990). Interleukin-1 in the noradrenergic chromaffin cells in the rat adrenal medulla. *Ann. N. Y. Acad. Sci.*, **594**, 207–213.
472.   Schultzberg, M., Andersson, C., Unden, A., Troye-Blomberg, M., Svenson, S. B., and Bartfai, T. (1989). Interleukin-1 in adrenal chromaffin cells. *Neuroscience*, **30**, 805–810.
473.   Schultzberg, M., Tingsborg, S., Nobel, S., Lundkvist, J., Svenson, S., Simoncsits, A. *et al.* (1995). Interleukin-1 receptor antagonist protein and mRNA in the rat adrenal gland. *J. Interferon Cytokine Res.*, **15**, 721–729.
474.   Nobel, C. S. and Schultzberg, M. (1995). Induction of interleukin-1 beta mRNA and enkephalin mRNA in the rat adrenal gland by lipopolysaccharides studied by *in situ* hybridization histochemistry. *Neuroimmunomodulation*, **2**, 61–73.

475. Conti, B., Jahng, J. W., Tinti, C., Son, J. H., and Joh, T. H. (1997). Induction of interferon-gamma inducing factor in the adrenal cortex. *J. Biol. Chem.*, **272**, 2035–2037.

476. Jaattela, M., Carpen, O., Stenman, U. H., and Saksela, E. (1990). Regulation of ACTH-induced steroidogenesis in human fetal adrenals by rTNF-alpha. *Mol. Cell. Endocrinol.*, **68**, R31–36.

477. Muramami, N., Fukata, J., Tsukada, T., Kobayashi, H., Ebisui, O., Segawa, H. *et al.* (1993). Bacterial lipopolysaccharide-induced expression of interleukin-6 messenger ribonucleic acid in the rat hypothalamus, pituitary, adrenal gland, and spleen. *Endocrinology*, **133**, 2574–2578.

478. Gonzalez-Hernandez, J. A., Ehrhart-Bornstein, M., Spath-Schwalbe, E., Scherbaum, W. A., and Bornstein, S. R. (1996). Human adrenal cells express tumour necrosis factor-alpha messenger ribonucleic acid: evidence for paracrine control of adrenal function. *J. Clin. Endocrinol. Metab.*, **81**, 807–813.

479. Judd, A. M. and MacLeod, R. M. (1992). Adrenocorticotropin increases interleukin-6 release from rat adrenal zona glomerulosa cells. *Endocrinology*, **130**, 1245–1254.

480. Judd, A. M. and MacLeod, R. M. (1995). Differential release of tumour necrosis factor and IL-6 from adrenal zona glomerulosa cells *in vitro*. *Am. J. Physiol.*, **268**, E114–120.

481. Karanth, S. and McCann, S. M. (1991). Anterior pituitary hormone control by interleukin 2. *Proc. Natl. Acad. Sci. USA*, **88**, 2961–2965.

482. Spangelo, B. L., Judd, A. M., Isakson, P. C., and MacLeod, R. M. (1989). Interleukin-6 stimulates anterior pituitary hormone release *in vitro*. *Endocrinology*, **125**, 575–577.

483. Pang, X. P., Hershman, J. M., Mirell, C. J., and Pekary, A. E. (1989). Impairment of hypothalamic–pituitary–thyroid function in rats treated with human recombinant tumour necrosis factor-alpha (cachectin). *Endocrinology*, **125**, 76–84.

484. Barak, V., Yanai, P., Treves, A. J., Roisman, I., Simon, A., and Laufer, N. (1992). Interleukin-1: local production and modulation of human granulosa luteal cells steroidogenesis. *Fertil. Steril.*, **58**, 719–725.

485. Best, C. L., Pudney, J., Anderson, D. J., and Hill, J. A. (1994). Modulation of human granulosa cell steroid production *in vitro* by tumour necrosis factor alpha: implications of white blood cells in culture. *Obstet. Gynecol.*, **84**, 121–127.

486. Nakamura, Y., Kato, H., and Terranova, P. F. (1990). Interleukin-1 alpha increases thecal progesterone production of preovulatory follicles in cyclic hamsters. *Biol. Reprod.*, **43**, 169–173.

487. Sjogren, A., Holmes, P. V., and Hillensjo, T. (1991). Interleukin-1 alpha modulates luteinizing hormone stimulated cyclic AMP and progesterone release from human granulosa cells *in vitro*. *Hum. Reprod.*, **6**, 910–913.

488. Roby, K. F. and Terranova, P. F. (1990). Effects of tumour necrosis factor-alpha *in vitro* on steroidogenesis of healthy and atretic follicles of the rat: theca as a target. *Endocrinology*, **126**, 2711–2718.

489. Adashi, E. Y., Resnick, C. E., Packman, J. N., Hurwitz, A., and Payne, D. W. (1990). Cytokine-mediated regulation of ovarian function: tumour necrosis factor alpha inhibits gonadotropin-supported progesterone accumulation by differentiating and luteinized murine granulosa cells. *Am. J. Obstet. Gynecol.*, **162**, 889–896.

490. Ogilvie, K. M., Held Hales, K., Roberts, M. E., Hales, D. B., and Rivier, C. (1999). The inhibitory effect of intracerebroventricularly injected interleukin 1beta on testosterone secretion in the rat: role of steroidogenic acute regulatory protein. *Biol. Reprod.*, **60**, 527–533.

491. Lin, T., Wang, D., and Stocco, D. M. (1998). Interleukin-1 inhibits Leydig cell steroidogenesis without affecting steroidogenic acute regulatory protein messenger ribonucleic acid or protein levels. *J. Endocrinol.*, **156**, 461–467.

492. Besedovsky, H. O. and del Rey, A. (1996). Immune–neuro-endocrine interactions: facts and hypotheses. *Endocr. Rev.*, **17**, 64–102.

493. Rothwell, N. J., Luheshi, G., and Toulmond, S. (1996). Cytokines and their receptors in the central nervous system: physiology, pharmacology, and pathology. *Pharmacol. Ther.*, **69**, 85–95.

494. Vallieres, L. and Rivest, S. (1997). Regulation of the genes encoding interleukin-6, its receptor, and gp130 in the rat brain in response to the immune activator lipopolysaccharide and the proinflammatory cytokine interleukin-1beta. *J. Neurochem.*, **69**, 1668–1683.

495. Schobitz, B., De Kloet, E. R., Sutanto, W., and Holsboer, F. (1993). Cellular localization of interleukin 6 mRNA and interleukin 6 receptor mRNA in rat brain. *Eur. J. Neurosci.*, **5**, 1426–1435.

496. Hopkins, S. J. and Rothwell, N. J. (1995). Cytokines and the nervous system. I: Expression and recognition. *Trends Neurosci.*, **18**, 83–88.

497. Schobitz, B., De Kloet, E. R., and Holsboer, F. (1994). Gene expression and function of interleukin 1, interleukin 6 and tumour necrosis factor in the brain. *Prog. Neurobiol.*, **44**, 397–432.

498. Hagan, P., Poole, S., and Bristow, A. F. (1993). Endotoxin-stimulated production of rat hypothalamic interleukin-1β *in vivo* and *in vitro*, measured by specific immunodiametric assay. *J. Mol. Endocrinol.*, **11**, 31–36.

499. Hillhouse, E. W. and Mosley, K. (1993). Peripheral endotoxin induces hypothalamic immunoreactive interleukin-1 beta in the rat. *Br. J. Pharmacol.*, **109**, 289–290.

500. Breder, C. D., Hazuka, C., Ghayur, T., Klug, C., Huginin, M., Yasuda, K. *et al.* (1994). Regional induction of tumour necrosis factor alpha expression in the mouse brain after systemic lipopolysaccharide administration. *Proc. Natl. Acad. Sci. USA*, **91**, 11393–11397.

501. Minami, M., Kuraishi, Y., Yamaguchi, T., Nakai, S., Hirai, Y., and Satoh, M. (1991). Immobilization stress induces interleukin-1 beta mRNA in the rat hypothalamus. *Neurosci. Lett.*, **123**, 254–256.

502. Suzuki, E., Shintani, F., Kanba, S., Asai, M., and Nakaki, T. (1997). Immobilization stress increases mRNA levels of interleukin-1 receptor antagonist in various rat brain regions. *Cell. Mol. Neurobiol.*, **17**, 557–562.

503. Shintani, F., Nakaki, T., Kanba, S., Sato, K., Yagi, G., Shiozawa, M. *et al.* (1995). Involvement of interleukin-1 in immobilization stress-induced increase in plasma adrenocorticotropic hormone and in release of hypothalamic monoamines in the rat. *J. Neurosci.*, **15**, 1961–1970.

504. Shizuya, K., Komori, T., Fujiwara, R., Miyahara, S., Ohmori, M., and Nomura, J. (1997). The influence of restraint stress on the expression of mRNAs for IL-6 and the IL-6 receptor in the hypothalamus and midbrain of the rat. *Life Sci.*, **61**, PL135–140.

505. Katsuura, G., Gottschall, P. E., Dahl, R. R., and Arimura, A. (1988). Adrenocorticotropin release induced by intracerebroventricular injection of recombinant human interleukin-1 in rats: possible involvement of prostaglandin. *Endocrinology*, **122**, 1773–1779.

506. LeMay, L. G., Vander, A. J., and Kluger, M. J. (1990). The effects of psychological stress on plasma interleukin-6 activity in rats. *Physiol. Behav.*, **47**, 957–961.

507. Morrow, L. E., McClellan, J. L., Conn, C. A., and Kluger, M. J. (1993). Glucocorticoids alter fever and IL-6 responses to psychological stress and to lipopolysaccharide. *Am. J. Physiol.*, **264**, R1010–1016.

508. Zhou, D., Kusnecov, A. W., Shurin, M. R., DePaoli, M., and Rabin, B. S. (1993). Exposure to physical and psychological stressors elevates plasma interleukin 6: relationship to the activation of hypothalamic–pituitary–adrenal axis. *Endocrinology*, **133**, 2523–2530.

509. Turnbull, A. V. and Rivier, C. (1995). Regulation of the HPA axis by cytokines. *Brain Behav. Immun.*, **9**, 253–275.

510. Mekaouche, M., Givalois, L., Barbanel, G., Siaud, P., Maurel, D., Malaval, F. et al. (1994). Chronic restraint enhances interleukin-1-beta release in the basal state and after an endotoxin challenge, independently of adrenocorticotropin and corticosterone release. *Neuroimmunomodulation*, **1**, 292–299.

511. Papanicolaou, D. A., Petrides, J. S., Tsigos, C., Bina, S., Kalogeras, K. T., Wilder, R. et al. (1996). Exercise stimulates interleukin-6 secretion: inhibition by glucocorticoids and correlation with catecholamines. *Am. J. Physiol.*, **271**, E601–605.

512. Spivak, B., Shohat, B., Mester, R., Avraham, S., Gil-Ad, I., Bleich, A. et al. (1997). Elevated levels of serum interleukin-1 beta in combat-related posttraumatic stress disorder. *Biol. Psychiatry*, **42**, 345–348.

513. Maier, S. F. and Watkins, L. R. (1995). Intracerebroventricular interleukin-1 receptor antagonist blocks the enhancement of fear conditioning and interference with escape produced by inescapable shock. *Brain Res.*, **695**, 279–282.

514. Donald, R. A., Redekopp, C., Cameron, V., Nicholls, M. C., and Bolton, J. (1983). The hormonal actions of CRF in sheep: effect of IV and ICV injection. *Endocrinology*, **113**, 866–870.

515. Katsuura, G., Gottschall, P. E., and Arimura, A. (1988). Identification of a high-affinity receptor for interleukin-1 beta in rat brain. *Biochem. Biophys. Res. Commun.*, **156**, 61–67.

516. Ericsson, A., Liu, C., Hart, R. P., and Sawchenko, P. E. (1995). Type 1 interleukin-1 receptor in the rat brain: distribution, regulation, and relationship to sites of IL-1-induced cellular activation. *J. Comp. Neurol.*, **361**, 681–698.

517. Nishiyori, A., Minami, M., Takami, S., and Satoh, M. (1997). Type 2 interleukin-1 receptor mRNA is induced by kainic acid in the rat brain. *Brain Res. Mol. Brain Res.*, **50**, 237–245.

518. Sei, Y., Vitkovic, L., and Yokoyama, M. M. (1995). Cytokines in the central nervous system: regulatory roles in neuronal function, cell death and repair. *Neuroimmunomodulation*, **2**, 121–133.

519. Cornfield, L. J. and Sills, M. A. (1991). High affinity interleukin-6 binding sites in bovine hypothalamus. *Eur. J. Pharmacol.*, **202**, 237–245.

520. Kinouchi, K., Brown, G., Pasternak, G., and Donner, D. B. (1991). Identification and characterization of receptors for tumour necrosis factor-alpha in the brain. *Biochem. Biophys. Res. Commun.*, **181**, 1532–1538.

521. Bebo, B. F. Jr and Linthicum, D. S. (1995). Expression of mRNA for 55-kDa and 75-kDa tumour necrosis factor (TNF) receptors in mouse cerebrovascular endothelium: effects of interleukin-1 beta, interferon-gamma and TNF-alpha on cultured cells. *J. Neuroimmunol.*, **62**, 161–167.

522. St Pierre, B. A., Granger, D. A., Wong, J. L., and Merrill, J. E. (1995). A study on tumour necrosis factor, tumour necrosis factor receptors, and nitric oxide in human fetal glial cultures. *Adv. Pharmacol.*, **34**, 415–438.

523. Tada, M., Diserens, A. C., Desbaillets, I., and de Tribolet, N. (1994). Analysis of cytokine receptor messenger RNA expression in human glioblastoma cells and normal astrocytes by reverse-transcription polymerase chain reaction. *J. Neurosurg.*, **80**, 1063–1073.

524. Boka, G., Anglade, P., Wallach, D., Javoy-Agid, F., Agid, Y., and Hirsch, E. C. (1994). Immunocytochemical analysis of tumour necrosis factor and its receptors in Parkinson's disease. *Neurosci. Lett.*, **172**, 151–154.

525. Banks, W. A., Kastin, A. J., and Durham, D. A. (1989). Bidirectional transport of interleukin-1 alpha across the blood–brain barrier. *Brain Res. Bull.*, **23**, 433–437.

526. Banks, W. A., Oritz, L., Plotkin, S. R., and Kastin, A. J. (1991). Human interleukin (IL)-1a, murine IL-1α, and IL-1β are transported from blood to brain in the mouse by a shared saturable mechanism. *J. Pharmacol. Exp. Ther.*, **259**, 988–996.

527. Gutierrez, E. G., Banks, W. A., and Kastin, A. J. (1994). Blood-borne interleukin-1 receptor antagonist crosses the blood–brain barrier. *J. Neuroimmunol.*, **55**, 153–160.

528. Banks, W. A., Kastin, A. J., and Gutierrez, E. G. (1994). Penetration of interleukin-6 across the murine blood–brain barrier. *Neurosci. Lett.*, **179**, 53–56.

529. Gutierrez, E. G., Banks, W. A., and Kastin, A. J. (1993). Murine tumour necrosis factor alpha is transported from blood to brain in the mouse. *J. Neuroimmunol.*, **47**, 169–176.

530. Komaki, G., Arimura, A., and Koves, K. (1992). Effect of intravenous injection of IL-1 beta on PGE2 levels in several brain areas as determined by microdialysis. *Am. J. Physiol.*, **262**, E246–251.

531. Watanobe, H. and Takebe, K. (1994). Effects of intravenous administration of interleukin-1-beta on the release of prostaglandin E2, corticotropin-releasing factor, and arginine vasopressin in several hypothalamic areas of freely moving rats: estimation by push–pull perfusion. *Neuroendocrinology*, **60**, 8–15.

532. Dunn, A. J. and Chuluyan, H. E. (1992). The role of cyclo-oxygenase and lipoxygenase in the interleukin-1-induced activation of the HPA axis: dependence on the route of injection. *Life Sci.*, **51**, 219–225.

533. Rivier, C. (1993). Effect of peripheral and central cytokines on the hypothalamic–pituitary–adrenal axis of the rat. *Ann. N. Y. Acad. Sci.*, **697**, 97–105.

534. Lacroix, S. and Rivest, S. (1997). Functional circuitry in the brain of immune-challenged rats: partial involvement of prostaglandins. *J. Comp. Neurol.*, **387**, 307–324.

535. Niimi, M., Sato, M., Wada, Y., Takahara, J., and Kawanishi, K. (1996). Effect of central and continuous intravenous injection of interleukin-1 beta on brain

cfos expression in the rat: involvement of prostaglandins. *Neuroimmunomodulation*, **3**, 87–92.

536. Sagar, S. M., Price, K. J., Kasting, N. W., and Sharp, F. R. (1995). Anatomic patterns of Fos immunostaining in rat brain following systemic endotoxin administration. *Brain Res. Bull.*, **36**, 381–392.

537. Niimi, M., Wada, Y., Sato, M., Takahara, J., and Kawanishi, K. (1997). Effect of continuous intravenous injection of interleukin-6 and pretreatment with cyclooxygenase inhibitor on brain cfos expression in the rat. *Neuroendocrinology*, **66**, 47–53.

538. Sharp, B. M. and Matta, S. G. (1993). Prostaglandins mediate the adrenocorticotropin response to tumour necrosis factor in rats. *Endocrinology*, **132**, 269–274.

539. Turnbull, A. V., Lee, S., and Rivier, C. (1998). Mechanisms of hypothalamic–pituitary–adrenal axis stimulation by immune signals in the adult rat. *Ann. N. Y. Acad. Sci.*, **840**, 434–443.

540. Bernardini, R., Calogero, A. E., Mauceri, G., and Chrousos, G. P. (1990). Rat hypothalamic corticotropin-releasing hormone secretion *in vitro* is stimulated by interleukin-1 in an eicosanoid-dependent manner. *Life Sci.*, **47**, 1601–1607.

541. Cameron, V. A., Nishimura, E., Mathews, L. S., Lewis, K. A., Sawchenko, P. E., and Vale, W. W. (1994). Hybridization histochemical localization of activin receptor subtypes in rat brain, pituitary, ovary, and testis. *Endocrinology*, **134**, 799–808.

542. Lyson, K. and McCann, S. M. (1992). Involvement of arachidonic acid cascade pathways in interleukin-6-stimulated corticotropin-releasing factor release *in vitro*. *Neuroendocrinology*, **55**, 708–713.

543. Navarra, P., Tsagarakis, S., Faria, M. S., Rees, L. H., Besser, G. M., and Grossman, A. B. (1991). Interleukins-1 and -6 stimulate the release of corticotropin-releasing hormone-41 from rat hypothalamus *in vitro* via the eicosanoid cyclooxygenase pathway. *Endocrinology*, **128**, 37–44.

544. Watanobe, H., Sasaki, S., and Takebe, K. (1995). Role of prostaglandins E1, E2 and F2 alpha in the brain in interleukin 1 beta-induced adrenocorticotropin secretion in the rat. *Cytokine*, **7**, 710–712.

545. Calza, L., Giardino, L., and Ceccatelli, S. (1993). NOS mRNA in the paraventricular nucleus of young and old rats after immobilization stress. *NeuroReport*, **4**, 627–630.

546. Lee, S., Barbanel, G., and Rivier, C. (1995). Systemic endotoxin increases steady-state gene expression of hypothalamic nitric oxide synthase: comparison with corticotropin releasing factor and vasopressin gene transcripts. *Brain Res.*, **705**, 136–148.

547. Rivier, C. (1995). Blockade of nitric oxide formation augments adrenocorticotropin released by blood-borne interleukin-1 beta: role of vasopressin, prostaglandins, and alpha 1-adrenergic receptors. *Endocrinology*, **136**, 3597–3603.

548. Wong, M. L., Bongiorno, P. B., al-Shekhlee, A., Esposito, A., Khatri, P., and Licinio, J. (1996). IL-1 beta, IL-1 receptor type I and iNOS gene expression in rat brain vasculature and perivascular areas. *NeuroReport*, **7**, 2445–2448.

549. Ceccatelli, S., Lundberg, J. M., Fahrenkrug, J., Bredt, D. S., Snyder, S. H., and Hokfelt, T. (1992). Evidence for involvement of nitric oxide in the regulation of hypothalamic portal blood flow. *Neuroscience*, **51**, 769–772.

550. Bredt, D. S., Glatt, C. E., Hwang, P. M., Fotuhi, M., Dawson, T. M., and Snyder, S. H. (1991). Nitric oxide synthase protein and mRNA are discretely localized in neuronal populations of the mammalian CNS together with NADPH diaphorase. *Neuron*, **7**, 615–624.

551. Ceccatelli, S., Hulting, A. L., Zhang, X., Gustafsson, L., Villar, M., and Hokfelt, T. (1993). Nitric oxide synthase in the rat anterior pituitary gland and the role of nitric oxide in regulation of luteinizing hormone secretion. *Proc. Natl. Acad. Sci. USA*, **90**, 11292–11296.

552. Rivier, C. and Shen, G. H. (1994). In the rat, endogenous nitric oxide modulates the response of the hypothalamic–pituitary–adrenal axis to interleukin-1 beta, vasopressin, and oxytocin. *Neuroscience*, **14**, 1985–1993.

553. Bluthe, R. M., Walter, V., Parnet, P., Laye, S., Lestage, J., Verrier, D. *et al.* (1994). Lipopolysaccharide induces sickness behaviour in rats by a vagal mediated mechanism. *C. R. Acad. Sci. (Paris)*, **317**, 499–503.

554. Watkins, L. R., Wiertelak, E. P., Goehler, L. E., Mooney-Heiberger, K., Martinez, J., Furness, L. *et al.* (1994). Neurocircuitry of illness-induced hyperalgesia. *Brain Res.*, **639**, 283–299.

555. Ishizuka, Y., Ishida, Y., Kunitake, T., Kato, K., Hanamori, T., Mitsuyama, Y. *et al.* (1997). Effects of area postrema lesion and abdominal vagotomy on interleukin-1 beta-induced norepinephrine release in the hypothalamic paraventricular nucleus region in the rat. *Neurosci. Lett.*, **223**, 57–60.

556. Laye, S., Bluthe, R. M., Kent, S., Combe, C., Medina, C., Parnet, P. *et al.* (1995). Subdiaphragmatic vagotomy blocks induction of IL-1 beta mRNA in mice brain in response to peripheral LPS. *Am. J. Physiol.*, **268**, R1327–1331.

557. Fleshner, M., Silbert, L., Deak, T., Goehler, L. E., Martin, D., Watkins, L. R. *et al.* (1997). TNF-alpha-induced corticosterone elevation but not serum protein or corticosteroid binding globulin reduction is vagally mediated. *Brain Res. Bull.*, **44**, 701–706.

558. Goehler, L. E., Relton, J. K., Dripps, D., Kiechle, R., Tartaglia, N., Maier, S. F. *et al.* (1997). Vagal paraganglia bind biotinylated interleukin-1 receptor antagonist: a possible mechanism for immune-to-brain communication. *Brain Res. Bull.*, **43**, 357–364.

559. Dunn, A. J., Powell, M. L., Moreshead, W. V., Gaskin, J. M., and Hall, N. R. (1987). Effects of Newcastle disease virus administration to mice on the metabolism of cerebral biogenic amines, plasma corticosterone, and lymphocyte proliferation. *Brain Behav. Immun.*, **1**, 216–230.

560. Meites, J. (1990). Aging: hypothalamic catecholamines, neuroendocrine–immune interactions, and dietary restriction. *Proc. Soc. Exp. Biol. Med.*, **195**, 304–311.

561. Miller, R. A. (1996). The aging immune system: primer and prospectus. *Science*, **273**, 70–74.

562. Pahlavani, M. A. and Richardson, A. (1996). The effect of age on the expression of interleukin-2. *Mech. Ageing Dev.*, **89**, 125–154.

563. ThyagaRajan, S., Madden, K. S., Kalvas, J. C., Dimitrova, S. S., Felten, S. Y., and Felten, D. L. (1998). L-deprenyl-induced increase in IL-2 and NK cell activity accompanies restoration of noradrenergic nerve fibres in the spleens of old F344 rats. *J. Neuroimmunol.*, **92**, 9–21.

564. ThyagaRajan, S., Madden, K. S., Stevens, S. Y., and Felten, D. L. (2000). Inhibition of tumour growth by L-deprenyl involves neural–immune interactions in

rats with spontaneously developing mammary tumours. *Anticancer Res.* **19**, 5023–5028.

565. ThyagaRajan, S., Meites, J., and Quadri, S. K. (1995). Deprenyl reinitiates estrous cycles, reduces serum prolactin, and decreases the incidence of mammary and pituitary tumours in old acyclic rats. *Endocrinology*, **136**, 1103–1110.

566. ThyagaRajan, S., Felten, S. Y., and Felten, D. L. (1998). Antitumour effect of L-deprenyl in rats with carcinogen-induced mammary tumours. *Cancer Lett.*, **123**, 177–183.

567. ThyagaRajan, S. and Quadri, S. K. (1999). L-deprenyl inhibits tumour growth, reduces serum prolactin, and suppresses brain monoamine metabolism in rats with carcinogen-induced mammary tumours. *Endocrine*, **10**, 225–232.

2

Anti-cancer mechanisms involving the immune system

P. W. SZLOSAREK AND A. G. DALGLEISH

1 Introduction

The past five years have witnessed a sustained period of growth in our understanding of the immune system and its interaction with solid tumours. The
continuing molecular revolution has undoubtedly been the single most important factor in these developments, enabling a redefinition of both the immune
mechanisms involved and the pathobiology of the disease at a structural and
functional molecular level. New methodologies, including cloning techniques
for tumour antigens and hence their characterization (the so-called human
cancer 'immunome' project), and new quantitative and functional assays
detailing the immune response such as ELISPOT and tetramer analysis have
been particularly important. This detailed knowledge has subsequently generated exciting new ideas and treatment strategies, which are based on a
rational, scientific approach to the problem of cancer (1–3).

Cancer is fundamentally a genetic disease, whether acquired or inherited, and
it has three important defining properties. The malignant tumour displays
abnormal growth kinetics, invasiveness, and has the capacity to metastasize.
All of these are dependent upon a continuous process of evolution from a
monoclonal cell into a genetically and phenotypically heterogeneous population. Hence, by definition the transformed cell should possess unique antigens (tumour-specific antigens or TSAs) and/or a differential display of antigens
(tumour-associated antigens or TAAs) which, if sufficiently immunogenic,
would provoke a specific immune response. The concept of immune surveillance of cancer was first proposed by McFarlane Burnet (4) and is not readily
supported by the facts as we know them, such as the lack of increase in incidence
of common malignancies in severe immunodeficiencies such as AIDS (5). Indeed,
the malignancies seen in patients with AIDS, being mainly non-Hodgkin's
lymphomas and Kaposi's sarcomas, are both associated with viruses (Epstein–
Barr virus (EBV) and human herpes virus 8 (HHV-8) respectively), where
immunological control is very well documented.

Furthermore, the fact that tumour-associated antigens are mainly self-antigens
that have often been expressed during foetal development means that the
tumour is not seen as foreign or as a danger signal to the immune system.
Nevertheless, a number of mutations in oncogenes and tumour suppressor
genes appear to be present in the majority of tumours, and if they were to
arise spontaneously it is likely that they would be instantly seen by the
immune system and killed as non-self. One of the fundamental understandings
of the immune system over the past few years is that functionally there are two
major types of response. The first is mainly a cell-mediated response, and the

second, a humoral or antibody immune response. These are known as T helper 1 (Th1) and Th2 responses, respectively. In patients with chronic infectious diseases, the cell-mediator response is suppressed, and the humoral response enhanced. This pattern also appears to occur in patients with cancer, and raises the possibility that for a cancer to evolve it must first learn to suppress the immune responses. However, until it has evolved it will itself be suppressed if it expresses any mutation. One way that cancer could evolve would be on a background of non-specific chronic inflammation/infection which is known to be associated with the suppression of the cell-mediated immune response as well as angiogenesis or new vessel formation as both these are properties associated with wound healing. Within this environment mutations could evolve without being immunologically detected. In this regard it is surprising how many of the common cancers do indeed evolve against a background of chronic inflammation and this is discussed in more detail later in this chapter.

The fact that so many cancers can escape the immune system by a variety of mechanisms, including the production of immunosuppressive factors which appear to have an effect on even peripheral circulating lymphocytes such as that seen in colorectal cancer (see Section 3.7), suggests that solid cancers not previously thought to be under immune control, such as colorectal cancer and lung cancer, may well be susceptible to new immunological approaches. The promising field of cancer vaccines, although developed mainly in the area of advanced melanoma and lymphoma, may be considerably more effective when applied to a variety of cancers at earlier stages of the disease, when the tumour load can be completely reduced by other modalities.

1.1   A BRIEF OVERVIEW OF THE IMMUNE RESPONSE

The human immune system has evolved as a highly flexible, multifunctional and integrated network of cells and molecules. The tendency to divide the system into two distinct categories is mostly artificial and based upon descriptive convenience, although in terms of evolution the adaptive system is a later development (Table 1). It is becoming clear that the specific or adaptive arm is critically dependent upon signals from the innate arm and there is immense crosstalk between the two systems. Furthermore, it is well known that major B- and T-cell abnormalities often do not prove fatal, whereas crippling of cells of the innate system (e.g. of neutrophils in neutropenia) heralds disaster for the host during an infection. The following sections outline the components of various anti-tumour host responses and emphasize their interdependence.

1.1.1   The innate immune system

The innate immune system is the first line of defence and has evolved as a fast and efficient mechanism for the neutralization of pathogens. It consists of natural surface barriers, secreted enzymes (e.g. lysozyme which triggers the

Table 1 Properties of the innate and adaptive immune systems

Innate immune system	Adaptive immune system
Monocytes, macrophages, neutrophils, NK cells	B and T lymphocytes
Rapid first line of defence	Slower onset of development
No memory to recall antigen	Memory to recall antigen
Non-specific immune mechanisms: Fc receptor, lectin receptors, complement receptors	Specific immune mechanisms: antibody–antigen complex, T-cell receptor and MHC-peptide engagement (trimolecular complex or signal 1)
Self-contained system	Dependent upon signals from the innate system
Early in evolution	Late in evolution

lysis of certain types of bacteria), a variety of cells (natural killer or NK cells, macrophages, and neutrophils), and molecules known as complement ('C') which function within a cascade activated via three distinct pathways.

Complement has a critical role in dealing with pathogens. The alternative (spontaneous) pathway of activation depends upon the presence of amino or hydroxyl groups, which are present within proteins and carbohydrates of foreign organisms. C3b, a central complement molecule, binds to these chemical groups and initiates a series of reactions culminating in the membrane attack complex (MAC), which punches a lethal hole into the surface structure of the pathogen (6), similar to the perforin proteins of T cells and NK cells (7). Inhibitory molecules, such as decay accelerating factor (DAF) and CD59, protect host cells from attack by inducing degradation of the C3bBb convertase and removing MAC from the cell surface, respectively (8). The classical pathway depends on the presence of IgM antibodies, which attract two or more molecules of C1, initiating the complement cascade via the activation of C3 convertase (9). Finally, the lectin activation pathway, which has recently been characterized, involves a mannose-binding lectin, which triggers the cascade by binding to carbohydrate molecules on the surface of pathogens (i.e. a type of 'smart bomb') (10).

The involvement of NK cells in host responses to tumours is now relatively well documented. These cells, also known as large granular lymphocytes (LGLs), are derived from the bone marrow and form a subset of lymphocytes in the blood and lymphoid tissues. Although NK cells lack the specific receptors found on T cells (the T-cell receptor or TCR complex, see Section 1.1.2) (11), they express a number of adhesion molecules (CD2, LFA-1, and CD56) and possess low-affinity receptors for the constant portion of the immunoglobulin molecule IgG1/3, also called FcγRIIIA/CD16, through which the majority of antibody-dependent cell-mediated cytotoxicity (ADCC) occurs (12).

Clustering of Fcγ RIIIA initiates downstream signalling events via the ξ chain (also found in the TCR activation pathway) with secretion of tumour necrosis factor alpha (TNF-α) and interferon gamma (IFN-γ) as well as granular exocytosis of perforins and granzyme B pathways leading to apoptosis. Cytokine receptor expression is varied, with incomplete interleukin 2 receptors (IL-2Rs) due to an absent α subunit (which means that high levels of IL-2 are required to induce NK proliferation) (13).

NK cells have both specific (requiring major histocompatibility complex or MHC) and non-specific (MHC-unrestricted) effector functions in relation to tumour cells. Although *in vitro* systems have provided compelling evidence for NK-mediated tumorlysis, NK presence in tumour-associated inflammatory infiltrates is usually insignificant (14). However, low NK cytotoxic activity correlates with the early appearance of metastases and decreased survival in patients with solid tumours (15). The importance of NK cells is also emphasized in mice of the 'beige' strain, which congenitally lack NK cells and succumb to spontaneously developing tumours at a high frequency (16). T-cell-deficient nude mice, however, with normal or elevated NK cells, do not display this high incidence of spontaneous tumours (17).

The NK–tumour cell interaction is modulated by both the qualitative and quantitative expression of MHC class I (see Section 1.1.2 for details on MHC biology), adhesion molecules (e.g. intercellular adhesion molecule-1 or ICAM-1), mucins and other surface glycoproteins, as shown using monoclonal antibodies and N-glycan processing inhibitors. Artificial sensitization using chemotherapeutic agents is also possible. Recent work suggests that the balance of MHC I signals (inhibition of NK cytotoxicity) and interactions with target cell carbohydrates (induction of NK cytotoxicity) determines whether the NK cell finally destroys a target cell. After binding to the tumour cell, NK cells display a marked increase in phosphoinositide hydrolysis and Ca^{2+} cycling. This does not occur with NK-resistant tumour lines, and MHC class I loss does not inhibit this cycling (18). Clearly, a signalling cascade further downstream is required for full development of NK cell-mediated cytotoxicity.

The NK cell is activated by a number of cytokines including IFN-γ, TNF-α, IL-2, and IL-12 and both necrotic and apoptotic mechanisms appear to mediate NK cell tumorlysis. NK cells use the perforin system (i.e. a membrane attack complex), and secrete enzymes directly into the target cell (19, 20). The FasL molecule that is expressed on the NK cell surface binds to Fas on target cells (expressed by a variety of tumours) and induces apoptosis (21). Certain molecules, for instance a serine protease in a rat NK cell line, induce tumoristasis and alter the phenotype of the malignant cells (22). NK cells, via their low-affinity receptors for IgG antibodies (FcγRIII), participate in ADCC of tumour cells.

Incubation of NK cells with IL-2 for 3–4 days boosts their innate activity and converts them to lymphokine-activated killer (LAK) cells, which have broader tumour specificity, including action against tumours refractory to NK lysis (23). This is probably mediated through the stimulation of other cytokines, such as TNF-α and IFN-γ. In contrast, transforming growth factor-beta or

TGF-β, a growth factor secreted by many tumour cells, antagonizes the activation of LAK cells by TNF-α. Thus, both positive and negative regulation operates *in vitro* and *in vivo*. LAK cells mediate numerous effects and produce many different cytokines; some of these may be detrimental to the host, as evidenced by the toxicity seen in patients given LAK cells with IL-2.

Another key cell of the innate system, the macrophage, is able to activate tumorlysis, and this state is denoted by several morphological, biochemical, and functional changes to the cells. The cytotoxic process involves cytolytic and cytostatic components, non-phagocytic, contact-dependent mechanisms, and ADCC (24). The former is thought to discriminate between normal and tumour cells by sensing alterations in membrane phospholipid composition (25).

TNF, as an example of a key member of the cytokine network, is a primary mediator of tumoricidal activities of macrophages. This is achieved via a number of mechanisms. The first involves two forms of TNF that can induce tumour cell apoptosis directly: a 26-kDa membrane-bound form (i.e. by juxtacrine signalling) (26), and the 17-kDa secretory form which initiates oxidative stress, inducing DNA and cytoskeletal fragmentation. The second is via indirect routes involving the activation of a number of host systems leading to tumour necrosis. These include the induction of endothelial cell apoptosis (and hence vessel destruction in tumours) by the selective deactivation of the $\alpha V\beta 3$ integrin (27), enhanced macrophage cytotoxicity (with IFN-γ synergism) (28), and modulation of specific anti-tumour immune responses (see below) (29).

Macrophages have an extremely important role in the immune system, being both scavenger cells and able to present new antigens to the immune system. When tumour cells are killed by T cells or chemotherapeutic agents, they are able to scavenge the dying tumour cells and may or may not present the relevant antigens to the immune system. This function is in addition to their ability to be involved in the active destruction of tumour cells. A number of complex cytokine networks (30) are clearly involved, and in experiments where tumours are inoculated into animal models they play a major role in the recognition and induction of relevant immune response by the immune system.

Macrophages stimulated by IFN-γ and TNF-α manufacture a flavoprotein that converts L-arginine to nitric oxide (NO) (31), initiating cytotoxicity by the formation of reactive nitrogen intermediates (e.g. NO_2^-). Possibly, of greater importance in relation to tumours is the superoxide pathway, resulting in the generation of reactive oxygen intermediates (e.g. O_2^-, H_2O_2), which is similarly induced by IFN-γ and TNF-α (32). Normal cells are protected from cytotoxic cytokines by the induction of certain scavenging proteins; for instance, TNF-α induces manganese-dependent superoxide dismutase (33).

It is important to realize that as well as responding to cytokines, macrophages will produce TNF-α and IFN-γ, among other cytokines, when non-specifically stimulated. Furthermore, this activity appears to be depressed in patients with colorectal cancer (34).

1.1.2 The adaptive immune system

Two characteristic features of adaptive immune mechanisms are the ability to
(a) recognize diverse antigenic forms with high specificity and (b) re-call antigen
(i.e. to show antigenic 'memory'). The two major cell types that make up the
adaptive immune system are the T cells and the B cells. The former are composed of cells involved in the initial recognition of an antigen (T helper or Th
cells) as well as suppressor cells (T suppressor or Ts cells) and effector cells
capable of effecting the required function (cytotoxic T-lymphocytes or CTLs).
Recognition cells are either naïve or classified as memory cells having previously seen a particular invading antigen and can respond to it much faster
than a naïve T cell would. Based on this initial interaction basic T cells can
provide help to B cells which respond by making antibodies against invading
organisms. Their ability to do so and the speed with which they can produce a
response depends greatly upon whether they have seen the invader previously.
(This is the main concept behind vaccination whereby the naïve cells are programmed to recognize an invader, which has yet to infect the body.) There is a
tremendous diversity of receptors expressed on these cell types particularly
with regards to the B cell, which is able to rearrange a pattern of variable
diverse and joining regions on the backbone of a constant region (Figure 1).
There is tremendous selection and diversity in these receptors so that cells may
recognize and manufacture extremely specific antibody responses.

Antigen recognition differs between B and T lymphocytes. The antibody
responses are primarily concerned with the inactivation, or neutralization, of
free or soluble antigen. B-cell antibodies directly associate with the antigen
and recognize generally the tertiary structure (or native form) of the antigen.
The parts of the antigen molecules that are recognized by B cells are called

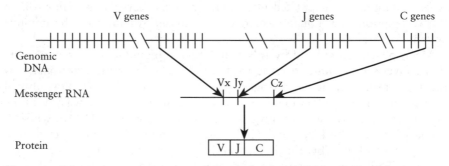

Figure 1 Schematic representation of the mechanisms which generate the immense
diversity seen in the immunoglobulins and the T-cell receptors repertoire. The diagram
represents the making of a light chain of an immunoglobulin. There are multiple V
genes in the genome but one will be translocated near a J gene and a C gene. The same
principle applies to the heavy chains of the immunoglobulins and the T-cell receptors.

epitopes and the availability, hydrophilicity, convexity, and flexibility of the antigen molecule are required for good recognition. On the other hand, T cells can only recognize an antigen that has been processed into small peptides of around 8 to 30 amino acids (35, 36) by an antigen-presenting cell (APC) or a target cell (in the case of cytotoxic T cells). The peptide is presented to a T cell in association with an MHC molecule (see below) expressed on the surface of an APC/target cell (signal 1). As such, MHC molecules are pivotal for T-cell recognition of antigens (37).

Although the major histocompatibility complex molecules have been called human histocompatibility antigens (HLAs) in humans, they are generally referred to as MHC, so this nomenclature will be used here. There are two types of MHC molecules: class I and class II. MHC class I molecules are formed by a single chain of three immunoglobulin-like domains and a beta-2 microglobulin molecule, whereas class II molecules are formed by two chains, alpha and beta, each formed by two immunoglobulin-like domains. When both domains are expressed on APCs such as macrophages and dendritic cells, both the class I and class II molecules form a pocket where the peptide antigen fits into in order to be presented to T cells. There are at least three loci of class I genes (A, B, C) and in the same way there are also at least three different types of gene-encoded class II molecules (DR, DQ, DP). Each individual possesses two class I A, B, and C molecules and two class II DR, DQ, and DP molecules (as there is one set of genes transmitted by the father and one transmitted by the mother) (see Figure 2 and ref. 38). MHC diversity among the general population is provided by different alleles coding for each of these molecules at each locus. The number of different alleles is limited. On the basis of the large diversity of TCRs recognizing the association MHC and antigen and on the basis of the huge number of possible foreign antigens available in nature, each MHC molecule can bind more than one antigen peptide depending on the contact of the peptide with the different amino acids of the pocket of the MHC molecule (Figure 2).

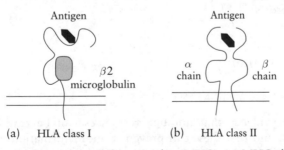

Figure 2 The major histocompatibility complex (MHC): (a) MHC class I⁺ processed peptide (8–10 amino acids, endogenous antigen) within the groove; (b) MHC class II⁺ processed peptide (12–25 amino acids, exogenous antigen) within the groove.

1.1.3 The dendritic cell—a differentiation bridge between pathogens and adaptive immunity

All cells express MHC class I molecules whereas only APCs and activated immune cells express MHC class II. MHC class I presents small peptides directly to effector lymphocytes (CD8⁺ CTLs) and generally these include only antigens derived from the cell or viral antigens following infection of a cell. MHC class II molecules, however, present much larger peptides and these are derived from the engulfment and processing of foreign antigens. The MHC class II molecules present the antigens as peptides to the CD4⁺ or helper inducer (Th) subset of lymphocytes. This process can occur on monocytes and macrophages but is most effective and sophisticated on dendritic cells (DCs), which are the most powerful APCs in the body, deriving from more than one source, including the thymus, skin, and myeloid cell progenitors. When an antigen is presented by a DC it has the capacity to induce a positive immune response or alternatively to induce tolerance to that antigen. The difference is dependent on the expression of co-stimulatory signals (signal 2) such as the B7/CD28 pathways or the CD40/CD40L (ligand) pathways. With regards to tumour recognition, the antigens of the tumour would need to be engulfed by these cells and presented in the presence of a co-stimulatory signal to the T helper cells in order to induce a strong immune response. The tumour cells, which may act as APCs, may present their own antigens in the absence of a co-stimulatory stimulus and thereby actively anergize the immune system against its antigens. This is one of the many ways employed by tumours to escape immune recognition (see Section 3). Finally, cytokines or polypeptide immunological hormones with paracrine and autocrine activity (signal 3) provide additional modulation of these cellular interactions and may either enhance or attenuate the final response (Figures 3a and 3b). Additional soluble players in the field of DC activation include heat-shock proteins, nucleotides, reactive oxygen intermediates, neuromediators, and extracellular-matrix breakdown products, which have collectively been termed danger signals (39) and are released during cellular stress (e.g. necrosis and apoptosis).

2   Tumour immunity

2.1   EVIDENCE OF AN IMMUNE RESPONSE

There is clear evidence that immune responses can be readily induced in animal models, and that these can prevent tumour formation in the event of rechallenge with tumour. More recently, similar specific and non-specific responses have been observed in the clinic with the use of whole cell and particulate vaccines mainly against melanoma antigens.

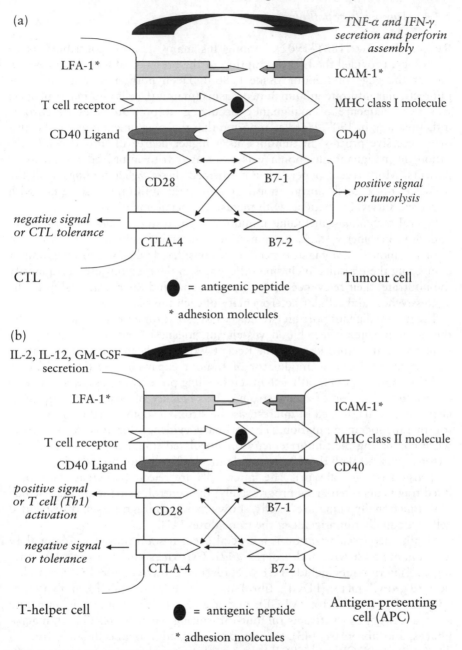

Figure 3 The MHC molecule presenting processed peptide to the T-cell receptor (the trimolecular complex or signal 1) with co-stimulatory interactions (signal 2) and release of cytokines (signal 3): (a) the cytotoxic T cell (CD8⁺)/tumour cell interaction; (b) the T helper cell (CD4⁺)/antigen-presenting cell interaction.

2.1.1   Tumour histopathology

Rudolf Virchow (1821–1902), among his many detailed contributions to pathology, provided the first description of the presence of host leukocytes in and at the edge of tumour tissue (1863). He hypothesized that the lymphorecticular infiltrate in human neoplasms (mainly T cells and macrophages) was a consequence of malignancy occurring at previous sites of chronic inflammation. In 1907, Hardley reported that this phenomenon was indicative of a 'recessive process' in tumours, as a higher degree of 'round cell infiltration' in malignant melanoma was associated with improved prognosis of patients. More recent papers have confirmed these earlier findings with the presence of a brisk intratumoral lymphocytic infiltrate associated with improved survival in patients with metastatic melanoma (40).

Several techniques, including immunocytochemistry, *in situ* hybridization, and flow cytometry, have been used to assess inflammatory infiltrates in human tumours. Many factors need to be considered when interpreting and/or comparing these results, including differences in the methods used to quantify the infiltrate, their relevance to disease outcome, and their relationship to the aggressiveness and cellular heterogeneity of each tumour.

The non-malignant portion (stroma) of the solid tumour is characterized by the development of new blood vessels (angiogenesis), an inflammatory cell infiltrate, and a fibrotic reaction. Recent work implicates the inflammatory component as a critical modulator of tumour expansion (Section 2.1.2). In addition, some cancers, rather than remodelling pre-existing tissue, are able to induce the formation of a new stroma. This balance of positive and negative elements is a major area of interest, as the stroma is considered to be a target for therapeutic manipulation. The primary evidence for this derives from work comparing the tumorigenicity of inoculated fragments of solid tumour (stroma present) with those from an identical cell line but instead injected as a suspension (stroma absent). The latter cells are rejected whereas the inoculated fragments often grow progressively; the control, using nude mice which have functionally immature T cells, shows that both fragments and suspended cells are equally tumorigenic at the same doses (41).

Finally, neovascularization is a crucial event if solid tumours greater than 2–3 mm are to survive and progress (42). Cytokines known to regulate angiogenesis in tumours include TGF-β, epidermal growth factor (EGF), platelet-derived growth factor (PDGF), fibroblast growth factor (bFGF), and vascular epidermal growth factor (VEGF), and are secreted by both malignant and stromal cells. TGF-β attracts tumour-infiltrating lymphocytes (TILs), macrophages, and fibroblasts (43), thereby providing additional cellular sources of TNF-α, IL-1, PDGF, and VEGF (many of these are also made by tumour cells in human tumours). TNF-α amplifies the system by stimulating IL-1 and PDGF release from endothelial cells; IL-1 induces autocrine proliferation of endothelial cells, whereas PDGF has a mitotic effect on the vascular smooth muscle; and VEGF stimulates angiogenesis *per se*. Many of the resulting vessels are structurally defective and highly permeable, and therefore facilitate metastasis of tumour cells. As will be outlined later (Section 2.1.4), an understanding of the interplay between the tumour neovasculature and the immune system is important for full therapeutic manipulation in favour of the host.

In terms of the immune infiltrate, an important player is the tumour-associated macrophage (TAM), which has been demonstrated in the stroma of malignant tumours derived from the colon (being particularly prominent in Dukes C stage), breast, lung, and skin (44). TAMs recognize tumour cells in a non-MHC-dependent manner and have been described as 'double-edged swords', since both tumour cytotoxicity and tumour growth have been described (45). Cytokines derived from the malignant and stromal cells in tumours (rather than specific T-cell activity) determine recruitment of TAMs. Several cytokines known to be chemotactic for macrophages (i.e. chemokines), including monocyte chemotactic proteins (MCPs) 1–3 and other chemotactic molecules, such as 5-lipoxygenase products, macrophage colony-stimulating factor (M-CSF), and TGF-β, have been reported to be upregulated in human tumours (46, 47).

Characterization of an *in vivo* concentration gradient of monocyte chemotactic activity (MCA) has been obtained by comparing the MCA in the pleural effusion and plasma of patients with lung adenocarcinoma (which has a high inflammatory component) and those with small-cell lung carcinoma (low inflammatory component) (48). The MCA gradient was found to be significantly greater in tumours with the higher inflammatory cell content, thus implicating a chemotactic gradient in the recruitment of TAMs.

In the case of lymphocytes, TILs have been isolated from many different forms of human tumour, and their characterization has yielded important information on their activity (e.g. type of tumour antigen recognized, the mechanisms of tumour escape involving the TCR complex and co-stimulatory molecules, and the role of cytokine networks in maintaining immunocompetence). For instance, in melanoma, short-term cultured TILs from HLA-A2 patients are normally lytic for malignant cells presenting an array of TAAs, including Melan-A/MART-1 and gp-100 (expressed on the majority of tumours) (49). Assessment of lymph node involvement revealed the presence of lymphocytes also lytic for clones presenting tyrosinase, MAGE-3 (70 per cent expression on tumours) and NA17-A (50 per cent expression on tumours) peptides (50). One explanation for the increased spectrum of recognized TAAs in lymph nodes as opposed to melanoma tumours is the enhanced antigen processing which may occur in the former (HLA class II-restricted pathway involving APCs, such as the DC). Furthermore, using sensitive assays involving DC priming, it has been possible to determine the frequency of specific CTLs directed against a known peptide used for vaccination (e.g. MAGE-3) (51). Comparative studies have shown that, unlike healthy individuals, cancer patients often display in their blood Melan-A-specific CTL precursors with a memory (CD45RO) phenotype, indicating an *in vivo* antigen priming phenomenon, during tumour progression (52). Moreover, data have emerged on the presence of CTLs specific for the HER2/neu antigen, which is overexpressed on breast, ovarian, and gastric carcinoma (53).

The dendritic cell, critical to antigen processing and activation of naïve T cells, has also been examined in solid tumours. A recent study of renal cell carcinoma explants revealed a 40-fold increase in tumour DC concentration compared with peripheral blood (54). Moreover, the tumour DCs are functionally mature, with upregulated MHC I and II and co-stimulatory molecules (CD86/B7–2), and the ability to stimulate naïve T cells from cord blood in mixed leukocyte reactions. Furthermore, a number of tumours, including gastric, oesophageal, colorectal, and lung carcinoma, have described a correlation between high DC infiltration and good prognosis. Immunological escape by tumour cells involves various mechanisms to reduce DC activity. These include the secretion of IL-10, which impairs T-cell co-stimulation by DC (55), and the induction of DC apoptosis (56) (see Section 3.7).

In the past few years, careful histopathological assessment of both metastases and primary vaccination sites in patients undergoing phase I/II gene therapy trials has indicated the role of various immune cells in the host response. Using a vaccine prepared from autologous cells retrovirally transduced with the gene for granulocyte–macrophage CSF (GM-CSF) (a promoter of antigen presentation by DCs) in patients with metastatic melanoma, Dranoff and colleagues (57) have shown an intense infiltration of lymphoid cells (B and T cells), dendritic cells, macrophages, and eosinophils with the formation of a fibrosing granulomatous-type reaction in the vaccination sites. Moreover, two-thirds of these patients developed inflammatory changes in distant metastases, with a fibrotic rim and an inner T-cell and plasma-cell infiltrate, with approximately 80 per cent tumour destruction (57). Both CD4$^+$ and CD8$^+$ T cells were present, and by direct contact induced tumour cell apoptosis in a highly specific manner. Other mechanisms considered to play a role include the release of antibodies by plasma cells, and the release of cytokines to induce recruitment of cells of the innate immune system. A final mechanism of tumour death involves immune-mediated vascular shutdown with subsequent necrosis. Again, lymphoid cells are implicated and it remains to be elucidated whether endothelial cells of the tumour neo-vasculature present tumour antigen and/or the lymphoid effector cells gain access due to the inherent leakiness of the vasculature. Chemokine release attracts eosinophils and neutrophils and the release of their toxic granules triggers disintegration of the endothelium. Preliminary data have also been presented in non-small-cell lung carcinoma with similar histopathological responses being observed (58), and in prostate carcinoma using an autologous cell vaccine transduced with GM-CSF, which also induces a host cell reaction (DCs, CD3$^+$ T cells, and eosinophils) at the primary vaccination site. In the latter study prostate specific antigen (PSA) velocities decreased in two-thirds of patients with the emergence of patient-specific, oligoclonal IgG1 antibodies to a range of prostate-specific antigens (59).

2.1.2 Chronic inflammation (immune deregulation) and carcinogenesis

Cancer is the end result of several mutations in tumour suppressor genes and oncogenes occurring sequentially in tumour cells. Cancer is thought to be initiated by a mutation in one of these genes by either chemicals or the inhibition of suppressor genes by viruses encoding inactivating genes (e.g. HPV, E6, and E7 which bind to p53 and Rb suppressor genes). However, in the presence of an active immune response both the mutated gene and viral epitopes will be recognized and targeted with specific CTLs. In order to progress to a tumour such changes in cells must be 'protected' from the T-cell immune response. Nature already protects certain areas from overenthusiastic T-cell responses. One such example is the care of wounds or acute inflammation where neutrophils and macrophages are encouraged to 'invade' and repel infections. However, if T-cell responses or Th1-associated cytokine responses were present during major healing, then in the presence of necrosis (and under certain conditions, apoptosis) some types of responses to self tissues (e.g. skin, muscle, vessels, etc.) would occur and result in unacceptable autoimmunity. It is of interest that another important component of cancer progression is also present and enhanced in wound healing and inflammation and that is angiogenesis. Indeed the two features go 'hand in hand' and may counterregulate each other (e.g. Th1 suppression is associated with increased angiogenesis (60)). It is speculated that in order for cancer to get even one step on the ladder, so to speak, it must escape the immune response. One way this would be possible is if it were to arise in sites of chronic inflammation with local Th1 suppression. A brief review of the major solid tumours is consistent with this (Table 2 and reviewed in refs 61 and 62).

Although no one hypothesis will explain the induction of all tumours (e.g. deletion of major suppressor genes during childhood development such as Rb and nephroblastoma), and does not necessarily need a history of chronic inflammation, it can be seen from Table 2 that the majority of adult malignancy is consistent with the chronic inflammation hypothesis. Indirect evidence comes from the large randomized aspirin studies which have been shown to have much lower ischaemic heart disease, rheumatoid arthritis, and colon cancer incidence in the aspirin-treated groups. Aspirin is of course an excellent anti-inflammatory agent and is supposedly attenuating enough with regards to chronic colon inflammation to inhibit progression to tumour. It would be of interest to know whether other regularly administered appropriate anti-inflammatory treatments have an effect on the major tumours. For example, do aerosol steroid anti-inflammatory agents (e.g. Becotide) lower the expected role of lung cancer in chronic smokers?

Table 2   Association between chronic inflammation and tumorigenesis

Malignancy	Type of chronic inflammation
Lung carcinoma	Chronic inflammation of the bronchi which is readily detectable pathologically even in those who do not have a good history of chronic bronchitis
Oesophageal carcinoma	Clearly associated with chronic oesophagitis and/or reflux
Gastric carcinoma	Strongly associated with gastritis and chronic helicobacter pylori infection (Grade I carcinogen)
Pancreatic carcinoma	Occurs more frequently in patients with chronic pancreatitis (may be histological and not overtly clinical)
Hepatocellular carcinoma	A background of chronic hepatitis caused by hepatitis B and C viruses
Colorectal carcinoma	Increased incidence in patients with ulcerative colitis is well recognized. Again subclinical inflammation is more common than formerly thought
Breast carcinoma	More frequent in previous mastitis. Male breast cancer associated with chronic irritation from braces
Prostate carcinoma	More frequently associated with chronic prostatitis and previous urinary tract infections
Cervical carcinoma	Most women are HPV positive in their twenties; however, HPV is only able to initiate cancer in those who develop chronic cervicitis. (May serve as a paradigm for other weak virus/tumour associations)
Lymphoma	Cause unclear but many are driven by EBV after 'escaping' immune surveillance. Can be induced in rodents by chronic inflammation and/or immune activation

Apart from anti-inflammatory treatments this hypothesis would suggest that cancer vaccines and treatment with anti-angiogenic agents should have a synergistic effect on early disease. Moreover, the effect of correcting a depressed Th1 immune response may have a far greater clinical effect than expected precisely because of the complex interactions between the tumour, its local environment, and systemic immunity. We have documented clear clinical responses in melanoma patients who recover their Th1 responses following vaccination or the addition of low-dose interleukin 2 and have observed that even patients with small Dukes A and B colorectal cancers have marked systemic Th1 suppression which returns to normal when the tumour is removed (34, 63). Studies examining a variety of other tumours, including renal and lung carcinomas, have also emphasized the striking relationship that exists between cell-mediated immunity and tumour control (64, 65).

2.1.3   Paraneoplastic phenomena

The cancer literature contains a number of case reports of the spontaneous regression of malignancy, in association with paraneoplastic neurological phenomena. Although a rare event (estimated to occur in fewer than 1 in 100 000 cases), the mechanism has been attributed to a successful immune response directed at shared epitopes on tumour and normal neuronal tissue (sequestered antigen). In the majority of patients, the neurological complications predate the diagnosis of the tumour by several months, or occasionally a few years, with the tumours being often small and radiologically silent. The syndromes may be debilitating, with a subacute onset, and commonly they are refractory to treatment. In the case of central neurological manifestations, cerebrospinal fluid immunoglobulin G (IgG) may be raised with characteristic immunopathology. Occasionally definitive treatment of the underlying malignancy has resulted in remission of the paraneoplastic syndrome, with tumour relapse being associated with recurrence of these symptoms (66).

Rare reports of spontaneous tumour regression have been linked to the generation of an immune effector response. Nevertheless, anecdotal examples of improved oncological outcome in association with the presence of a paraneoplastic disorder are mostly due to the earlier diagnosis and management of the underlying tumour. However, in a recent study in small-cell lung carcinoma (SCLC), patients with low titres of anti-Hu antibody without paraneoplastic manifestations had a better prognosis than those who did not harbour such antibodies (67).

The best evidence for the immune-mediated hypothesis is seen with the failure of neuromuscular transmission that occurs with the Lambert–Eaton myasthenic syndrome or LEMS (68). Here, antibodies with specificity for multiple epitopes bind to voltage-gated calcium channels (VGCCs) of the P/Q type (found on the presynaptic cholinergic synapse, cerebellar Purkinje cells, and SCLC cells) and inhibit the entry of calcium to initiate the release of acetylcholine. Using immunoelectron microscopy, antibodies reacting to the alpha-1 subunit, which forms the channel of this transmembrane protein, can be demonstrated at the active zone of the presynaptic neuromuscular junction. Moreover, elimination of these IgG antibodies using plasma exchange, immunosuppression, or tumour-targeted therapy results in improvement in the patient's symptoms. Similarly, it is possible to transfer the syndrome to an experimental animal system by transferring the IgG. Antibodies to VGCCs have also been observed in patients with paraneoplastic cerebellar degeneration (PCD) in association with SCLC. Patients who develop these phenomena tend to have a longer survival than those who do not, suggesting a containment effect on the tumour.

The data for the remaining central paraneoplastic syndromes are not as compelling, and despite the presence of high titres of antibodies their pathogenicity remains to be demonstrated. However, in the case of PCD linked to ovarian and breast carcinoma, a pathogenic cellular immune response has been proposed (69). Although anti-Purkinje antibodies (anti-Yo, with specificity for the tumour and brain cdr2 antigen) have been recognized for several years, their presence is most likely to be an epiphenomenon, since treatments reducing antibody titres are ineffective and the transfer of the antibody does not reproduce the disorder in animals. A recent study has isolated and expanded autoreactive MHC class I-restricted cdr2-specific CTLs in the blood of HLA-A2[+] patients with PCD. In addition, cross-presentation of apoptotic tumour cells by dendritic cells was capable of inducing a potent CTL response, indicating that peripheral activation of cdr2-specific CTLs may subsequently generate autoimmune neuronal degeneration (a selective loss of Purkinje cells with Bergmann astrogliosis).

Clearly, the ability to generate autoimmunity in patients with malignancy has important implications in our efforts to break host tolerance using immunotherapeutic manoeuvres. Such phenomena may thus become more widespread, although for a number of tumour types, autoimmunity to the normal tissue from which the tumour evolved may be an added bonus (e.g. prostate, breast, and gynaecological tumours). Recent animal experiments, however, indicate that it may be possible to uncouple autoimmunity from tumour immunity. Using a syngeneic mouse model and DNA encoding the human gp75 antigen (tyrosinase-related protein-1) it was possible to break tolerance to the native mouse gp75 with the production of gp75 autoantibodies and significant tumour protection (70). Immunization with the mouse gp75 DNA had no effect. Moreover, the tumour protection was dependent upon intact CD4[+], NK1.1[+] cells and the Fc receptor gamma-chain pathway. The autoimmune phenomenon (vitiligo-like coat depigmentation), however, was independent of these cellular mechanisms, suggesting that such an approach may be safe in the clinic.

2.1.4 Tumour dormancy and spontaneous cancer regression

The clinical phenomenon of tumour dormancy or latency is well recognized, and recent hypotheses emphasize a close interplay between tumour neoangiogenesis and the immune system. Thus, tumours can downregulate the expression of various endothelial adhesion molecules (ICAM-1 and -2), by the action of several angiogenic factors (bFGF and VEGF), thereby resulting in an ineffective inflammatory infiltrate. Moreover, these endothelial cells become resistant to cytokines such as TNF-α, which normally induce the expression of adhesion molecules. Recent attempts, using inhibitors of angiogenesis, indicate that this endothelial cell anergy may be reversed. Thus, it is possible to envisage a dynamic state in which the outcome (tumour growth or regression) is determined by the dominance of these opposing biological influences. Other factors considered to play a role include psychological influences, hormonal modulation, and the persistence or absence of a carcinogen.

Lymphomas have been used to study tumour dormancy both in humans and animal systems. For instance, a recent review of five patients with durable complete remissions (after 4–10 years of follow-up) following anti-idiotype antibody vaccination has demonstrated residual disease using a number of techniques: enzyme-linked immunosorbent assays (ELISA) for idiotype protein (serum), flow cytometry for idiotype positive cells, and the polymerase chain reaction (PCR) for clonal gene rearrangements of immunoglobulin CDR3 sequences or t(14; 18) translocations (blood and bone marrow) (71). Thus, immunologically targeted therapy is able to induce long-term tumour control, without completely eliminating the malignant clone. Escape from dormancy has been explored using animal models. Initially, vaccination with a lymphoma-derived idiotype (Id$^+$) immunoglobulin in mice produces protection against tumour challenge, although with a state of dormancy. Relapse is subsequently a frequent occurrence and is accompanied by the emergence of both Id$^-$ variants and Id$^+$ cells, which continue to progress despite the presence of anti-Id antibodies. In the latter case, functional abnormalities of several signalling molecules downstream of the immunoglobulin receptor have been characterized. Interestingly, there is a negative correlation between the rate of escape from dormancy and the post-vaccination levels of anti-Id antibodies (i.e. before tumour challenge).

In some instances of experimental dormancy, a cell-mediated immune mechanism has been proposed. This has been extrapolated from the adoptive transfer of lymphoma-containing splenocytes into syngeneic recipients, and immunodeficient mice (e.g. SCID, CD8$^+$ depleted) exposed to lymphoma cells, with specific homing to bone marrow and lymph nodes. In the latter type of experiment, immunosuppression induced tumour outgrowth from the bone marrow, indicating that the reticuloendothelial organs, in particular, are privileged sites, maintaining dormancy.

Using a tumour expressing HIV gp160 as a model viral tumour antigen, with a pattern of tumour growth–regression–recurrence, it has been possible to investigate immunosurveillance more closely (72). In this system, tumour regression was dependent upon CD8$^+$ T cells, with recurrent tumours being resistant to CTL lysis. Tumour recurrence was also associated with deficiencies of both IL-4 and IFN-γ (more pronounced), and inhibited with CD4 T-cell depletion. In the case of CD4 depletion following tumour regression, analysis of the CD8$^+$ CTL population revealed both upregulation of their IFN-γ mRNA and lytic capability (*ex vivo* stimulation not required). Indeed, IFN-γ appears critical to maintaining immunocompetence in the mouse, with both chemically induced and spontaneously arising tumours occurring with IFN-γ insufficiency. Thus, IFN-γ receptor-deficient and Stat-1 (all IFN)-deficient mice develop tumours more rapidly and with greater frequency compared with wild-type mice, when exposed to methylcholanthrene (73). Additional mutations such as p53 on a background of IFN-γ insensitivity promote further tumorigenesis. The effect of IFN-γ appears to be mediated partly through increasing tumour immunogenicity. The relevance to human tumours is underscored by the fact that a number of tumours become selectively unresponsive to IFN-γ during progression. Intriguingly, recent progress in this area has demonstrated that both lymphocytes and IFN-γ collaborate to protect against chemically induced sarcomas and spontaneously arising epithelial carcinomas, and concomitantly selecting for tumours with reduced immunogenicity. This unforeseen immunoselection helps to explain why tumours continue to develop in individuals with an intact immune system (74).

A thorough understanding of the mechanisms involved in tumour dormancy and tumour regression may allow application of these principles in the clinic. Spontaneous tumour regression has been reported with greatest frequency in patients with neuroblastoma, renal cell carcinoma, malignant melanoma, and lymphomas/leukaemias. Immunological data in the human are particularly well developed in melanoma. Analysis of melanoma tumours undergoing spontaneous regression has revealed in a number of cases (Section 2.1.1) expanded populations of CTLs specific for certain TAAs (75). Assessment of the cytokine profile, using reverse transcription-PCR and *in situ* hybridization, has revealed a Th1 cytokine mRNA pattern (TNF-α, IFN-γ, IL-2, IL-12, GM-CSF, and IL-15) in regressive melanoma lesions and a Th2 cytokine mRNA pattern (IL-4 and IL-5) in progressive tumours. Animal data in the case of neuroblastoma, whereby IL-2 was used to generate an immune cell infiltrate (predominantly NK and LAK), resulted in a characteristic scar-free anatomy (76). This is akin to patients with advanced disease who undergo spontaneous regression, suggesting that a similar mechanism may be operational.

2.1.5   Immunomodulation

In 1891 William Coley, a New York surgeon at the Memorial Sloan-Kettering Cancer Center, began research into malignancy after observing the complete recovery of a patient who had both a metastatic sarcoma and a severe inter-current erysipelas infection. He concluded that the bacterial infection had been instrumental to the regression of the cancer, and pursued the development of a crude, inactivated filtrate from bacterial cultures (*Streptococcus pyogenes* and *Serratia marcescens*), which became widely known as 'Coley's mixed toxins' (77). This filtrate was until the mid-1930s the only approved systemic treatment for cancer by the American Medical Association, and over two hundred patients out of over a thousand benefited from this approach. Although a number of these cures were dramatic and cited evidence for immune activation by the vaccine, Coley's mixed toxins were made redundant with the advent of more quantitative, less toxic, and efficient therapies (chemotherapy and radiotherapy)—although by no means more scientific.

Despite a lack of clinical enthusiasm, experimentation continued in the field and culminated with the discovery of the principal active component of Coley's mixed toxins: lipopolysaccharide (LPS) or endotoxin. This constituent of the outer membrane of gram-negative bacterial organisms induced *in vivo* the synthesis of TNF-α or cachectin by macrophages. Despite the ability of TNF-α to induce marked haemorrhagic necrosis of a range of transplantable tumours in mice, this cytokine also mediates this intrinsic toxicity of LPS in humans (endotoxic shock). Although this prototypical cytokine remains to find its place clinically, cytokine-based immunotherapy has revolutionized the practice of a number of areas within oncology and although progress is slow, many avenues remain completely untapped. Interferon-alpha, which in part has direct anti-proliferative effects on tumours, was the first cytokine to be licensed in clinical practice for hairy cell leukaemia (1986), with interleukin 2 (IL-2) being approved several years later in renal cell carcinoma (1992) and malignant melanoma (1997) (78).

IL-2, essentially a T-cell growth factor, maintains the immunocompetence of antigen-activated IL-2 receptor positive lymphocytes (both T and B cells). This effect is possible with the administration of low doses, both with continuous intravenous infusion or subcutaneously. With higher systemic doses NK cell activity is upregulated, and this is responsible for triggering secondary, pro-inflammatory cytokines (TNF-α, IFN-γ, and GM-CSF), which in turn activate macrophages and monocytes, releasing yet more mediators of inflammation (IL-1, IL-6, IL-12, TNF-α, and GM-CSF). Clinically this manifests as a cytokine syndrome, characterized by severe hypotension, oedema, and organ failure. Nevertheless, well-documented durable tumour regressions have been observed in patients with renal cell carcinoma and metastatic melanoma, and the focus is currently on combining IL-2 with tumour antigen in various forms to improve upon the anti-tumour immune response and reduce systemic toxicity.

The use of allogeneic irradiated whole-cell vaccines as a source of tumour antigen has provided evidence, particularly in melanoma, of efficacy in the metastatic setting—a threefold increase in survival (79, 80). Responding patients are associated with a positive delayed-type hypersensitivity (DTH) reaction, an increase in IgM antiganglioside antibodies, and a positive mixed lymphocyte tumour reaction. Interestingly, a negative correlation has been shown with the presence of Anti-TA90 IgG complexes, which may reflect tumour escape through a 'blocking' mechanism (Section 3.4). Although a more practical approach than the use of autologous cells, several problems may arise. First, there is the effect of cell culture and the passaging of tumour cells with the potential for the growth of clones, which diverge from the antigenic profile of the original cancer; second, antigenic modulation may induce tolerance; and third, there is the possibility of contamination on a large scale.

Another allogeneic area, which is rapidly gaining ground, looks at the use of donor immune cells in combating the malignant process (81). From observations in patients with bone marrow transplantation in leukaemic disorders, it was shown that patients who developed the graft-versus-host disease (GVHD) were also more likely to have a beneficial graft-versus-tumour (GVT) effect. Donor leukocyte infusions (DLIs) have been used successfully in the treatment of relapsed chronic-phase chronic myelogenous leukaemia or CML (complete remission in 60–80 per cent of patients) and in post-transplantation EBV-related lymphoproliferative disease (PTLD). This form of adoptive immunotherapy is currently being assessed in 'mini-allograft' protocols (i.e. without traditional myeloablative therapy) to tease out a therapeutic GVT effect and thus reduce the incidence of GVHD.

The ability of the immune system to target and eradicate tumour cells at the level of minimal residual disease has recently been described in patients with follicular lymphoma (82). Here, the vaccine consisted of the immunoglobulin variable portion expressed on the cell surface (idiotype) with conjugation to KLH (keyhole limpet haemocyanin) adjuvant. GM-CSF, which has a number of adjuvant properties including DC proliferation, maturation, and migration, in addition to the upregulation of ADCC and secretion of a number of cytokines (IL-1, TNF, and IL-6), was administered in conjunction with this anti-idiotype vaccine (i.e. Id-KLH$^+$GM-CSF). The authors demonstrated that 8 out of 11 patients displaying the classic follicular lymphoma translocation (14;18) 6 months following chemotherapy and in complete response (i.e. indicative of minimal residual disease) became t(14;18) negative on PCR after a subsequent course of vaccination with Id-KLH$^+$GM-CSF. Moreover, a positive response to the vaccination, as shown by the induction of tumour-specific CD8$^+$ and CD4$^+$ T cells (a humoral response was also induced but was not seen in all cases) correlated with a prolonged disease-free survival, and at the time of the study no evidence of relapse in the patients who became PCR negative.

A more 'generic' approach was described in a recent study using a synthetic immunodominant peptide (with increased binding to HLA-A2) based on the melanoma antigen gp100, a non-mutated differentiation protein expressed by cells of melanocytic lineage (83). In this phase I study of patients with advanced metastatic melanoma, a 42 per cent response rate was observed in patients where the immunodominant peptide was combined with IL-2. Immunological reactivity was evaluated by *in vitro* sensitization of peripheral blood mononuclear cells (PBMCs) to the peptide pulsed onto APCs. High levels of reactivity were obtained after only a single exposure of PBMCs to peptide, and furthermore, precursor frequencies were in the range of 1 in 2800 and 1 in 5900, which compares favourably with levels achieved against viral or allogeneic antigens.

The increasing success of immunomodulation (see Table 3), with the ability to break tolerance to tumour-associated antigen, has led to concerns regarding the development of autoimmune phenomena. Indeed, there is some evidence to support this in the clinic, perhaps best illustrated with the increasing frequency of vitiligo in patients with melanoma, responding to IL-2 based strategies. Similarly in the IL-2 treatment of renal cell carcinoma, responding patients who are commonly HLACw7$^+$ have a risk of reversible thyroid dysfunction (mainly hypothyroidism), which correlates with the induction of thyroid autoantibodies and an improved survival (84). Interestingly, at baseline, patients with renal cell carcinoma have a twofold increase in these antibodies compared with the general population. Fortunately, to date, serious

Table 3 Summary of tumour immunotherapies in clinical practice

Type	Some examples in clinical use
BCG	Intravesical therapy in bladder carcinoma Metastatic malignant melanoma (i.e. cutaneous deposits)
SRL172 (M. vaccae) (s.c.)	Variety of tumours (melanoma, lung and renal cancer)
Cytokine therapy (i.v.)	IL-2 induces both complete responses (6%), and partial responses (12%) in patients with metastatic melanoma (4% durable response rate) and renal cell carcinoma
Biochemotherapy (i.v.)	Increases the overall response to 60% (10% durable rate)
Allogeneic tumour cells with adjuvant (e.g. BCG)	Morton's polyvalent melanoma cell vaccine (PMCV)
Autologous cells modified genetically to enhance signals 1–3 (see text)	Melanoma cells lipofected with HLA-B7 (signal 1)
	Melanoma cells transduced with B7 (signal 2)
	Various tumours transduced with GM-CSF (signal 3)
Monoclonal therapy (i.v.)	Anti-CD20 (Mabthera): follicular B cell lymphoma
	Anti-CDw52 (CAMPATH-1): lymphoma
	Anti-HER2/neu (Herceptin): breast carcinoma (trials in progress in a variety of other tumours)
Anti-idiotype vaccine[+] GM-CSF adjuvant	Idiotype[+] KLH: in follicular lymphoma
Subunit peptide vaccine[+] IL-2/GM-CSF adjuvant	Metastatic melanoma + IL-2
Adoptive cell immunotherapy	Donor leukocyte infusions ('Graft-versus-tumour effect') in relapsed CML and EBV–PTLD disorders
Dendritic cells pulsed with peptide or autologous cells[+] IL-2 adjuvant (s.c./ i.v.)	Various tumours (metastatic melanoma, lymphoma, renal cell carcinoma, and prostate carcinoma)
Genetic modification of immune cells	T cells expressing chimeric immune receptors
Gene therapies with an immunological component	HSVtk retroviral transduction in glioblastoma multiforme and melanoma ('bystander effect', see text)

autoimmune reactions have not been described. However, with the prediction that immunotherapies will become more effective at breaking tolerance, such sequelae may rise in importance (see also Section 2.1.3).

Alternative methods of skewing a favourable cytokine milieu involve the use of specific bacterial adjuvants, and in some respects this represents refinement of the original Coley's mixed toxins. BCG has been used more successfully in the treatment of superficial bladder cancer (85) and in the local therapy of cuta-neous deposits of melanoma. Other preparations using mycobacterial deriva-tives, such as *mycobacterium vaccae*, a heat-killed preparation of limited toxicity, are also being developed as immunomodulators in melanoma, renal cell carcinoma, and lung carcinoma. Survival data from randomized clinical trials currently in progress are eagerly awaited. OK-432, another bacterial adjuvant derived from the streptococcus has been employed in both lung and gastric carcinoma with a switch to Th1 and improved survival, respectively (86). It appears from previous immunotherapy trials in lung carcinoma, in particular, that employing bacterial adjuvants on their own to realign the cytokine milieu is insufficient to produce an effective, durable anti-tumour response. Thus, a potent, immunogenic tumour antigen must be provided in addition, and the dendritic cell is currently the focus of a number of immuno-therapeutic strategies, as the best-placed candidate to provide this signal.

DC manipulation aims to overcome both tumour-induced tolerance and immunological ignorance (87). Pathological assessment of a number of tumours has linked DC infiltration with an improved patient prognosis (Section 2.1.1). Moreover, recent clinical studies in patients with malignant melanoma, lymphoma, and prostate carcinoma have emphasized a potential role for DC-based vaccine immunotherapy. Early work focused on lymphoma (88), with three out of four patients obtaining a response upon intravenous infusion of autologous DC pulsed with idiotypic protein. DC immunotherapy has also been extended to melanoma with interesting results from a recent European trial (89). In this study DCs generated in the presence of GM-CSF and IL-4 were pulsed with either tumour lysate or specific peptides and injected into clinically uninvolved lymph nodes, achieving a response rate of 30 per cent. Other promising approaches under investigation include tumour–DC fusion, which in early phase I trials is achieving stabilization of disease in a propor-tion of patients over a significant period of time.

A number of monoclonal antibodies are available which target cell-surface tumour antigens (see Section 2.2) and whose mechanism of action is thought to be based partly upon the activation of immune pathways such as ADCC, complement-dependent cytotoxicity, idiotype–anti-idiotype networks, and the generation of CTLs (90, 91). Other mechanisms may include modulation at the level of signal transduction pathways (e.g. the inhibition of cyclin-depend-ent kinases and the upregulation of their inhibitors) and the induction of apoptosis; however, the exact contribution of these processes remains an area of active research.

The efficacy of these antibodies is dependent upon a number of factors: specificity, the concentration of tumour antigen, immunogenicity (i.e. the human anti-mouse and anti-chimera antibodies or HAMA and HACA, respectively), and physiochemical factors such as accessibility (physical barriers and poor vascularization). Antibodies used clinically which may trigger an immune effector response include: anti-CD20 in B cell lymphomas (Rituximab) (92), anti-CDw52 (CAMPATH-1) in both B- and T-cell lymphomas, anti-17–1A (anti-Ep-CAM or 'Panorex') in colonic carcinoma (93), and more recently anti-p185HER2 (anti-HER2/neu or 'Herceptin') used in breast carcinoma (94). Antibody-based immunotherapy has also been used effectively in the treatment of non-metastatic manifestations of malignancy. A recent paper described the successful treatment of hypercalcaemia secondary to parathyroid hormone (PTH) release by a parathyroid carcinoma, which was unresponsive to conventional treatment (95). An anti-PTH antibody response, with a concomitant breakdown in B-cell tolerance to PTH, was generated with the use of both human and bovine PTH peptides and human PTH in Freund's complete adjuvant, with the application of further booster doses. This novel approach may have wider application to a host of other syndromes in which a tumour-derived product is directly implicated.

Lastly, as alluded to earlier (see Section 2.1.2), immunotherapy employing genetic strategies is providing tantalizing data on the initiation and maintenance of an effective anti-tumour immune response (96). There is currently an embarrassment of riches with regard to approach (i.e. from a mechanistic perspective) and as yet a lack of efficacy; and efforts are thus being refocused upon the engineering of technologies of transfer and expression of pharmacological doses of immunostimulatory genes. However, a number of clinical trials have been completed (summarized in Table 3) and of the more promising include attempts to enhance the pathway of immune cell activation from signal 1 at the level of the trimolecular complex to the triggering of signal 3 or cytokine release (e.g. GM-CSF in autologous cells from melanoma and prostate carcinoma). Other approaches being investigated include the genetic modification of immune cells, by providing chimeric receptors for tumour antigen linked to T-cell signalling pathways (97) or the introduction of cytokines and chemokines to T cells and DCs (98, 99).

A method which recruits the immune system for part of its therapeutic 'bystander effect' (i.e. unexpected therapeutic activity when a small fraction of tumour cells is transduced), the so-called suicide gene strategy (also known as GDEPT or Gene-Directed Enzyme Prodrug Therapy), has also been studied in patients with malignancy, especially glioblastoma multiforme and melanoma (100). Here, a gene coding for an enzyme, such as the herpes simplex virus thymidine kinase (HSVTK), is delivered using a retroviral strategy into malignant cells with selective destruction occurring after the administration of the prodrug ganciclovir (converted by HSVTK into the active ganciclovir triphosphate). Specificity is ensured by both the retrovirus, as it targets proliferating and hence malignant cells, and the viral form of thymidine kinase which metabolizes ganciclovir in preference to the human form of thymidine kinase. The net result of suicide gene therapy is the activation of both apoptotic and necrotic death, the latter being a strong inducer of a Th1 immune response, leading not only to tumour regression but also to the induction of memory as demonstrated by the rejection of tumour upon rechallenge (101, 102).

Table 4   Tumour antigens

Tumour-specific antigens (TSAs)

Potent tumour-rejection antigens, with high T-cell affinity and absence of tolerance

1	*Mutational antigens* specific to the tumour and not present on other tissues
	Examples: ras, p53, bcr/abl, CDK-4, Caspase-8
2	*Viral antigens* linked to tumour aetiopathogenesis
	Examples: Epstein–Barr virus (EBV), human papilloma virus (HPV-E7)

Tumour-associated antigens (TAAs)

Wide spectrum of potency, T-cell affinity, and tolerance

1	*Cancer-testis (CT) antigens* restricted to primitive germ cells of the testis, and following oncogenesis, activation of CT expression occurs in a variety of tumours
	Examples: MAGE-1/2, GAGE-1/2, BAGE, RAGE, NY-ESO-1
2	*Differentiation antigens* found in normal tissue with altered expression (i.e. under- or overexpressed) in the tumour
	Examples: MART-1/MelanA, gp100, tyrosinase, TRP-1/2, GM2 ganglioside, HER-2/neu, CEA

2.2   TUMOUR-SPECIFIC ANTIGENS

Two main cloning approaches have resulted in the isolation of genes which code for tumour antigens recognized by the immune system—the human cancer immunome project. The first, so-called 'classical', method employs TILs to select targets from a cDNA tumour expression library, and the second defines antibody-recognized antigens, or SEREX (serological identification of antigens by recombinant expression cloning). Other confirmatory strategies include the detection of multiple antigenic peptides eluted from tumour-derived MHC class I molecules. Apart from a minority of truly unique antigens (mutational antigens, e.g. p53, ras, and viral antigens, e.g. EBV, HPV, and HBV), the majority are tumour-associated antigens that, because of their altered expression in cancer, become immunogenic and for this reason may be considered to have inherent cancer specificity (Table 4). This latter group has been subclassified as: (a) differentiation antigens (e.g. the components of melanin processing in malignant melanoma, such as tyrosinase, gp100, and Melan-A/ MART-1; Her-2/neu and GM2 ganglioside), and (b) cancer-testis (CT) antigens (e.g. MAGE, BAGE, NY-ESO-1, SSX, CT7, and SCP-1).

The CT antigens, in particular, have attracted a considerable degree of interest. During malignant transformation, antigens that are normally restricted to primitive germ cells (spermatogonia) and the placenta become expressed in a variety of cancers, and currently there are 10 known gene families, of which six are coded on the X chromosome (103). It is important to note that tumours are a highly heterogeneous population of cells, and antigens may be expressed in all or only a small proportion of the cells. Moreover, dissection of the immune response to the various tumour antigens is also showing variability. Thus, some antigens elicit mainly CTL activity (e.g. gp100 and Melan-A/MART-1), other antigens a strong humoral response (e.g. GM2 and p53), and a proportion stimulate both a strong $CD8^+$ T-cell and an antibody response (e.g. NY-ESO-1).

A major endeavour of tumour immunology into the next millennium will be to determine whether the induction of an immune response to a defined tumour antigen correlates with an improved clinical outcome. Some persuasive data have been obtained from ganglioside and polyvalent allogeneic vaccination studies in patients with malignant melanoma, which associate prolonged survival with the presence of anti-GM2 IgG antibodies and anti-TA90 IgM antibodies, respectively, and from current vaccine studies in patients with lymphoma (see Section 2.1.5). A recent innovation involves synthetic peptides, which often are based on a single amino acid substitution to enhance immunogenicity, with the result that cross-reactivity is effected against the native peptide. Increasingly, the challenge will be to develop cancer vaccines which are tailor-made to the phenotype of the patient's tumour.

2.3   ANTIGEN PRESENTATION

The dendritic cell is critical to antigen presentation, with the unique capacity to induce both primary and secondary immune responses *in vivo*, directed against both foreign and self-antigens (104). Delivery of tumour antigen may take various forms, and several studies have indicated that antigen drives DC maturation and the subsequent orchestration of tumour immunity. DCs, with their huge surface area, have a phenomenal capacity to sample their environment and ingest antigens via their veil-like projections (dendrites) ready for processing. In this immature state, surface expression of MHC molecules (class I and class II) and co-stimulatory molecules (B.7.1/CD80, B7.2/CDF86, and CD40) is low, whereas the presence of receptors for antigen uptake is upregulated (mannose receptor, DEC-205, Fcγ receptors). The cells display marked endocytotic activity and poor motility. Following antigen uptake, and in the presence of local inflammatory mediators (e.g. LPS or TNF-α), the MHC and co-stimulatory molecules undergo maximal upregulation, resulting in a mature DC phenotype which is capable of high motility and presenting processed antigen to activate cellular immune responses. In addition, CD40–CD40L interactions amplify the levels of CD80 and CD86, and trigger IL-12 secretion, which promotes the development of Th1 cells and CTLs. Although no DC-specific cell marker has been isolated, the CD83 is relatively specific (a member of the immunoglobulin superfamily).

Several other DC modulators have been described, including IL-2, FLT3 Ligand, immunostimulatory DNA sequences or CpG motifs, and lymphotactin, a chemokine, which has been shown to stimulate an immune infiltrate into primary tumours upon gene transfer into the DC. FLT-3 Ligand, in particular, has several interesting qualities, enabling both tumour protection and tumour regression in animal models (105), and the ability to mobilize DCs without the need for GM-CSF or IL-4.

The role of B cells in tumour antigen processing in comparison to DCs is poorly understood. Recent work, however, suggests that B cells, by presenting tumour antigen to CD4$^+$ T cells, may in fact divert immunity towards a Th2 pathway resulting in inhibition of tumour immunity.

2.4 HUMORAL IMMUNITY

Immunoglobulin produced by B cells may play a role in controlling tumour growth (tumour-reactive antibodies are being defined increasingly in the serum of cancer patients and provide the basis for SEREX, Section 2.2), and in binding, processing, and presenting tumour antigens for induction of T-cell responses to the tumour. Antibodies mediate tumorlysis by three mechanisms: (a) complement fixation; (b) ADCC, mediated via NK, macrophages, and granulocytes; and (c) a blocking effect upon growth factor receptors. The subtype of immunoglobulin has been shown to correlate with a beneficial tumour response in patients with melanoma in studies of both allogeneic whole-cell and anti-ganglioside vaccines (Section 2.1.5).

Switching of the immunoglobulin class is cytokine-driven, and this principle is operational within animal systems. For instance, using tumour cell vaccines expressing a genetically transduced cytokine (IL-12 and IL-4) and a defined tumour antigen (the human gp38 folate receptor), a characteristic antibody profile (IgG2a) predicted tumour regression, which occurred in 50 per cent of the animals (106). This correlation was seen only with the IL-12 gene-modified tumour vaccine, and not with the IgG1 antibody induced by the IL-4-producing tumour. IL-12 is a potent adjuvant for eliciting humoral immunity, and in a number of model systems can upregulate IgG2a, IgG2b, and IgG3 levels, while suppressing IgG1 and IgE responses. It promotes the Th1 pathway by eliciting IFN-γ production, compared with IL-4 that drives a Th2 pathway with isotype switching to IgG1 and IgE. Moreover, both antibody responses were dependent upon the presence of CD4$^+$ T cells, with CD8 depletion having no effect. The mechanism of action of IgG2a involved a high-affinity type I Fc receptor (CD64, found on macrophages), whereas the IgG1 effect was mediated through interaction with the type II (CD32) and type III (CD16) Fc receptors located on macrophages, monocytes, neutrophils, and NK cells. IL-4-producing tumour cells clearly mediate their effect via alternative pathways, which may involve eosinophil aggregation and activation of the CD8⁺ Tc2 cell population, which interacts with granulocytes to induce tumorlysis. The dissection of the immune response into both humoral and cellular components provides a unique view of the elements critical to an effective anti-tumour response, and should provide prognostic data during vaccination follow-up.

Finally, the idiotype–anti-idiotype network, first proposed by Jerne, has been explored in experimental systems. Thus, a given antibody (Ab1) is able to react both to its target antigen and with a second antibody (Ab2), with Ab2 mimicking the antigen epitope recognized by Ab1. Similarly, Ab2 may be recognized by a third antibody (Ab3), of which some will have the same specificity as Ab1. This network of idiotypes is dependent upon T cells. For instance, using p53 (overexpressed on a wide variety of human tumours) antibodies for vaccination, an idiotype network was induced, with tumour protection correlating with the presence of anti-p53 Ab3, and dependence on the T cell for production (107).

2.5 CELL-MEDIATED IMMUNITY

It is evident, using *in vivo* immunodepletion experiments, that successful tumour eradication and maintenance of long-term immunity requires both intact CD8⁺ and CD4⁺ T cells. Early work concentrated on the CTL, with its ability to recognize and lyse tumours expressing both MHC class I and an immunogenic peptide. The lytic machinery of the CTL is an area of intense research and at least three mechanisms are involved: a calcium-dependent (perforin pathway) and an independent process (Fas Ligand–Fas Receptor interaction), and the secretion of cytotoxic cytokines, such as TNF-α and IFN-γ (108).

Tumorlysis by CTLs is critically dependent upon the effective presentation of processed tumour antigens to the TCR. Both IFN-γ and TNF-α are important inducers of MHC class I, as well as increasing the tumoricidal activity of the CTLs. The principal cytokine involved in maintaining the immunocompetence of T lymphocytes is IL-2. Isolated in 1976 and described as a T-cell growth factor, it has generated a similar level of interest to that of TNF-α in the innate immune system. In fact, from a clinical perspective it now dominates cytokine immunotherapy in certain solid tumours (malignant melanoma and renal cell carcinoma). IL-2 induces the maturation of the T-cell subsets, B cells, LGL (NK/LAK); it stimulates CTL activity and augments immunoglobulin production. A range of cytokines is induced via the cytokine network, including IFN-γ, TNF-α, TNF-β, differentiation factors (IL-4, IL-6), haemopoietic factors (IL-3, IL-5, GM-CSF), and TGF-β.

The CD4⁺ T helper cell has a number of functions in conducting an effective anti-tumour response. First, by the provision of help for CTLs, via the activation of APCs through a mechanism of CD40–CD40L interaction (see below), which results in cross-priming of the CTL by the activated APC. Second, by a CTL-independent mechanism, whereby the CD4$^+$ T cell is activated by a TAM or DC (positive for MHC class II), with the triggering of Th1 and Th2 pathways which in turn activate macrophages to produce reactive oxygen species or eosinophils and antibody production by plasma B cells. Third, the CD4$^+$ T cell can directly kill tumour cells by lysis or cytokine secretion. Other aspects such as memory and a subpopulation of cells which appear to have non-classical MHC molecules (such as CD1) involved in target recognition require further characterization. Currently, efforts are in progress to define the tumour antigens recognized by CD4$^+$ T cell, in the hope that these may provide more effective tumour vaccines (109).

Finally, certain co-stimulatory molecule interactions, namely B7/CD28 (110, 111) and CD40/CD40L, are critical to maintaining an efficient anti-tumour immune response. Indeed, lack of B7 expression (either on APCs or tumour cells) induces a state of tolerance, with immunological escape (Section 3.8). Analysis of the CD40/CD40L system has revealed a high degree of complexity in tumour immunosurveillance. CD40L is expressed mainly on activated CD4$^+$ and CD8$^+$ T cells, DCs and B cells, and CD40 on B cells, DCs, and a range of tumours. The CD40–CD40L interaction induces functional changes in a wide range of cells (increased MHC, co-stimulatory and adhesion molecules), with the net result of enhanced T- and B-cell-mediated immune responses (112). Moreover, CD40 ligation has been shown to inhibit tumour growth and induce apoptosis. In melanoma, a recent study suggested this effect was mediated by upregulation of the NF-κB signalling pathway, with stimulation of a range of cytokines (IL-6, IL-8, TNF-α, and GM-CSF) and immunorelevant molecules (intercellular adhesion molecule-1 and MHC class I and II molecules) (113). Similarly, CD40 ligation of lymphoma cells activates CTL to eradicate the tumour without the requirement of CD4$^+$ Th cells (114).

3   Immunological escape

The major obstacle to immune-mediated tumour destruction is, without doubt, the intrinsic ability of the tumour to evade, subvert, and paradoxically capitalize upon its opponent's immune system. This perversion of the host's defences is both ingenious and frustrating. Some of the underlying mechanisms have only recently been elucidated and clearly the development of a successful immunotherapy will entail understanding and bypassing these processes.

3.1   TUMOUR KINETICS

Tumour cells may not be recognized until growth is established, by which time the tumour has 'sneaked through'. Tumours with fast doubling times may evade an immune response, which normally takes several weeks to achieve full activation. Furthermore, in immunized animals, tumour cells will develop into cancers when sufficient doses of tumour are administered. Such a mechanism may account for immunological escape in both clinical and experimental systems.

3.2 THE PHYSICOCHEMICAL ENVIRONMENT

The physicochemical conditions present within solid tumours may directly influence immunocompetence. Studies have shown that the proliferative response of murine lymphocytes to IL-2 in cultures subjected to low oxygen tension, low glucose concentrations, and acidic pH is markedly reduced, compared with simulated physiological conditions. In contrast, *in vivo*, using a mammary tumour model expressing IL-2, it is possible to overcome the effects of hypoxia by stimulating increased tumour vasculature formation, and with a concomitant influx of immune cells (115). Thus, although the host may recognize a particular TAA, the immune response will not be sustained. This may also account for the relatively poor success rate of IL-2/LAK immunotherapy.

3.3 IMMUNOSELECTION

Analysis of cells present in a tumour mass reveals heterogeneity with respect to morphology and surface phenotype. Since the tumour may be viewed as an evolutionary biological system, with selection an integral component, cell variants resistant to immunosurveillance may become the dominant population. Thus resistance may be conferred by the modulation of a variety of proteins, from scavenging enzymes for reactive oxygen intermediates (ROIs), absence of pivotal adhesion molecules in cytotoxicity, to the loss of immunodominant antigens (Section 3.5) and HLA class I molecules (Section 3.6) (116). Furthermore, by the time the tumour is detected clinically, the original immune response would no longer be detectable.

Other genetic factors, such as the association of HLA haplotypes with certain malignancies (nasopharyngeal carcinoma with HLA-A2, 8w46, RR = 2.31; and breast carcinoma with Bw35, RR = 1.35), may be important not only in susceptibility to a particular tumour but also in resistance once the tumour is established.

3.4 BLOCKING FACTORS

A number of blocking factors have been isolated in the sera of patients with progressive tumours that specifically inhibit both cell-mediated cytotoxicity and ADCC. Thus, excess circulating antigen or antigen–antibody immune complexes may subvert immunity by occupying antigen-specific receptors, or by acting as decoys away from the tumour site. Both innate and adaptive effectors may be affected in this way. Perturbation in the idiotype–anti-idiotype network and other forms of immune deregulation (i.e. T-suppressor cells) may also be important.

Analysis of the immune response to a polyvalent melanoma cell vaccine ('Cancervax') has revealed the induction of both cell-mediated and humoral activity (79). Although prolonged survival was associated with an anti-TA90 (a glycoprotein TAA, present on the surface of most melanoma cells) IgM response, the induction of an anti-TA90 IgG titre correlated with decreased survival. The ability of anti-TA90IgG to reduce the *in vitro* complement-dependent cytotoxicity of anti-TA90 IgM has been described in animal systems, and may operate via blocking of the epitope recognized by the IgM antibody.

3.5   ANTIGENIC MODULATION

The elimination of tumour antigens that are recognized by the immune system may be achieved through antigen shedding (upon binding with antibodies), antigen masking (e.g. sialomucin denies access to the immune effector cell (117)), and a form of immunoselection that results in the expansion of TAA-negative clones (118, 119). Animal data from the early 1980s, using the murine mastocytoma P815 system, suggested that tumour escape following initial rejection was a consequence of the emergence of antigen-loss variants rather than the presence of immunosuppression. Furthermore, analysis of the TIL population within human melanoma is predominantly oligoclonal rather than polyclonal in nature, as shown by the patterns of TCR gene rearrangement. Thus, the concept of immunoselection with antigen escape mutants was proposed and this has now been confirmed in malignant melanoma, with a number of studies in patients correlating tumour progression with a gradual loss of tumour antigens, such as Melan-A/MART-1 and tyrosinase. However, assessment of antigen-positive tumours which undergo tumour escape often indicates an alternative mechanism, such as HLA loss (Section 3.6).

Similarly, in immunotherapeutic trials, patients initially responding to a specific melanoma peptide vaccine have demonstrated antigen-loss variants at subsequent relapse. This emphasizes, in the case of peptide vaccines, as with TIL-based approaches, the importance of a polyvalent strategy in vaccination protocols. However, serological analysis of melanoma tumours has revealed highly heterogeneous patterns of antigen expression, with both antigen-negative and positive clones, with the former resistant to CTL lysis. There appears to be a direct correlation between the degree of homogeneous antigen expression and the effectiveness of target lysis by antigen-specific CTLs, thereby preventing immunoselection of antigen-loss variants *in vivo*. Methods of modulating tumour antigen expression may be critical to immunotherapy, and *ex vivo* data suggest that cytokine pretreatment (e.g. IFN-γ and TNF-α) can upregulate TAA and sensitize relatively resistant tumour cells to TIL lysis (120). In addition, combination protocols involving DCs pulsed with tumour peptide appear to be effective in avoiding the possibility of enhancing tumour outgrowth via CTL tolerization, which is known to occur with peptide vaccination alone.

3.6 DEFECTIVE ANTIGEN PRESENTATION

Although there are several examples of human CD8$^+$ T cells that specifically recognize tumour cells, recent studies indicate that aberrant processing of antigen by the tumour can compromise the trimolecular complex (121). Pulse-chase experiments revealed that MHC class I molecules were not transported from the endoplasmic reticulum to the cell surface. Moreover, northern blot analysis demonstrated low to non-detectable levels of both proteasome (LMP-2 and LMP-7) and putative peptide transporter (TAP-1 and TAP-2) units, thereby providing an explanation for the absence of antigenic peptides required for the proper assembly of the class I alpha chain with beta-2 microglobulin, and hence their transfer to the cell surface. Both the functional and biochemical parameters were reversed with IFN-γ. Further studies of the regulatory mechanisms of TAP-1 and LMP2, in small-cell lung carcinoma, indicate that the tumour cells lack trans-regulatory nuclear proteins. These normally bind to the IFN-γ response element (ISRE) in the TAP-1 and LMP-2 bidirectional intergenic promoter and induce expression of these genes. Thus, exogenous IFN-γ reverses this defect with a concomitant increase in the expression of HLA class I molecules. An alternative approach involves replacing the defective antigen-processing machinery by transfecting the gene for TAP1.

Independent downregulation of MHC class I is also a viable mechanism for escaping immunosurveillance (122). This has been demonstrated in a range of tumours, including melanoma, renal cell carcinoma, lung carcinoma, gynaecological tumours (breast and ovary), colorectal and pancreatic carcinoma. Multiple mechanisms appear to be involved. For instance, in melanoma, large deletions and point mutations in the β2-microglobulin gene have been described (particularly an 8 base-pair CT repeat region of exon 1), most of which occur at the level of translation. Cytokine modulation with IL-12 is able to reverse the antigenic loss in melanoma (most cell lines express at least one chain of the IL-12R), with upregulation of HLA class I, class II, and ICAM-1 molecules. IL-12, delivered both in its native form and using gene therapy technology, is presently the theme of ongoing clinical trials. There is additional evidence of a positive interaction with B7 to induce effective anti-tumour immunity. Alternatively, transfection of the wild-type β2-microglobulin gene is able to restore HLA class I expression and recognition by tumour antigen-specific CTLs. It appears in some melanomas that the loss of HLA is an early event in progression to the malignant phenotype. In contrast, recent work involving NK immunosurveillance indicates that expression of an NK inhibitory molecule, HLA-G, is overexpressed on melanoma cells resulting in tumour escape (123). Occasionally HLA class II, which is usually located only on immune cells, becomes expressed on tumour cells during progression and may paradoxically enable a host response.

The central role of DCs in directing an effective anti-tumour response has also been sabotaged, with tumours inducing DC inactivation (124). The mechanisms of tolerance involve the secretion of a variety of downregulatory molecules, including cytokines (Th-2 profile), growth factors (VEGF), and prostaglandins (PGE_2). Two cytokines, IL-6 and M-CSF, secreted by certain tumours (e.g. renal cell carcinoma), affect directly DC development from $CD34(^+)$ progenitors, by triggering their commitment towards monocytic cells, with a potent phagocytic but non-antigen-presenting function. This inhibition of DC differentiation is preceded by M-CSF receptor expression and loss of GM-CSF receptor, both effects being reversed by the use of IL-6/IL-6R and M-CSF antibodies. The growth factor VEGF is also able to inhibit the maturation of DCs from $CD34(^+)$ precursors. Studies of patients with gastric carcinoma show an inverse relationship between the level of VEGF expression and the extent of DC infiltration, which itself is associated with prognosis. Thus VEGF may induce tumour escape by both promoting neoangiogenesis and downregulating the immune response. In addition, both the deregulation of co-stimulatory molecules and the induction of apoptosis have been described with DCs derived from tumour environments (125). Thus, it is critical that a clearer understanding of the mode of action that DCs utilize to generate specific anti-tumour immune responses is elaborated. Indiscriminate use of DCs may instead generate tolerance and tumour escape variants.

3.7 TUMOUR AND STROMAL PRODUCTS

Cytokines, inflammatory mediators, and structural proteins have all been shown to affect various immunological parameters (e.g. chemotaxis, activation and proliferation of cells). For example, the prostaglandin PGE_2, released by a number of tumour lines, including breast, non-small-cell lung, and head and neck squamous cell carcinomas, inhibits NK/LAK lytic function and TIL proliferation respectively. This may be overcome *in vitro* by the use of indomethacin, and by using higher amounts of IL-2 or phytohaemagglutinin (PHA). NK-cell activity declines markedly with progressive tumours, and becomes refractory to certain cytokine manipulations (e.g. IFN-γ). The role of PGs in tumour progression and immunosuppression is currently being reviewed in the light of specific cyclooxygenase-2 (COX-2) inhibitors. Evidence from both animal and human studies (patients with familial adenomatous polyposis or FAP) suggests that non-steroidal anti-inflammatory drugs reduce prostaglandin pro-tumorigenic activity, and that this effect involves several mechanisms including an improved immune response and reduced neoangiogenesis. In a study of spontaneous mammary tumours in mice, chronic indomethacin (a non-selective COX inhibitor) therapy was associated with a twofold increase in spontaneous tumour regression, significantly prolonged survival, and a twofold reduction in pulmonary metastases compared with control animals. Furthermore, immunostaining for COX-2 revealed positivity in tumour cells, stromal cells, and TAMs, with indomethacin-treated animals exhibiting mononuclear cell infiltration, increased differentiation, a reduction in vascularity, and significant tumour cell death (126).

A number of cytokines produced by the tumour, stroma, and inflammatory cells have potent immunosuppressive effects. IL-10 functions at several levels to downregulate the immune response. It inhibits DC accumulation and antagonizes the effects of GM-CSF, thereby blocking the initiation rather than the effector phase of the immune response, reduces NK sensitivity, and decreases the expression of MHC class I antigen. Moreover, despite the presence of an inflammatory infiltrate in tumours, such as breast carcinoma, the TILs are usually functionally defective. Analysis of mRNA for IL-10 and IL-2 has shown skewing in favour of the former, suggesting perhaps the reason for the immunoparesis. In studies on lung carcinoma cell lines, the IL-10 transcription rate in lymphocytes appears to be enhanced by the release of PGE_2, and this may be abrogated with the use of indomethacin. Similarly, the defective production of IFN-γ by peripheral blood lymphocytes when co-cultured with tumour supernatant can be restored with the use of anti-IL-10 monoclonal antibody (mAb). Other cytokines implicated in tumour escape mechanisms include IL-15 in melanoma (a negative controller of HLA class I molecule expression), TNF-α in ovarian carcinoma (a potent inducer of MCP-1 and matrix metalloprotease-9 with an emphasis on stromal reorganization to the tumour's advantage) (62,127), deregulation of TGF-β in colonic, ovarian, and breast carcinoma, and melanoma progression, and MCP-1 in cervical intraepithelial neoplasia and cervical carcinomas. In breast carcinoma, for instance, TGF-β is overexpressed during the development of resistance to the anti-oestrogen, tamoxifen. Using both nude and nude/beige mice (additional NK-cell deficiency) and human xenografts, it was possible to show that TGF-β inhibits NK-cell activity, which may be reversed using TGF-β antibodies. Moreover, it appears that part of the tamoxifen effect is mediated via sensitization of NK cells to tumorlysis (128).

Several studies have endeavoured to profile *in vivo* cytokine levels with the malignant process (Section 2.1.2). In one study, cellular immune status was defined according to cytokine production in mitogen-induced lymphocyte proliferation tests for patients with varying clinical stages of malignant melanoma, BCC, and normal individuals (129). Significantly lower levels of IFN-γ and IL-2 were found in the blood cultures of patients with melanoma, with the former correlating with clinical stage. In contrast, patients with BCC did not differ from normal controls, suggesting that this is possibly a more immunogenic tumour. Thus, one form of melanoma-induced immunosuppression is mediated via disturbances in the cytokine network, and this may favour metastasis of this tumour (see also Section 2.1.2).

Other studies have looked at pre- and postoperative cytokine levels in cancer patients. It is hypothesized that the growth of malignant cells may involve cytokine-mediated downregulation of the immune response. For instance, TNF-α, IL-1, GM-CSF, and IL-6 produced by resident macrophages, and via autocrine loops involving tumour cells themselves, synergize to promote mitogenesis of the tumour. Surgical removal of the tumour results in profound changes in cytokine levels, which are temporally distributed and reinforce the concept of a cytokine network. Some tumour-induced cytokines not only modulate immune parameters for the benefit of the tumour (e.g. the recruitment of macrophages favouring a symbiotic relationship) but also mediate systemic phenomena. IL-6 is a good example, being implicated in a number of the clinical features associated with renal cell carcinoma (fever, the acute phase response, and several of the paraneoplastic syndromes).

Structural proteins on the surface of malignant cells remain a major barrier to immune-mediated destruction. The sialomucin complex (SMC), a large glycoprotein structure in the rat, is a homologue of the human mucin gene MUC4, both of which are highly expressed on adenocarcinoma cell lines (117). Mucin-type glycoproteins, due to their extended morphology, have suppressive effects on cell–cell and cell–matrix interactions, and for this reason are postulated to promote tumour escape. Indeed, both SMC overexpression and an increase in the number of mucin repeats block killer-cell binding and effectively remove the tumour antigen signal. Complement regulatory proteins on the surface of a number of human tumours, such as lung and ovarian carcinoma, are another dominant hurdle to be overcome (130). Thus, 'C' regulators, membrane cofactor protein (MCP, CD46), and protectin (CD59) are strongly expressed on a range of ovarian tumours (both benign and malignant), with a more heterogeneous expression of DAF, which correlates inversely with vulnerability of the cells to 'C'-mediated lysis. This resistance may be reversed experimentally with the use of anti-CD59 antibodies, and may be an important strategy in combination with the current use of 'C'-activating mAb targeted at epithelial TAA.

Several studies have shown that absent or decreased zeta and epsilon chain expression of the TCR complex, decreased Ca^{2+} flux, impaired kinase activity following triggering with anti-CD3 antibodies, and altered expression of the downstream protein tyrosine kinase p56lck occur in the TILs of patients with advanced malignancy (malignant melanoma, renal cell carcinoma, ovarian cancer, and colorectal cancer) (131). Similar defects have been reported in the Fc gamma RIII of NK cells. Phenotypically these tumour-associated lymphocytes (TALs) proliferate poorly in response to PHA or phorbol esters (T-cell stimulatory agents), have depressed anti-tumour toxicity, and fail to produce the usual cytokine profile associated with activation. Recent data suggest there is a correlation between the extent of these defects and prognosis, particularly in head and neck cancer and melanoma. Co-incubation of normal activated T cells with tumour targets (either freshly isolated or tumour cell lines) has been shown to induce degradation of the zeta chain as well as apoptosis in a percentage of lymphocytes. The mechanism probably involves several pathways, including direct contact via Fas–FasL interactions, and the secretion of altered cytokine profiles and as yet unidentified molecules. Significantly, it is possible to reverse some of these changes by applying various cytokines (e.g. IL-2), although this is more effective for TALs derived from the primary rather than the metastatic site.

Lastly, immunotherapy ironically may promote immunological escape via modulation of the cytokine network. For example, Ts cells and soluble IL-2 receptors increase during IL-2 cancer immunotherapy; the latter may decrease IL-2 bioavailability. This has important implications for biological approaches to disease in general, and emphasizes the complexity of the immune system.

3.8   TOLERANCE

Various homeostatic mechanisms actively maintain a state of immune unresponsiveness to self-antigen. This ensures that autoimmunity is a comparatively rare event. Tumours, however, have adopted these tolerizing mechanisms thereby resulting in an effective form of immunological escape. Recent experiments in animal system are providing interesting data, suggesting that employing counteractive strategies may break tolerance. It is notable that many of these pathways have a dual nature with both amplification and abrogation of the immune response (see B7 co-stimulators and IL-2 below). A thorough understanding of the interaction between the different tolerizing strategies and the nature of the tumour antigen (type, concentration, and level of persistence), as well as the critical adjuvants, is required to produce more effective immunotherapies.

Thus, antigen expression by the tumour in the absence of co-stimulatory factors may induce anergy in T-effector cells to TSAs. For instance, tumours or APCs deficient in B7-1/2 expression (or CD80/86, a principal co-stimulatory molecule) do not bind the CD28 molecule present on the T cell, and thus induce a state of unresponsiveness in the T cell. Under physiological conditions engagement of CD28 with B7-1/2 triggers a survival signal to the T cell by inducing the expression of anti-apoptotic proteins of the Bcl family (e.g. Bcl-xL) and the secretion of IL-2. Melanoma cells have been transfected with the B7 molecule, resulting in rejection of the tumour in animal models (132). This not only emphasizes the importance of co-stimulation (i.e. signal 2 in T-cell activation) but is also currently under investigation in a number of immunotherapy trials. A second co-receptor for B7, known as CTLA-4, has the opposite effect and dampens down immune activation. The exact biochemical basis remains to be elucidated, although both the inhibition of IL-2 transcription and the antagonism of CD28 are probably involved. Moreover, knockout mice for CTLA-4 demonstrate immune hyperactivation with an early death due to lymphoproliferative and autoimmune disease. Similarly, in animal systems downregulation of CTLA-4 using an inhibitory antibody has resulted in the rejection of tumours (133).

Another mechanism of inducing tolerance employs Fas(CD95)–FasL-induced apoptosis in FasL-expressing T cells, the so-called Fas-mediated activation-induced cell death. This is potentiated by IL-2 and the constitutive expression of Bcl-2 proteins has no effect. Mouse experiments suggest that T cells which encounter persistent antigen are deleted via this strategy, since mutations in Fas or FasL result in autoimmune disease, with no apparent effect of responses to alloantigen or virus. A number of tumours have been shown to express both non-functional Fas and FasL, which 'counterattack' activated Fas-sensitive T-cells (134, 135).

The tumour–host interaction may promote the induction of both effector T cells and regulatory or Ts cells. Indeed, cells cloned from patients with malignant melanoma suggest that Ts cells exist in the TIL population which specifically downregulate the host response (136). The effect is probably mediated by the release of cytokines such as TGF-β1 (inhibits lymphocyte proliferation) and IL-10 (inhibits macrophage activation and the expression of co-stimulatory molecules). IL-2 itself appears to function within a feedback loop to downregulate T-cell activity. This has been aptly demonstrated with targeted disruption of the IL-2 gene, and using mice lacking the high-affinity IL-2R, resulting in the appearance of uncontrolled lymphocyte activation and autoimmune events. The importance and complexity of this pathway in tumour systems has yet to be delineated.

Lastly, an important and fundamentally different strategy is based upon loss of lymphocytes due to 'death by neglect' (137). Apoptosis is triggered passively due to lymphocyte deprivation of survival signals, such as co-stimulation and cytokines, which under normal conditions may upregulate a cellular response from a background level of 1×10^6 to 1×10^3 or more within a week with a return to baseline within 4–12 weeks. Tumours, which commonly lose antigen, B7, and HLA molecules, may thus terminate an initially effective immune response.

4   Summary and conclusions

Immune-mediated tumour destruction is multifaceted, involving all the cellular and small-molecule components of the immune system. Thus, cell–cell interactions, the release of cytotoxic and cytostatic cytokines, proteolytic enzymes, free radicals, and cell-membrane disruption (e.g. the perforins) are all important in defence. The success of the host depends not only on the opposing escape mechanisms, which are activated by the tumour, but also on the ability to contain these interactions at the tumour site (138). Otherwise, the systemic appearance of potent cytokines, such as IL-2 or TNF-α, may provoke end-organ failure and death.

The recent detailed characterization of tumour antigens (signal 1), co-stimulatory molecules (signal 2), and cytokine networks (signal 3) and the characterization of key cells such as the CD4+, CD8+ T cells, and the APCs such as dendritic cells, are enabling more rational attempts at immunotherapy to be explored *in vivo*.

Both cancer and the immune system are highly complex and non-linear (chaotic) systems, whose interactions cannot be predicted from linear analysis. Like weather patterns and their prediction, if the correct information on both sides can be gathered and the minor changes in the starting conditions calculated, it is theoretically possible to alter the dynamics of the immune response to contain the heterogeneous evolutionary properties of an early tumour (139).

5 References

1. Boon, T. (1993). Teaching the immune system to fight cancer. *Sci. Am.*, **268**, 32–39.
2. Dalgleish, A. G. and Browning, M. (1996). *Tumour Immunology: Immunotherapy and Cancer Vaccines*. Cambridge University Press.
3. Smyth, M. J., Godfrey, D. I., and Trapani, J. A. (2001). A fresh look at tumor immunosurveillance and immunotherapy. *Nat. Immunol.*, **4**, 293–299.
4. Burnet, F. M. (1970). *Immunological Surveillance*. Pergamon Press, Oxford.
5. Penn, I. (1988). Tumors of the immunocompromised patient. *Annu. Rev. Med.*, **39**, 63–73.
6. Muller-Eberhard, H. J. (1986). The membrane attack complex of complement. *Annu. Rev. Immunol.*, **4**, 503–528.
7. Lowin, B., Beermann, F., Schmidt, A. *et al.* (1994). A null mutation in the perforin gene impairs cytolytic T lymphocyte- and natural killer cell-mediated cytotoxicity. *Proc. Natl. Acad. Sci. USA*, **91**, 11571–11575.
8. Liszewski, M. K., Farries, T. C., Lublin, D. M. *et al.* (1996). Control of the complement system. *Adv. Immunol.*, **61**, 201–283.
9. Porter, R. R. and Reid, K. B. (1978). The biochemistry of complement. *Nature*, **275**, 699–704.
10. Turner, M. W. (1998). Mannose-binding lectin (MBL) in health and disease. *Immunobiology*, **199**, 327–339.
11. Lanier, L. L., Cwirla, S., Federspiel, N.A. *et al.* (1986). Human natural killer cells isolated from peripheral blood do not rearrange T cell antigen receptor beta chain genes. *J. Exp. Med.* **163**, 209–214.
12. Trinchieri, G. and Valiante, N. (1993). Receptors for the Fc fragment of IgG on natural killer cells. *Nat. Immunol.*, **12**, 218–234.
13. Lissoni, P. (1997). Effects of low-dose recombinant interleukin-2 in human malignancies. *Can. J. Sci. Am.*, **3**, S115–S120.
14. Abbas, A. K., Lichtman, A. H., and Pober, J. S. (1997). *Cellular and Molecular Immunology* (3rd edn), Chapter 13. W. B. Saunders Company.
15. Garzetti G.G., Cignitti, M., Marchegiani, F. *et al.* (1992). Natural killer cell activity in patients with gynecologic malignancies: correlation with histologic grading and stage of disease. *Gynecol. Obstet. Invest.*, **34**, 49–51.

16. Talmadge, J. E., Meyers, K. M., Prieur, D. J. *et al.* (1980). Role of NK cells in tumour growth and metastasis in beige mice. *Nature*, **284**, 622–624.

17. Hanna, N. (1982). Role of natural killer cells in control of cancer metastasis. *Cancer Metastasis Rev.*, **1**, 45–64.

18. Kaufman, D. S., Schoon, R. A., and Leibson, P. J. (1993). MHC class I expression on tumour targets inhibits natural killer cell-mediated cytotoxicity without interfering with target recognition. *J. Immunol.*, **150**, 1429–1436.

19. Liu, C. C., Perussia, B., Cohn, Z. A. *et al.* (1986). Identification and characterization of a pore-forming protein of human peripheral blood natural killer cells. *J. Exp. Med.*, **164**, 2061–2076.

20. Shresta, S., Maclvor, D. M., Heusel, J. W. *et al.* (1995). Natural killer and lymphokine-activated-killer cells require granzyme B for the rapid induction of DNA fragmentation and apoptosis in susceptible target cells. *Proc. Natl. Acad. Sci. USA*, **92**, 5679–5683.

21. Oshimi, Y., Oda, S., Honda, Y. *et al.* (1996). Involvement of Fas ligand and Fas-mediated pathway in the cytotoxicity of human natural killer cells. *J. Immunol.*, **157**, 2909–2915.

22. Sayers, T. J., Wiltrout, T. A., Knappe, W. A. *et al.* (1992). Purification of a factor from the granules of a rat NK cell line (RNK) that reduces tumour cell growth and changes tumour morphology. Molecular identity with a granule serine protease (RNKP-1). *J. Immunol.*, **148**, 292–300.

23. Rosenberg, S. A. (1992). Karnofsky memorial lecture. The immunotherapy and gene therapy of cancer. *J. Clin. Oncol.*, **10**, 180–199.

24. Munn, D. H. and Cheung, N. K. (1989). Antibody-dependent antitumor cytotoxicity by human monocytes cocultured with recombinant macrophage colony stimulating factor. *J. Exp. Med.*, **170**, 511–526.

25. Chapman, H. A. and Hibbs, J. B. (1978). Modulation of macrophage tumoricidal capability by polyene antibiotics: support for membrane lipid as a regulatory determinant of macrophage function. *Proc. Natl. Acad. Sci. USA*, **75**, 4349–4353.

26. Perez, C., Albert, I., DeFay, K. *et al.* (1990). A nonsecretable cell surface mutant of tumor necrosis factor (TNF) kills by cell-to-cell contact. *Cell*, **63**, 251–258.

27. Ruegg, C., Yilmaz, A., Bieler, G. *et al.* (1998). Evidence for the involvement of endothelial cell integrin alphaVbeta3 in the disruption of the tumor vasculature induced by TNF and IFN-gamma. *Nat. Med.*, **4**, 408–414.

28. Brouckaert, P. G. G., Leroux-Roels, G. G., Guisez, Y. *et al.* (1986). *In vivo* antitumour activity of recombinant human and murine TNF, alone and in combination with murine IFN-gamma, on a syngeneic murine melanoma. *Int. J. Cancer*, **38**, 763–769.

29. Yokota, S., Geppert, T., and Lipsky, P. (1988). Enhancement of antigen- and mitogen-induced human T lymphocyte proliferation by tumour necrosis factor-alpha. *J. Immunol.*, **140**, 531–536.

30. Balkwill, F. R. and Burke, F. (1990). The cytokine network. *Immunol. Today*, **10**, 299–303.

31. Drapier, J. C., Wietzerbin, J., and Hibbs, J. B. (1988). Interferon-gamma and tumor necrosis factor induce the L-arginine-dependent cytotoxic effector mechanism in murine macrophages. *Eur. J. Immunol.*, **18**, 1587–1592.

32. Vassalli, P. (1992). The pathophysiology of tumor necrosis factors. *Annu. Rev. Immunol.*, **10**, 411–452.

33. Wong, G. H. W. and Goeddel, D. V. (1988). Induction of manganous superoxide dismutase by tumour necrosis factor: possible protective mechanism. *Science*, **242**, 941–943.

34. Heriot, A. G., Marriott, J. B., Cookson, S. *et al.* (2000). Immunosuppression in patients with colorectal cancer is associated with Duke's stage and is reversed by tumour resection. *Br. J. Cancer*, **5**, 1009–1012.

35. Rock, K. L. and Goldberg, A. L. (1999). Degradation of cell proteins and the generation of MHC class I-presented peptides. *Annu. Rev. Immunol.*, **17**, 739–780.

36. Watts, C. (1997). Capture and processing of exogenous antigens for presentation on MHC molecules. *Annu. Rev. Immunol.*, **15**, 821–850.

37. Garcia, K. C., Teyton, L., and Wilson, I. A. (1999). Structural basis of T cell recognition. *Annu. Rev. Immunol.*, **17**, 369–397.

38. Jones, E. Y. (1997). MHC class I and II structures. *Curr. Opin. Immunol.*, **9**, 75–79.

39. Gallucci, S. and Matzinger, P. (2001). Danger signals: SOS to the immune system. *Curr. Opin. Immunol.*, **13**, 114–119.

40. Clemente, C. G., Mihm, M. C., Bufalino, R. *et al.* (1996). Prognostic value of tumor infiltrating lymphocytes in the vertical growth phase of primary cutaneous melanoma. *Cancer*, **77**, 1303–1310.

41. Singh, S., Rosa, S. R., Acena, M. *et al.* (1992). Stroma is critical for preventing or permitting immunological destruction of antigenic cancer cells. *J. Exp. Med.*, **175**, 139–146.

42. Folkman, J. (1995). Angiogenesis in cancer, vascular, rheumatoid, and other disease. *Nat. Med.*, **1**, 27–31.

43. Letterio, J. J. and Roberts, A. B. (1998). Regulation of immune responses by TGF-β. *Annu. Rev. Immunol.*, **16**, 137–161.

44. Mantovani, A., Bottazzi, B., Colotta, F. *et al.* (1992). The origin and function of tumour-associated macrophages. *Immunol. Today*, **13**, 265–270.

45. Hennemann, B. and Andreesen, R. (1996). Monocyte/macrophage activation by immunostimulators. *Clin. Immunother.*, **5**, 294–308.

46. Wang, J. M., Deng, X., Gong, W. *et al.* (1998). Chemokines and their role in tumor growth and metastasis. *J. Immunol. Methods*, **220**, 1–17.

47. Rossi, D. and Zlotnik, A. (2000). The biology of chemokines and their receptors. *Annu. Rev. Immunol.*, **18**, 217–242.

48. Martinet, N., Beck, G., Bernard, V. *et al.* (1992). Mechanism for the recruitment of macrophages to cancer site. *Cancer*, **70**, 854–859.

49. Bakker, A. B., Schreurs, M. W., De Boer, A. J. *et al.* (1994). Melanocyte lineage-specific antigen gp-100 is recognized by melanoma-derived tumor-infiltrating lymphocytes. *J. Exp. Med.*, **179**, 1005–1009.

50. Labarriere, N., Pandolfino, M. C., Raingeard, D. *et al.* (1998). Frequency and relative fraction of tumor antigen-specific T cells among lymphocytes from melanoma-invaded lymph nodes. *Int. J. Cancer*, **78**, 209–215.

51. Chaux, P., Vantomme, V., Coulie, P. *et al.* (1998). Estimation of the frequencies of anti-MAGE-3 cytolytic T-lymphocyte precursors in blood from individuals without cancer. *Int. J. Cancer*, **77**, 538–542.

52. D'Souza, S., Rimoldi, D., Lienard, D. *et al.* (1998). Circulating Melan-A/MART-1 specific cytolytic T lymphocyte precursors in HLA-A2$^+$ melanoma patients have a memory phenotype. *Int. J. Cancer*, **78**, 699–706.

53. Peoples, G. E., Goedegebuure, P. S., Smith, R. *et al.* (1995). Breast and ovarian cancer-specific cytotoxic T lymphocytes recognize the same Her2/neu-derived peptide. *Proc. Natl. Acad. Sci. USA*, **92**, 432–436.

54. Thurhner, M., Radmayr, C., Ramoner, R. *et al.* (1996). Human renal cell carcinoma tissue contains dendritic cells. *Int. J. Cancer*, **67**, 1–7.

55. Steinbrink, K., Jonuleit, H., Müller, G. *et al.* (1999). Interleukin-10 treated human dendritic cells induce a melanoma-antigen specific anergy in CD8⁺ T cells resulting in a failure to lyse tumor cells. *Blood*, **93**, 1634–1642.

56. Shurin, M. R., Lokshin, A., Esche, C. *et al.* (1999). Tumors induce apoptosis of dendritic cells: role of FLT3-Ligand and IL-12 in tumor-associated dendritic cell function. *Proc. Am. Assoc. Cancer Res.*, **39**, abstract 3745.

57. Soiffer, R., Lynch, T., Mihm, M. *et al.* (1998). Vaccination with irradiated autologous melanoma cells engineered to secrete human granulocyte–macrophage colony stimulating factor generates potent antitumor immunity in patients with metastatic melanoma. *Proc. Natl. Acad. Sci. USA*, **95**, 13141–13146.

58. Sone, S., Yano, S., Hanibuchi, M. *et al.* (1999). Heterogeneity of multiorgan metastases. *Cancer Chemother Pharmacol.*, **43**, S26–31.

59. Simons, J. W., Mikhak, B., Chang, J. F. *et al.* (1999). Clinical activity and broken immunologic tolerance from vaccination with *ex vivo* GM-CSF gene transduced prostate cancer vaccines. *Cancer Res.*, **59**, 5160–5168.

60. Scahhfer, M. and Barbul, A. (1998). Lymphocyte function in wound healing and following injury. *Br. J. Surg.*, **85**, 444–460.

61. O'Byrne, K. J., Dalgleish, A. G., Browning, M. J. *et al.* (2000). Angiogenesis and suppression of cell mediated immunity precede and play a central role in the pathogenesis of malignant disease. *Eur. J. Cancer*, **36**, 151–169.

62. Balkwill, F. and Mantovani, A. (2001). Inflammation and cancer: back to Virchow? *Lancet*, **357**, 539–545.

63. Maraveyas, A., Baban, B., Kennard, D. *et al.* (1999). Possible improved survival of patients with stage IV AJCC melanoma receiving SRL 172 immunotherapy: correlation with induction of increased levels of intracellular interleukin-2 in peripheral blood lymphocytes. *Ann. Oncol.*, **10**, 1–8.

64. Angevin, E., Kremer, F., Gaudin, C. *et al.* (1997). Analysis of T-cell immune response in renal cell carcinoma: polarisation to type 1-like differentiation pattern, clonal T-cell expansion, and tumour-specific cytotoxicity. *Int. J. Cancer*, **72**, 431–440.

65. Norimasa, I., Nakamura, H., Tanaka, Y. *et al.* (1999). Lung carcinoma: analysis of T helper 1 and 2 cells and T cytotoxic type 1 and 2 cells by intracellular cytokine detection with flow cytometry. *Cancer*, **85**, 2359–2367.

66. Posner, J. B. and Dalmau, J. (1997). Paraneoplastic syndromes. *Curr. Opin. Immunol.*, **9**, 723–729.

67. Graus, F., Dalmau, J., and Rene, R. (1997). Anti-Hu antibodies in patients with small-cell lung cancer: association with complete responses to therapy and improved survival. *J. Clin. Oncol.*, **15**, 2866–2872.

68. Motomura, M., Lang, B., Johnston, I. *et al.* (1997). Incidence of serum anti-P/Q-type and anti-N-type calcium channel autoantibodies in the Lambert–Eaton myasthenic syndrome. *J. Neurol. Sci.*, **147**, 35–42.

69. Albert, M. L., Darnell, J. C., Bender, A. *et al.* (1998). Tumor-specific killer cells in paraneoplastic cerebellar degeneration. *Nat. Med.*, **4**, 1321–1324.

70. Weber, L. W., Bowne, W. B., Wolchok, J. D. *et al.* (1998). Tumor immunity and autoimmunity induced by immunization with homologous DNA. *J. Clin. Invest.*, **102**, 1258–1264.

71. Davis, T. A., Maloney, D. G., Czerwinski, D. K. *et al.* (1998). Anti-idiotype antibodies can induce long-term complete remissions in non-Hodgkin's lymphoma without eradicating the malignant clone. *Blood*, **92**, 1184–1190.

72. Matsui, S., Ahlers, J. D., Vortmeyer, A. O. *et al.* (1999). A model for CD8⁺ CTL tumor immunosurveillance and regulation of tumor escape by CD4 T cells through an effect on quality of CTL. *J. Immunol.*, **163**, 184–193.

73. Kaplan, D. H., Shankaran, V., Dighe, A. S. *et al.* (1998). Demonstration of an interferon gamma-dependent tumor surveillance system in immunocompetent mice. *Proc. Natl. Acad. Sci. USA*, **95**, 7556–7561.

74. Shankaran, V., Ikeda, H., Bruce, A. T. *et al.* (2001). IFNgamma and lymphocytes prevent primary tumour development and shape tumour immunogenicity. *Nature*, **410**, 1107–1111.

75. Zorn, E. and Hercend, T. (1999). A MAGE-6-encoded peptide is recognised by expanded lymphocytes infiltrating a spontaneously regressing human primary melanoma lesion. *Eur. J. Immunol.*, **29**, 602–607.

76. Ishizu, H., Bove, K. E., Ziegler, M. M. *et al.* (1994). Immune-mediated regression of 'metastatic' neuroblastoma in the liver. *J. Pediatr. Surg.*, **29**, 155–60.

77. Starnes, C. O. (1992). Coley's toxins in perspective. *Nature*, **357**, 11–12.

78. Gillis, S. and Williams, D. E. (1998). Cytokine therapy: lessons learned and future challenges. *Curr. Opin. Immunol.*, **10**, 501–503.

79. Morton, D. L., Foshag, L. J., Hoon, D. S. B. *et al.* (1993). Polyvalent melanoma vaccine improves survival of patients with metastatic melanoma. *Ann. N. Y. Acad. Sci.*, **690**, 120.

80. Hsueh, E., Gupta, R. K., Qi, K. *et al.* (1998). Correlation of specific immune responses with survival in melanoma patients with distant metastases receiving polyvalent melanoma cell vaccine. *J. Clin. Oncol.*, **16**, 2913–2920.

81. Porter, D. L. and Antin, J. H. (1999). The graft-versus-leukaemia effects of allogeneic cell therapy. *Annu. Rev. Med.*, **50**, 369–386.

82. Bendandi, M., Gocke, C. D., Kobrin, C. B. *et al.* (1999). Complete molecular remissions induced by patient-specific vaccination plus granulocyte-monocyte colony-stimulating factor against lymphoma. *Nat. Med.*, **5**, 1171–1177.

83. Rosenberg. S. A., Yang, J. C., Schwartzentruber, D. J. *et al.* (1998). Immunologic and therapeutic evaluation of a synthetic peptide vaccine for the treatment of patients with metastatic melanoma. *Nat. Med.*, **4**, 321–327.

84. Franzke, A., Peest, D., Probst-Kepper, M. *et al.* (1999). Autoimmunity resulting from cytokine treatment predicts long-term survival in patients with metastatic renal cell carcinoma. *J. Clin. Oncol.*, **17**, 529–533.

85. Alexandroff, A. B., Jackson, A. M., O'Donnell, M. A. *et al.* (1999). BCG immunotherapy of bladder cancer: 20 years on. *Lancet*, **353**, 1689–1694.

86. Fujimoto, T., Duda, R. B., Szilvasi, A. *et al.* (1997). Streptococcal preparation OK-432 is a potent inducer of IL-12 and a T helper cell 1 dominant state. *J. Immunol.*, **158**, 5619–5626.

87. Timmerman, J. M. and Levy, R. (1999). Dendritic cell vaccines for cancer immunotherapy. *Annu. Rev. Med.*, **26**, 507–529.

88. Hsu, F. J., Benike, C., Fagoni, F. *et al.* (1996). Vaccination of patients with B-cell lymphoma using autologous antigen-pulsed dendritic cells. *Nat. Med.,* **2**, 52–58.

89. Nestle, F. O., Alijagic, S., Gilliet, M. *et al.* (1998). Vaccination of melanoma patients with peptide- or tumor lysate-pulsed dendritic cells. *Nat. Med.,* **4**, 328–332.

90. Cragg, M. S., French. R. R., and Glennie, M. J. (1999). Signalling antibodies in cancer therapy. *Curr. Opin. Immunol.,* **11**, 541–547.

91. White, C. A., Weaver, R. L., and Grillo-Lopez, A. J. (2001). Antibody-targeted immunotherapy for treatment of malignancy. *Annu. Rev. Med.,* **52**, 125–145.

92. McLaughlin, P., Grillo-Lopez, A. J., Link, B. K. (1998). Rituximab chimeric anti-CD20 monoclonal antibody therapy for relapsed indolent lymphoma: half of patients respond to a four-dose treatment programme. *J. Clin. Oncol.,* **16**, 2825–2833.

93. Riethmuller, G., Holz, E., Schlimok, G. *et al.* (1998). Monoclonal antibody therapy for resected Dukes' C colorectal cancer: seven year outcome of a multicenter randomized trial. *J. Clin. Oncol.,* **16**, 1788–1794.

94. Slamon, D., Leyland-Jones, B., Shak, S. *et al.* (1998). Addition of Herceptin (humanized Anti-HER2 antibody) to first line chemotherapy for HER2 over-expressing metastatic breast cancer (HER2$^+$/MBC) markedly increases anticancer activity: a randomised, multinational controlled phase III trial. *Proc. Am. Soc. Clin. Oncol.,* **17**, 98a (abstract 377).

95. Bradwell, A. R. and Harvey, T. C. (1999). Control of hypercalcaemia of para-thyroid carcinoma by immunisation. *Lancet,* **353**, 370–373.

96. Szlosarek, P. W. and Dalgleish, A. G. (2000). The potential applications of gene therapy in the patient with cancer. *Drugs Aging,* **17**, 121–132.

97. McGuiness, R. P., Ge, Y., Patel, S. D. *et al.* (1999). Anti-tumor activity of human T cells expressing the CC49-zeta chimeric immune receptor. *Hum. Gene Ther.,* **10**, 165–173.

98. Rosenberg, S. A., Aebersold, P., Cornetta, K. *et al.* (1990). Gene transfer into humans: immunotherapy of patients with advanced melanoma using tumor infiltrating lymphocytes modified by retroviral gene transduction. *N. Engl. J. Med.,* **323**, 570–578.

99. Cao, X., Zhang, W., He, L. *et al.* (1998). Lymphotactin gene-modified bone marrow dendritic cells act as more potent adjuvants for peptide delivery to induce specific antitumor immunity. *J. Immunol.,* **161**, 6238–6244.

100. Perry, M. A., Todryk, S. and Dalgleish, A. G. (1999). The role of HSVtk in the treatment of solid tumours. *Exp. Opin. Invest. Drugs,* **8**, 777–785.

101. Vile, R. G., Castleden, S. C., Marshall, J. *et al.* (1997). Generation of an anti-tumour immune response in a nonimmunogenic tumour: HSVtk-killing *in vivo* stimulates a mononuclear cell infiltrate and a Th1-like profile of intratumoral cytokine expression. *Int. J. Cancer,* **71**, 267–274.

102. Consalvo, M., Mullen, C. A., Modesti, A. *et al.* (1995). 5-Fluorocytosine eradi-cation of murine adenocarcinomas engineered to express the cytosine deaminase suicide gene requires host immune competence and leaves an efficient memory. *J. Immunol.,* **154**, 5302–5312.

103. Chen, Y. T., Gure, A. O., Tsang, S. *et al.* (1998). Identification of multiple cancer/testis antigens by allogeneic antibody screening of a melanoma cell line library. *Proc. Natl. Acad. Sci. USA*, **95**, 6919–6923.

104. Banchereau, J. and Steinman, R. M. (1998). Dendritic cells and the control of immunity. *Nature*, **392**, 245–252.

105. Lynch, D. H., Andreasen, A., Maraskovsky, E. *et al.* (1997). Flt3 ligand induces tumor regression and antitumor immune responses *in vivo*. *Nat. Med.*, **3**, 625–631.

106. Rodolfo, M., Melani, C., Zilocchi, C. *et al.* (1998). IgG2a induced by interleukin (IL) 12-producing tumor cell vaccines but not IgG1 induced by IL-4 vaccine is associated with the eradication of experimental metastases. *Cancer Res.*, **58**, 5812–5817.

107. Erez-Alon, N., Herkel, J., Wolkowicz, R. *et al.* (1998). Immunity to p53 induced by an idiotypic network of anti-p53 antibodies: generation of sequence-specific anti-DNA antibodies and protection from tumor metastasis. *Cancer Res.*, **58**, 5447–5452.

108. Shresta, S., Pham, C. T. N., Thomas, D. A. *et al.* (1998). How do cytotoxic lymphocytes kill their targets. *Curr. Opin. Immunol.*, **10**, 581–587.

109. Pardoll, D. M. and Topalian, S. L. (1998). The role of CD4+ T cell responses in antitumor immunity. *Curr. Opin. Immunol.*, **10**, 588–594.

110. Schwartz, R. H. (1992). Costimulation of T lymphocytes: the role of CD28, CTLA-4, and B7/BB1 in interleukin-2 production and immunotherapy. *Cell*, **71**, 1065–1068.

111. Bretcher, P. and Cohn, M. (1970). A theory of self–nonself discrimination. *Science*, **169**, 1042–1049.

112. Heath, W. R. and Carbone, F. R. (1999). Cytotoxic T lymphocyte activation by cross-priming. *Curr. Opin. Immunol.*, **11**, 314–318.

113. Von Leoprechting, A., Van der Bruggen, P., Pahl, H. L. *et al.* (1999). Stimulation of CD40 on immunogenic human malignant melanomas augments their cytotoxic T lymphocyte-mediated lysis and induces apoptosis. *Cancer Res.*, **59**, 1287–1294.

114. French, R. R., Chan, H. T., Tutt, A. L. *et al.* (1999). CD40 antibody evokes a cytotoxic T-cell response that eradicates lymphoma and bypasses T-cell help. *Nat. Med.*, **5**, 548–553.

115. Lee, J., Fenton, B. M., Koch, C. J. *et al.* (1998). Interleukin 2 expression by tumor cells alters both the immune response and the tumor microenvironment. *Cancer Res.*, **58**, 1478–1485.

116. Jager, E., Ringhoffer, M., Altmannsberger, M. *et al.* (1997). Immunoselection *in vivo* independent loss of MHC Class I and melanocyte differentiation antigen expression in metastatic melanoma. *Int. J. Cancer*, **71**, 142–147.

117. Komatsu, M., Yee, L., and Carraway, K.L. (1999). Overexpression of sialomucin complex, a rat homologue of MUC4, inhibits tumor killing by lymphokine-activated killer cells. *Cancer Res.*, **59**, 2229–2236.

118. Hornung, M. O., Krementz, E. T., Sullivan, K. A. *et al.* (1986). Immunological heterogeneity in human melanoma: immunogenic alloantigen expression in autologous host. *Cancer Res.*, **46**, 3704–3710.

119. Topalian, S. L., Kasid, A., and Rosenberg, S. A. (1990). Immunoselection of a human melanoma resistant to specific lysis by autologous tumor-infiltrating lymphocytes. *J. Immunol.*, **144**, 4487–4495.

120. Vanky, F., Hising, C., Sjowall, K. *et al.* (1995). Immunogenicity and immuno-sensitivity of *ex vivo* human carcinomas: interferon gamma and tumour necrosis factor alpha treatment of tumour cells potentiates their interaction with auto-logous blood lymphocytes. *Cancer Immunol. Immunother.*, **41**, 217–226.

121. Restifo, P. N., Esquivel, F., Kawakami, Y. *et al.* (1993). Identification of human cancers deficient in antigen processing. *J. Exp. Med.*, **177**, 265–272.

122. Ruiz-Cabello, F. and Garrido, F. (1998). HLA and cancer: from research to clinical impact. *Immunol. Today*, **19**, 539–542.

123. Paul, P., Rouas-Freiss, N., Khalil-Daher, I. *et al.* (1998). HLA-G expression in melanoma: a way for tumor cells to escape from immunosurveillance. *Proc. Natl. Acad. Sci. USA*, **95**, 4510–4515.

124. Enk, A. H., Jonuleit, H., Saloga, J. *et al.* (1997). Dendritic cells as mediators of tumor-induced tolerance in metastatic melanoma. *Int. J. Cancer*, **73**, 309–316.

125. Ludewig, B., Graf, D., Gelderblom, H. R. *et al.* (1995). Spontaneous apoptosis of dendritic cells is efficiently inhibited by TRAP (CD4O-Ligand) and TNF-alpha, but strongly enhanced by interleukin-10. *Eur. J. Immunol.*, **25**, 1943–1950.

126. Lala, P. K., Al-Mutter, N., and Orucevic, A. (1997). Effects of chronic indomethacin therapy on the development and progression of spontaneous mammary tumors in C3H/HEJ mice. *Int. J. Cancer*, **73**, 371–380.

127. Malik, S. T. A., Griffin, D. B., Fiers, W. *et al.* (1989). Paradoxical effects of tumour necrosis factor in experimental ovarian cancer. *Int. J. Cancer*, **44**, 918–925.

128. Arteaga, C. L., Koli, K. M., Dugger, T. C. *et al.* (1999). Reversal of Tamoxifen resistance of human breast carcinomas *in vivo* by neutralising antibodies to transforming growth factor-β. *Natl. Cancer Inst.*, **91**, 46–53.

129. Elsässer-Beile, U., von Kleist, S., Stähle, W. *et al.* (1993). Cytokine levels in whole blood cell cultures as parameters of cellular immunologic activity in patients with malignant melanoma and basal cell carcinoma. *Cancer*, **71**, 231–236.

130. Maio, M., Brasoveanu, L. I., Coral, S. *et al.* (1998). Structure, distribution, and functional role of protectin (CD59) in complement-susceptibility and in immuno-therapy of human malignancies. *Int. J. Oncol.*, **13**, 305–318.

131. Finke, J. H., Zea, A. H., Stanley, J. *et al.* (1993). Loss of T-cell receptor zeta-chain and p56lck in T-cells infiltrating human renal cell carcinoma. *Cancer Res.*, **53**, 5613–5616.

132. Townsend, S. E. and Allison, J. P. (1993). Tumour rejection after direct cost-imulation of CD8⁺ T cells by B7-transfected melanoma cells. *Science*, **259**, 368–370.

133. Leach, D. R., Krummel, M. F., and Allison, J. P. (1996). Enhancement of anti-tumor immunity by CTLA-4 blockade. *Science*, **271**, 1734–1736.

134. Walker, P. R., Saas, P., and Dietrich, P. Y. (1997). Role of Fas ligand (CD95L) in immune escape: the tumor cell strikes back. *J. Immunol.*, **158**, 4521–4524.

135. Von Bernstorff, W., Spanjaard, R. A., and Chan, A. K. (1999). Pancreatic cancer cells can evade immune surveillance via nonfunctional Fas (APO-1/CD95) recep-tors and aberrant expression of functional Fas ligand. *Surgery*, **125**, 73–84.

136. Mukherji, B., Guha, A., Chakraborty, N. G. *et al.* (1989). Clonal analysis of cytotoxic and regulatory T cell responses against human melanoma. *J. Exp. Med.*, **169**, 1961–1976.

137. Van Parijs L., and Abbas, A. K. (1998). Homeostasis and self-tolerance in the immune system: turning lymphocytes off. *Science*, **280**, 243–248.

138. Wojtowicz-Praga, S. (1997). Reversal of tumor-induced immunosuppression: a new approach to cancer therapy. *J. Immunother.*, 20, 165–177.

139. Dalgleish, A. G. (1999). The relevance of non-linear mathematics (chaos theory) to the treatment of cancer, the role of the immune response and the potential for vaccines. *Q. J. Med.*, 92, 347–359.

PART II

The clinical context: studies and speculations on human cancer

3

The role of psychological factors in cancer onset and progression: a critical appraisal

J. L. LEVENSON AND K. McDONALD

1 Introduction

Many professionals and lay people believe that psychological factors play a major role in cancer onset and progression. The media have promoted popular ideas of overcoming cancer through 'mind over body', and there are self-help books and retreat centres where patients can learn imagery and relaxation techniques to fight their cancer. Guided imagery (visualizing white cells attacking cancer cells), cognitive restructuring (thinking positive thoughts), and assertiveness training have all been promoted alongside traditional health care for the cancer patient to 'combat' the disease.

Enthusiasm for these optimistic theories and practices should be tempered by acknowledgement of the fact that scientific evidence supporting a relationship between psychological factors and cancer lags far behind. In part, this may be due to the complexities involved in studying cancer, for a host of factors may contribute to onset and progression. This chapter reviews the scientific evidence pertaining to the major psychological factors that have been studied. Flaws in research design and analysis of many existing reports will also be discussed.

From a historical perspective, the 1950s witnessed a surge in public interest in psychosomatic medicine and in research linking psychological, social, and environmental factors to disease onset and progression. A major finding was the association between smoking and lung cancer. In the following decade, personality traits, conflicts, and affects were examined as possible contributors to the onset and progression of many diseases, including cancer. Exposure to certain environmental and occupational toxins was also linked to several types of cancer. The 1960s likewise witnessed the growth of experiments using animals in the hope of better understanding the effects of psychological and behavioural factors on cancer, while controlling confounding variables that are difficult or impossible to control in humans. Extrapolating conclusions from animal studies to human cancer remains problematic and will be discussed later. The 1970s saw rapid advances in immunology and neurochemistry, and psychiatry became more involved with the biological basis of mental disorders. Intriguing associations between certain affective states and the neuroendocrine system were demonstrated. Further research in psychoneuroimmunology in the 1980s and 1990s explored the relationship between immunological and psychosocial variables, as well as the implications for cancer vulnerability and progression.

In this chapter, we will look at the hypothesis, along with positive and negative studies associated with it, that cancer onset and progression are affected by psychosocial variables. Psychosocial variables examined here include affective states; coping, defensive styles, and personality traits; bereavement; social support; and stressful life events.

While extensive research in psycho-oncology has appeared over recent decades, much of it is methodologically flawed. Flaws have included use of small and biased samples, heterogeneous sample groups of mixed patients with very different cancer types and/or cancers at different stages, limited or no statistical analysis, poor controls, and retrospective subject recall bias. Several studies that seemed to show significant effects were inconclusive because of non-equivalence in groups at baseline, either in disease severity or in the therapy received (many studies did not even monitor this possibility). Some studies failed to attend to important potential confounding factors such as smoking or diet. A number of studies measured too many psychological variables and then overly emphasized the few 'discovered' positive associations in published results. Very few studies examining psychological effects on cancer progression control for psychopathology prior to cancer. Failure to standardize measures of baseline psychological factors and measures of medical outcome has also been frequent.

Extensive previously published reviews of this topic are available to the reader and we have supplemented these with MEDLINE searches through early 1999. Studies were not included in the present review if they were judged to be seriously flawed methodologically (according to the criteria noted above). We have emphasized recent research (1992–1999). Space does not permit citation of many of the earlier studies referenced in the first edition of this book, to which the interested reader is referred (1).

2   Affective states

2.1   PREVALENCE OF DEPRESSION IN CANCER PATIENTS

McDaniel *et al.*'s meta-analysis of prevalence studies of depression in cancer patients found rates ranging from 1.5 to 50 per cent with a mean of 24 per cent and median of 22 per cent (2). Recent studies of the prevalence of depression in cancer patients have found similar rates. The highest rates were found in pancreatic cancer patients, with as many as 50 per cent of these patients presenting with depression prior to a diagnosis of cancer (3). There has been speculation that there is some shared pathophysiology between affective disorders and pancreatic cancer, but more clinical research is needed, especially to determine the chronological order of the phenomenology (i.e. which came first?). It is difficult to generalize from the majority of prevalence studies because they were retrospective, had very small numbers, used different instruments and definitions of depression, and used cohorts from different cancer sites (1). However, it is clear that there is significant psychological distress in patients with a variety of cancers (4–6). The level of distress is most dramatically exemplified by the fact that the suicide rate in head and neck cancer patients is 1.2 per cent (7). Depression in cancer patients has been shown to have similar symptomatology as depression in psychiatric patients (8), and similar benefits from diagnosis and treatment in cancer patients have been clearly demonstrated (9).

2.2   DEPRESSION AND CANCER ONSET

The linking of affective states, particularly depression, with the onset of cancer has been an active area of investigation. Early epidemiological studies showed significantly increased risk with depression but attempts to replicate this have been largely negative (1). In a meta-analysis of studies relating to cancer onset, McGee *et al.* (10) report a small but significant association between the two but further state that there is little practical significance of such a relationship of that magnitude. Another recent study found that elderly adults who were depressed for 6 or more years had double the risk of developing cancer as non-depressed adults even after adjusting for ethnicity, physical ability, number of hospital admissions, smoking, and alcohol intake (11).

In general, most studies examining depressive states are flawed by their lack of specification. Most investigators have not differentiated between various depressive disorders and have not examined depression from the perspective of past history, duration, chronicity, or treatment pursued. Whether or not differences in depressive states might influence cancer outcome (for example characterologic depression vs. melancholic depression) remains unknown. Many reports have regarded feelings of hopelessness and helplessness as equivalent to the presence of depression. Additionally, it is problematic to compare studies that use different instruments to measure the presence of depression. Instruments vary in whether they are designed to measure depressive states, traits, or clinical depression, which further confounds cross-comparison of studies. Few studies have systematically examined the prevalence of psychiatric disorders among cancer patients, and, of these, many have been limited by biased samples and instruments that measure symptoms rather diagnoses. Another problem is that studies often do not control for other relevant psychosocial variables. For example, depression precipitated by loss of a significant other may be confounded by changes in coping styles, changes in habits such as excessive alcohol intake, poor diet, or increased social isolation. A more complete review of depression and cancer can be found in McDaniel *et al.* (2).

2.3 DEPRESSION AND CANCER OUTCOME

Besides epidemiological studies, other research has focused on the impact of affective states on outcome in cancer patients. Studies examining the effect of depression on cancer outcome in clinical samples most often have focused on breast cancer. Many of the data have been retrospective and can be criticized not only for lack of controls but also for the bias that exists when patients who know their diagnoses are queried about lifestyle and affective states. Another problem with most studies of depression and cancer has been that few studies have measured lifetime prevalence of depression.

Depression could be reasonably expected to result in increased levels of pain (12), decreased functional status (13), more medical comorbidity, increased health care utilization (14), changes in compliance with treatment (15, 16), decreased desire for life-sustaining treatment (17), and increased mortality from cancer (18, 19). Although many investigators have found depression associated with a variety of poor outcomes in cancer patients, even some of the more recent research studies are beset by some of the same methodological issues as earlier studies, such as a lack of adequate control or cohort, and failure to control for confounding variables. Even if one ignores any methodological shortcomings, the picture painted by research is not a clear one. Ayres *et al.* (15) found an *increase* in treatment compliance for cancer patients with depression (a counterintuitive finding) but did not control for severity of disease. In addition, there are several studies that found no or not significant relationships between cancer outcomes and depression (1). Garssen and Goodkin (20) cite several studies providing contradictory conclusions regarding the association between psychological distress and length of survival, with 14 of 17 studies finding a positive (i.e. high distress predicted increased length of survival) or no relationship. Tross *et al.* (21) found a negative relationship between psychological distress and survival (high distress predicted shorter survival). However, they used a general measure of distress in a sample of breast cancer patients with stage II disease who received chemotherapy, making generalization difficult. Although Glover *et al.* (12) found that depression in cancer patients was associated with higher levels of pain, they did not control for stage of disease.

Several studies did seem to adequately control for confounding variables. Takeida *et al.* (18) followed elderly patients for 5 years and found increased mortality for cancer (among other disorders) in a cohort with severe depression compared to non-depressed and moderately depressed cohorts. In an innovative study, McDonough *et al.* (16) looked at the interaction of variables, including depression, anxiety, and disability, with diet and medication compliance. A wide variety of interactions between the three variables was associated with poor compliance. Recent research by the authors found that men diagnosed with prostate cancer and a mental illness (including depression) were half as likely to receive any form of treatment as those with no mental illness diagnosis. Race, marital status, age at diagnosis, stage of disease, socioeconomic status, and education level were all controlled for. A mediating effect of age and marital status was also apparent, with older individuals who were single being more likely to have a diagnosis of mental illness (22).

3 Coping, defensive style, and personality traits

A large body of literature has described the cancer patient's degree of emotional expressiveness and its purported effect on prognosis. Descriptive case reports began appearing in the 1950s, noting shorter survival in patients with depressed, resigning characteristics compared with patients who were able to express more negative emotions, such as anger. However, many studies were flawed by a failure to control for staging and other confounding variables. Studies in the 1980s both supported and refuted the belief that certain coping, defensive style, or personality traits were associated with different risks for cancer onset or mortality (1).

More recent investigators continue to explore various personality variables and their relation to cancer onset and progression. The research has been diverse and scattered over a multitude of variables and has provided very contradictory conclusions. Most recent studies examined each variable separately with very few looking at the effect of the interaction of variables. There has been little confirmation of personality variables that relate to cancer onset but more promising results regarding cancer progression. Garssen and Goodkin provide an excellent review (20) of the literature to date on the relationship of personality variables to cancer onset and progression. Some of the more common variables found to be associated with progression of disease include repression of emotion and difficulty coping with stress, which are the main components of the Type C personality (23), lack of fighting spirit (24), external locus of control (25), hopelessness (26), and helplessness. Garssen and Goodkin found four studies reporting a significant relationship between repression of emotion and cancer progression and decreased survival (20). The majority of studies of helplessness have found that helplessness predicted more cancer progression (20). Early research by Greer *et al.* (27) indicated that women with a coping style of fighting spirit or denial had survived breast cancer significantly longer than those displaying stoic acceptance or helplessness.

Scheier and Bridges (28) cite age and place in disease course as mediators between personality variables and health outcomes. Some studies found that positive relationships between personality measures and cancer were stronger for younger persons. In early stages of disease, personality variables may have more impact on health status and treatment than biological ones, whereas in later stages of disease biological factors appear to be more important in determining health outcomes. In addition to the direct impact that personality variables and affective states have on cancer, they may play a mediating role by their impact on self-care behaviour and preferences (29).

4   Bereavement

Bereavement has been recognized as a significant stressor and has often been assumed to be a risk factor in cancer onset and progression. Most early studies did not show a relationship between bereavement and cancer onset or progression (1, 27). However, a more recent study by Prigerson *et al.* (30) found that subjects with symptoms of traumatic grief 6 months after the death of a spouse had a variety of negative health outcomes including more diagnosis of cancer. Another study (31) found that moderate increases in mortality from chronic ischaemic heart disease and lung cancer were associated with bereavement. There was an interaction with gender in this study. Men who experienced bereavement showed increased cancer mortality but women who experienced bereavement had no such increase in cancer mortality. This finding was greater at time periods less than 6 months and also among younger patients. Considering all studies to date, bereavement has not been convincingly shown to be a factor in cancer onset or progression.

Other promising avenues for a possible link between bereavement and cancer onset are the relationships between immune function and grief. As previously reviewed (1), levels of immune function were not pathologically low in these studies. Irwin *et al.* (32) found that NK-cell activity was significantly lower in women experiencing bereavement from the loss of a spouse and also those anticipating death of their husband from lung cancer. A more recent study found similar effects with lymphokine-activated killer cell activity reduced in patients with depressive symptoms and high anxiety states (33) (see Chapters 1, 2, and 6).

5 Social support

Lack of social support has been shown to be a risk factor for all-cause mortality, and many studies have examined the effects of social support on cancer incidence and mortality. Social relations and support and their effects on cancer patients (as with other diseases) are complex phenomena and may vary with cancer site and extent of disease (34). Social support varies with regard to type, stability, quality, and quantity, and is likely to have different effects depending on cancer type, stage, and treatment. Most studies to date have found positive prognostic effects associated with social support for cancer patients, but others have found no such association (35, 36). Maunsell *et al.* (37) studied 224 women with breast cancer over 7 years. Women who used two or more types of confidants in the 3 months after surgery had half the mortality of those who used no confidants. Marriage was also found to have a protective effect, as others have found for men with prostate cancer (38). Tominaga *et al.* (39) found being a widow increased the risk of death in breast cancer patients (hazard ratio 3.29), while having female adult children reduced the risk (hazard ratio 0.64). While most recent studies of the impact of social support on cancer have been careful to control for other demographic and disease factors, some are open to criticism for using multiple measures of social support without prospectively predicting which is expected to have the greatest effect on disease progression or mortality. Nevertheless, the literature to date does provide evidence that social support via marriage or other relationships is associated with lower mortality from cancer, as it has with other diseases.

6 Stressful life events

Interest in this area has been particularly stimulated by animal studies that have shown that stress in animals can hasten the onset of viral-induced cancer (mainly using susceptible mouse strains). Other studies have shown that stress can enhance the carcinogenic potential of several known mutagens in animal subjects. Animal studies demonstrating negative findings also exist and have shown that under certain conditions stress can reduce susceptibility or delay the 'take' of implanted tumours. Fox (40) has provided a critical analysis of both the positive and negative findings in animal studies.

Several human studies have shown an increased incidence of stressful life events preceding the onset of cervical, pancreatic, gastric, lung, colorectal, and breast cancer (1). Many other studies have failed to find any association between preceding stressful life events and cancer onset (1). Most recent studies have focused on breast cancer, using case control designs, and have both supported (41, 42) or not supported (43) an increased risk of breast cancer after stressful life events. Most studies have used aggregate measures of stressful life events; there are fewer studies of the impact of specific types of stressful life events (with the exception of bereavement as reviewed earlier in this chapter). Recent research has implicated involuntary job changes (44) and unemployment (45) as increasing the risk of lung cancer, and serious problems with work were found to be strongly associated with the occurrence of colorectal cancer (46).

A much smaller number of studies have examined the effect of stressful life events on cancer recurrence or progression. Most of the samples have been small and the results equivocal. Most recent studies have tended to be of breast cancer with no effect found of stressful life events on relapse or progression of breast cancer (35, 47).

In 1983 on the basis of the sum of human and animal studies, Fox (48) concluded that if stressful life events have an effect on cancer incidence, it is small. We believe that this conclusion is just as valid today, and applicable to effect of stressful life events on cancer recurrence or progression as well.

7   Behavioural mechanisms

If psychosocial variables influence cancer onset and progression, how are their effects mediated? Psychoimmunologic and neuroendocrine theories and data are discussed elsewhere in this volume. Behavioural explanations may also account for effects of some psychological factors on cancer development and outcome. The effect of some psychological factors on mortality (for example cynicism) may be mediated by smoking and alcohol (49), although such relationships are likely to be interactive rather than unidirectional (50). Failure to control for known oncogenic behaviours like smoking and alcohol is an important source of confounding, potentially magnifying or masking the real effects on cancer of other psychological variables. Psychological factors have been shown to affect whether and when patients seek medical attention for their initial cancer symptoms in some (51), but not all, studies (52). Cancer prevention is also influenced by psychosocial factors. In families with hereditary non-polyposis cancer, who are at elevated risk of developing colon cancer, barriers to acceptance of genetic testing were identified as the presence of depression symptoms and less education (53). This too may be a complex relationship, since offering genetic testing (for breast cancer) increased symptoms of depression from 26 to 47 per cent of those who declined testing (54) while reducing depression in non-carriers and leaving it unchanged in identified carriers. In older black Americans, better social support is associated with increased use of mammography and occult blood stool examinations (55). High anxiety has been directly related to poor attendance at a breast examination clinic and poor adherence to breast self-examination in high-risk patients (56). In medically ill elderly in general, patients' assessment of their quality of life is the most powerful predictor of desire for life-saving interventions (17). Depression and other psychological dysfunction has often been associated with non-compliance with treatment and recommended modifications in lifestyle across a wide variety of chronic medical illnesses. Psychological factors contribute to patients' choices of treatment options (57), which in turn impact on psychological status (58). Investigators should keep in mind that even what appear to be purely medical factors, for example oestrogen receptor status in breast cancer, may be confounded through associations with psychosocial factors such as age and stressful life events (59).

8   Clinical implications

Depression and anxiety remain common but often underdiagnosed and undertreated in cancer patients. We believe that the question of whether mood or anxiety disorders affect the incidence, course, or clinical outcomes of cancer has yet to be definitively answered by systematic research. Nevertheless, depression and anxiety warrant clinical attention because of their clear adverse effects on the quality of life of cancer patients. Behaviour with obviously harmful effects for cancer patients (smoking, alcohol abuse, non-compliance with treatment) should also be targeted for intervention.

Psychotherapeutic interventions may be of great benefit to cancer patients. If it is suggested, however, in an overly optimistic manner that psychological therapies will deliver cure or remission, there is a risk of deeply disappointing patients and their families and distracting them from the direct benefits of psychiatric treatment to enhance the quality of life. Psychiatrists and psychologists should keep in mind that psychosocial interventions are more likely to contribute to quality than to quantity of life in cancer patients. Psychiatric interventions are primarily justified if they reduce distress and dysfunction, such as when depressive or anxiety disorders are diagnosed in the context of oncological illness.

8.1   ALTERNATIVE THERAPIES

This book summarizes many intriguing findings on the relationship between mind and body in cancer. To most investigators, these relationships appear complex and resistant to facile explanation. This chapter supports a cautious, rational, and sceptical approach towards the clinical applications of this work. In contrast, a large and growing popular literature of 'mind/body medicine' or 'alternative medicine' has taken inspiration from the scientific literature and made the leap to specific interventions.

The popular treatments in existence propose to act on some or all of the psychosocial factors addressed in this chapter: affective state, coping style and personality, life stress and anxiety, as well as immune mechanisms. Full discussion of the popular literature is beyond the scope of this chapter. While these 'alternative' approaches may be helpful for some, their efficacy in combating cancer has yet to be objectively demonstrated. Some traditional psychotherapists have also encouraged high expectations. However, a prescription to change one's life or one's attitude is not without potential risks or harms. Foremost among these is guilt. Some patients may be led to feel responsible for their disease (or relapse) because they were unable to develop the 'right attitude' or personality characteristics to 'beat' cancer. People may feel an inordinate amount of responsibility to heal themselves, and may feel that they have not loved enough or visualized correctly if their efforts fail.

Another potential harm of alternative therapies is their pursuit in place of conventional medical treatment. This is less relevant in cases where conventional treatment also has little proven benefit (and unpleasant side-effects), but becomes a concern when patients forego effective chemotherapy, surgery, or radiation therapy. Similarly, alternative therapies may be counterproductive if they are used instead of potentially helpful conventional psychiatric treatment for treatable conditions such as major depression or anxiety disorders.

More subtle concerns arise when proponents of interventions that are appealing and benevolent make them universal prescriptions. A focus on personality change may provide a constructive form of redirection for one patient, while generating frustration and alienation for another. The scientific literature attempts to delineate various psychological factors and confounding variables affecting cancer, while the popular literature draws sweeping conclusions that generally ignore the differences. Clinicians should be open to discussing patients' reactions to the popular literature and to giving guidance and support on what may or may not be helpful to the individual patient.

Alternative therapies are now being studied to assess objectively whether they influence outcomes. One must be cautious in interpreting results of non-randomized studies, as alternative medicine is more likely to be chosen by certain patients. Contrary to expectations, a recent study found that among women with early breast cancer who had received standard therapies, those who also turned to alternative medicine were more likely to have depression, fear of recurrence of cancer, and more physical and mental distress (59). Thus, initial use of alternative medicine may be a marker of worse quality of life and greater psychosocial distress.

9 Summary

In summary, a number of studies have lent some support to the relationship between a variety of psychological factors and the onset, excerbation, and/or outcome of neoplastic disease. At the present time, no clear associations (let alone causal relationships) have been proven, both because of methodological limitations in the positive studies and because of other studies of comparable methodology that have failed to find such relationships.

Compared with other known risk factors, psychosocial factors may themselves (other than via cigarette smoking or alcoholism) make a small contribution to cancer onset and influence cancer progression. However, as the body of research has grown, the overall picture has become complex, and no straightforward relationships have emerged implicating specific psychological factors as oncogenic. Better, systematically designed research is needed to further elucidate the impact of psychological factors on cancer. Future studies will need to control for staging, the type of cancer and treatment, and confounding variables such as smoking, and other risk-associated behaviours. They also will need to include well-matched controls.

The gap that currently exists between our scientific knowledge base and popular beliefs about cancer onset and progression can be problematic for individuals with cancer and their health care providers. How can cancer patients distinguish between the popular ideas based on fact and those founded on myth? Are cancer patients responsible for their disease because they did not have the 'right attitude' or personality characteristics that would have enhanced their disease resistance? Does seeking a cure for cancer in 'love and miracles' complement or undermine standard cancer care? There are some beliefs that exist about cancer onset and progression that may not be empirically supported but that nevertheless can contribute to a patient's sense of wellbeing and control, while others may have an adverse impact.

While psychosocial interventions are more likely to contribute to the quality, rather than the quantity, of life of cancer patients, their proper scope of application remains to be worked out. Scarce resource allocation needs to be directed at psychosocial interventions that have empirical support. With the application of improved, systematic studies, it is hoped that we will obtain a clearer understanding of where resources should be directed in the future.

10 References

1. Levenson, J.L., Bemis C., and Presberg, B.A. (1994). The role of psychological factors in cancer onset and progression: a critical appraisal. In *The Psychoimmunology of Cancer* (eds C.E. Lewis, C. O'Sullivan, and J. Barraclough), pp. 246–264. Oxford University Press, Oxford.

2. McDaniel, J., Musselman, D. L., Porter, M. R., Reed, D. A., and Nemeroff, C. B. (1995). Depression in patients with cancer. *Arch. Gen. Psychiatry*, 52, 89–99.

3. Green, A. I. and Austin, C. P. (1993). Psychopathology of pancreatic cancer: a psychobiologic probe. *Psychomatics*, 34, 208–221.

4. Payne, D. K., Hoffman, R. G., Theodoulou, M., Dosic, M., and Massie, M. J. (1999). Screening for anxiety and depression in women with breast cancer. Psychiatry and medical oncology gear up for managed care. *Psychosomatics*, 40, 64–69.

5. Kissane, D. W., Clarke, D. M., Ikin, J., Bloch, S., Smith, G. C., Vitetta, L. *et al.* (1998). Psychological morbidity and quality of life in Australian women with early-stage breast cancer: a cross-sectional study. *Med. J. Aust.*, 169, 192–196.

6. Hahn, R. C. and Petitti, D. B. (1988). Minnesota Multiphasic Personality Inventory-rated depression and the incidence of breast cancer. *Cancer*, 61, 845–848.

7. Henderson, J. M. and Ord, R. A. (1997). Suicide in head and neck cancer patients. *J. Oral Maxillofac. Surg.*, 55, 1217–1221.

8. Middleboe, T., Ovesen, L., and Mortensen, E. L. (1994). Depressive symptoms in cancer patients undergoing chemotherapy: a psychometric analysis. *Psychother. Psychosom.*, 61, 171–177.

9. Van Heeringen, K. and Zivkov, M. (1996). Pharmacological treatment of depression in cancer patients. A placebo-controlled study of mianserin. *Br. J. Psychiatry*, 169, 440–443.

10. McGee, R., Williams, S., and Elwood, M. (1994). Depression and the development of cancer: a meta-analysis. *Soc. Sci. Med.*, 38, 187–192.

11. Penninx, B. W., Guralnik, J. M., Pahor, M., Ferrucci, J. R., Cerhan, J. R., Wallace, R. B. *et al.* (1998). Chronically depressed mood and cancer risk in older persons. *J. Natl. Cancer Inst.*, 90, 1888–1893.

12. Glover, J., Dibble, S. L., Dood, M. J., and Miaskowski, C. (1995). Mood states of oncology outpatients: does pain make a difference? *J. Pain Symptom Manage.*, 10, 120–128.

13. Covinsky, K. E., Justice A. C., Rosenthal, G. E., Palmer, R. M., and Landefeld, C. S. (1997). Measuring prognosis and case mix in hospitalized elder. The importance of functional status. *J. Gen. Intern. Med.*, 12, 203–208.

14. Callahan, C. M., Kesterson, J. G., and Tierney, W. M. (1997). Association of symptoms of depression with diagnostic test charges among older adults. *Ann. Intern. Med.*, 126, 426–432.

15. Ayres, A., Hoon, P. W., Franzoni, J. B., and Matheny, K. B. (1994). Influence of mood and adjustment to cancer on compliance with chemotherapy among breast cancer patients. *J. Psychosom. Res.*, 38, 393–402.

16. McDonough, E. M., Boyd, J. H., Varvares, M. A., and Maves, M. D. (1996). Relationship between psychological status and compliance in a sample of patients treated for cancer of the head and neck. *Head Neck*, 18, 267–269.

17. Lee, M. A. and Ganzini, L. (1992). Depression in the elderly: effect on patient attitudes toward life-sustaining therapy. *J. Am. Geriatr. Soc.*, 40, 983–988.

18. Takeida, K., Nishi, M., and Miyake, H. (1997). Mental depression and death in elderly persons. *J. Epidemiol.*, 7, 210–213.

19. Shekelle, R. B., Raynor, W. J. Jr., Ostfeld, A. M., Garron, D. C., Bieliauskas, L. A., Liu, S. C. *et al.* (1981). Psychological depression and 17-year risk of death from cancer. *Psychosom Med.*, 43, 117–125.

20. Garssen, B. and Goodkin, K. (1999). On the role of immunological factors as medicators between psychosocial factors and cancer progression. *Psychiatry Res.*, 85, 51–61.
21. Tross, S., Herndon, J. II, Korzun, A., Kornblith, A. B., Cella, D. F., Holland, J. F. *et al.* (1996). Psychological symptoms and disease-free and overall survival in women with stage II breast cancer. Cancer and Leukemia Group B. *J. Natl. Cancer Inst.*, 88, 661–667.
22. McDonald, K. M., Penberthy, L. T., and Levenson, J. L. The role of mental health status on patterns of cancer treatment (unpublished data).
23. Eysenck, H. J. (1994). Cancer, personality and stress: prediction and prevention. *Adv. Behav. Res. Prevent.*, 16, 167–215.
24. Classen, C., Koopman, C., Angell, K., and Spiegel, D. (1996). Coping styles associated with psychological adjustment to advanced breast cancer. *Health Psychol.*, 15, 434–437.
25. Grassi, L. and Rosti, G. (1996). Psychiatric and psychosocial concomitants of abnormal illness behaviour in patients with cancer. *Psychother. Psychosom.*, 65, 256–262.
26. Everson, S. A., Goldberg, D. E., Kaplan, G. A., Cohen, R. D., Pukkala, E., Tuomilehto, J. *et al.* (1996). Hopelessness and risk of mortality and incidence of myocardial infarction and cancer. *Psychosom Med.*, 58, 113–121.
27. Greer, S., Morris, T., and Pettingale, K. W. (1979). Psychological response to breast cancer: effect on outcome. *Lancet*, 2, 785–787.
28. Scheier, M. F. and Bridges, M. W. (1995). Person variables and health: personality predispositions and acute psychological states as shared determinants for disease. *Psychosom Med.*, 57, 255–268.
29. Greimel, E. R., Padilla, G. V., and Grant, M. M. (1997). Self-care responses to illness of patients with various cancer diagnoses. *Acta Oncol.*, 36, 141–150.
30. Prigerson, H. G., Bierhals, A. J., Kasl, S. V., Reynolds, C. F. III, Shear, M. K., Day, N. *et al.* (1997). Traumatic grief as a risk factor for mental and physical morbidity. *Am. J. Psychiatry*, 154, 616–623.
31. Martikainen, P. and Valkonen, T. (1996). Mortality after the death of a spouse: rates and causes of death in a large Finnish cohort. *Am. J. Public Health*, 86, 1087–1093.
32. Irwin, M., Daniels, M., and Weiner, H. (1987). Immune and neuroendocrine changes during bereavement. *Psychiatr Clin North Am.*, 10, 449–465.
33. Sachs, G., Rasoul-Rockenschaub, S., Aschauer, J., and Spiess, K. (1995). Lytic effector cell activity and major depressive disorder in patients with breast cancer: a prospective study. *J. Neuroimmunol.*, 59, 83–89.
34. Ell, K., Mishimoto, R., Mediansky, L., Mantell, J., and Hamovitch, M. (1992). Social relations, social support and survival among patients with cancer. *J. Psychosom. Res.*, 36, 531–541.
35. Barraclough, J., Pinder, P., Cruddas, M., Osmond, C., Taylor, I., and Perry, M. (1992). Life events and breast cancer prognosis. *Br. Med. J.*, 304, 1078–1081.
36. Bleiker, E. M., van der Ploeg, H. M., Hendriks, J. H., and Ader, H. J. (1996). Personality factors and breast cancer development: a prospective longitudinal study. *J. Natl. Cancer Inst.*, 88, 1478–1482.
37. Maunsell, E., Brisson, J., and Deschenes, L. (1995). Social support and survival among women with breast cancer. *Cancer*, 76, 631–637.

38. Krongrad, A., Lai, H., Burke, M. A., Goodkin, K., and Lai, S. (1996). Marriage and mortality in prostate cancer. *J. Urol.*, **156**, 1670–1696.
39. Tominaga, K., Andow, J., Koyama, Y., Numao, S., Kurokawa, E., Ojima, M. *et al.* (1998). Family environment, hobbies and habits as psychosocial predictors of survival for surgically treated patients with breast cancer. *Jpn. J. Clin. Oncol.*, **28**, 36–41.
40. Fox, B. H. (1995). The role of psychological factors in cancer incidence and prognosis. *Oncology*, **9**, 245–253.
41. Chen, C. C., David, A. S., Nunnerley, H., Mitchell, M., Dawson, J. L., Berry, H. *et al.* (1995). Adverse life events and breast cancer: case-control study. *Br. Med. J.*, **311**, 1527–1530.
42. Ginsberg, A., Price, S., Ingram, D., and Nottage, E. (1996). Life events and the risk of breast cancer: a case-control study. *Eur. J. Cancer*, **32A**, 2049–2052.
43. Roberts, F. D., Newcomb, P. A., Trentham-Dietz, A., and Storer, B. E. (1996). Self-reported stress and risk of breast cancer. *Cancer*, 77, 1089–1093.
44. Jahn, I., Becker, U., Jockel, K. H., and Pohlabein, H. (1995). Occupational life course and lung cancer risk in men. Findings from a socio-epidemiological analysis of job-changing histories in a case-control study. *Soc. Sci. Med.*, **40**, 961–975.
45. Lynge, E. and Andersen, O. (1997). Unemployment and cancer in Denmark, 1970–1975 and 1986–1990. *IARC Sci. Publ.*, **138**, 353–359.
46. Courtney, J. G., Longnecker, M. P., Theorell, T., and Gerhardsson de Verdier, M. (1993). Stressful life events and the risk of colorectal cancer. *Epidemiology*, **4**, 407–414.
47. Giraldi, T., Rodani, M. G., Cartei, G., and Grassi, L. (1997). Psychosocial factors and breast cancer: a 6-year Italian follow-up study. *Psychother. Psychosom.*, **66**, 229–236.
48. Fox, B. H. (1983). Current theory of psychogenic effects on cancer incidence and prognosis. *J. Psychosoc Oncol.*, **1**, 17–31.
49. Almada, S. J., Zonderman, A. B., Shekelle, R. B., Dyer, A. R., Daviglus, M. L., Costa, P. T. Jr *et al.* (1991). Neuroticism and cynicism and risk of death in middle-aged men: the Western Electric Study, *Psychosom. Med.*, **53**, 165–175.
50. Grossarth-Maticek, R. and Eysenck, H. J. (1990). Personality, smoking, and alcohol as synergistic risk factors for cancer of the mouth and pharynx. *Psychol. Rep.*, **67**, 1024–1026.
51. Vracko-Tusevljak, M. and Kambic, V. (1989). The significance of psychological factors in the early diagnosis of laryngeal and hypopharyngeal tumors. *Laryngorhinootologie*, **68**, 118–121.
52. Keinan, G., Carmil, D., and Rieck, M. (1991–1992). Predicting women's delay in seeking medical care after discovery of a lump in the breast: the role of personality and behavior patterns. *Behav. Med.*, **17**, 177–183.
53. Lerman, C., Hughes, C., Trock, B. J., Myers, R. E., Main, D., Bonney, A. *et al.* (1999). Genetic testing in families with heredity nonpolyposis colon cancer. *J. Am. Med. Assoc.*, **281**, 1618.
54. Lerman, C., Hughes, C., Lemon, S. J., Main, D., Snyder, C., Durham, C. *et al.* (1998). What you don't know can hurt you: adverse psychologic effects in members of BRCA1-linked and BRCA2-linked families who decline testing. *J. Clin. Oncol.*, **16**, 1650–1654.

55. Kang, S. H. and Bloom, J. R. (1993). Social support and cancer screening among older black Americans. *J. Natl. Cancer Inst.*, **85**, 737–742.
56. Kash, K. M., Holland, J. C., Halper, M. S., and Miller, D. G. (1992). Psychological distress and surveillance behaviors of women with a family history of breast cancer. *J. Natl. Cancer Inst.*, **84**, 24–30.
57. Margolis, G. J., Goodman, R. L., Rubin, A., and Pajac, T. F. (1989). Psychological factors in the choice of treatment for breast cancer. *Psychosomatics*, **30**, 192–197.
58. Lasry, J. C. and Margolese, R. G. (1992). Fear of recurrence, breast-conserving surgery, and the trade-off hypothesis. *Cancer*, **69**, 2111–2115.
59. Tjemsland, L., Soreide, J. A., and Malt, U. F. (1995). Psychosocial factors in women with operable breast cancer. An association to estrogen receptor status? *J. Psychosom. Res.*, **39**, 875–881.

4

Psychospiritual healing and the immune system in cancer

R. J. BOOTH

1 Introduction

'Psychospiritual healing' combines three terms often nebulously understood or at least interpreted in a variety of ways by different people. What is clear, however, is that when people use the terms 'psychological', 'spiritual', or 'healing', they are referring to aspects of human experience that are beyond purely physical dimensions. In order to discuss psychospiritual aspects of healing and the immune system in relation to cancer, we therefore need to address human experience. We will begin by considering something of the nature of human biological existence and then explore how a concept of 'self' emerges from the ways in which we interact in the world and make distinctions. This will lead us to a concept of body and mind as mutually influential domains of self-expression which are shaped by spiritual factors. Finally, we will discuss psychospiritual healing and its possible impact on cancer and cancer therapy and treatment.

2 The self-generating human

We humans, like all other living things, are biological entities. That means our physical forms consist of agglomerations of chemicals organized into complex, nested networks such as cells, organs, and organ systems. What is unique about living things, however, is not the chemical components of which they are made but the manner in which those components are organized. Sometimes we think of our bodies as complex machines but they are much more than that. Certainly our bodies contain many parts that operate in seemingly mechanical ways if considered in certain contexts, but there is a fundamental difference between living things and machines in the way they are generated and maintained. Machines are assembled and maintained from outside themselves (usually by people). In contrast, our bodies (and all other living things) constantly generate and maintain themselves. We can understand this most easily if we think of a cell. It is a bag of chemicals forming a network of chemical reactions that produce the very components of the cell itself. While it is living, a cell constantly takes in small molecules, incorporates them into its self-construction networks, and excretes other small molecules that it no longer needs. On a grander scale our bodies do exactly the same thing. They build and maintain themselves out of what we take in (food, water, air) and excrete what we no longer require.

This process of continual self-generation has been termed autopoiesis (self-poetry) (1, 2) and is a constitutive characteristic of all living things. Yet the autopoietic process of living always arises in a particular context or environment. A living organism and its environment are structurally coupled. Although they are separate from one another, they remain in intimate contact such that, as one changes, so the other changes and a mutually satisfactory relationship is maintained between them. This process, called adaptation, is a second essential requirement for living. Through their continually changing rebuilding process of autopoiesis, living things are able to maintain an adequately harmonious relationship with the environments in which they live. As environments change, living things change (or adapt) to maintain an adequate relationship with their environments. When they cannot do this, they die. Living, therefore, is an ever-changing process of self-renewal in relation to an ever-changing environment. It is a little like a surfer riding a wave on a surfboard;

always moving and rebalancing in order to maintain a satisfactory relationship
with the ever-changing wave.

3   Self and context

In order for living things to remain adapted to their environments they must
be sensitive to changes in those environments. Different living things do this in
different ways. For example, at a very simple level, many species of bacteria
are able to sense changes in the concentrations of chemicals at their surface
membranes and alter their structure accordingly. Sometimes these structural
alterations result in movement, and the bacteria can be seen to swim in a
particular direction in response to those chemical 'signals'. As humans, we are
sensitive to our environments in a wide variety of ways. For example, we are
sensitive to the temperature, pressure, humidity, and oxygen concentration of
our environment and 'automatically' alter the structure of our bodies as these
change. Sweating when our environmental temperature rises and shivering
when the temperature falls are adaptive changes in us that endeavour to maintain a relatively constant internal body temperature.

We also possess the five senses of sight, sound, smell, taste, and touch.
These allow us to respond to other aspects of our environment both automatically and voluntarily. For example, if our eyes sense an object approaching them
very fast they will trigger an automatic blink reaction to protect our eyeballs
from damage. Alternatively, if we see something terrifying we can voluntarily
close our eyes to shut out the sight but our bodies will also automatically
respond with changes in endocrine secretions, digestive system, musculature,
breathing, heart rate, and blood circulation. All these changes occur in a
coherent manner within us in order that we can continue to generate ourselves
as distinct entities and maintain an adequate relationship with the environment
in which we are living at the time. They help us to continue generating ourselves as separate from but in concert with our environments. This means that,
in its living processes, each living thing must generate some sense of itself and
what is not itself and, through autopoiesis and adaptation, maintain an appropriate boundary between that self and non-self. How is this achieved in the
human body and what coordinates the structural changes within us that occur
as a consequence of changes that we sense in our environment?

4   Distinguishing self within the body—the nervous system and the immune system

The sensory parts of our bodies are usually quite physically remote from some
of the parts they affect. Neither my feet nor my heart are close to my eyes and

yet if I see a child run out onto the roadway while I am driving, I will instantly step on the brake pedal and my heart will pump faster. This is possible because I have a nervous system. Nervous systems, therefore, serve to link sensory and effector parts of our bodies and to coordinate their activities. They act to maintain coherent relationships among our bodily components so that they all act cohesively. At the centre of the nervous system is the brain. This serves to modulate and moderate the connections between all the different parts of the body so that actions in response to sensed changes are appropriate with respect to context, history, and current bodily structure. In effect, the brain and the nervous system coordinate the autopoietic and adaptive processes in the living body to maintain a 'self' that is distinct from, but in adequate relationship with, its 'non-self' environment or context.

Because of the modulating and moderating property of the nervous system, both the manner of our sensing environmental changes and our capacity to respond to those changes alter over time and in response to circumstances. For example, when we first move from a light to a dark place we can see very little, but gradually, by reorganizing structural elements in our eyes and receptivity within our nervous system, our bodies adapt our visual acuity to the conditions and we begin to see in the dark. Alternatively, if we are awoken in the night by an unfamiliar sound, aural receptivity is instantly cranked up, we are fully alert and perceive the slightest tremors of which a few moments earlier we would not have been aware. Moreover, sounds that alert us in the middle of the night are irrelevant to us at other times and so they have little or no influence upon us. This highlights the fact that what we sense is always sensed in the context of our situation. Sensations affect our bodies according to their *meaning* for us. The manner and degree of structural change that take place within us in response to a sensation are determined by the relevance to our 'selves' of what we sense, and the contexts in which we generate and maintain the integrity of those 'selves'.

Furthermore, unless we have some means of sensing changes we cannot respond to them. Some environmental changes with the capacity to compromise our integrity are not readily detected by our traditional five senses. These include many microorganisms within our environments that we cannot see, hear, taste, or smell. Yet because of the nature and lifestyle of these organisms, if we had no means of sensing them they would readily be able to compromise our biological integrity. Fortunately, within our bodies we have a 'sensory system' receptive to such microorganisms—it is the immune system. The immune system is a network of organs, cells, and molecules that operates within our bodies by constantly monitoring molecular shapes (which we call antigens). As a whole, it can discriminate between shapes that are acceptable parts of our bodies and shapes that are not. When it senses unacceptable shapes it triggers a variety of mechanisms to limit, modulate, assimilate, or destroy the bearers of those shapes. We call these mechanisms immune responses. Thus, in discriminating between acceptable and unacceptable shapes, the immune system has the capacity to distinguish 'biological self' from 'biological non-self' and to take steps to maintain the integrity of that self.

As with all other sensibilities, immune sensibility depends on the context and history of the individual in which it arises. Our immune systems change as a consequence of what they are exposed to. Just as darkness leads to structural changes in our bodies that produce night vision, so exposure to the shapes of a particular microorganism (measles virus, for example) leads to changes in immune system structure that produce enhanced receptivity and responsiveness in future to those particular shapes, resulting in phenomena we call immunological memory and specific immunity. Also, because immune systems operate within living bodies, they are integrated with the myriad of other bodily processes. Of particular importance here is the relationship between the immune system and the nervous system. Given that both are involved in coordinating and maintaining integrity of 'self' in the context of 'non-self', it would make sense if these two systems were intimately connected with one another. That is indeed the case. When the immune system recognizes and responds to some foreign pathogen (for example, a viral or bacterial infection), it affects the operation of the nervous system in ways that facilitate the body's ability to recover from the pathogen. We experience these effects in a variety of ways that we identify as the characteristics of being unwell—increased body temperature (fever), increased propensity for sleep, decrease in physical activity, diminished desire for social activity, etc. Immune system activity affects the nervous system to alter the structure and behaviour of our bodies in order to promote recovery.

Conversely, changes that occur in our nervous systems also alter immune system behaviour. For example, when we are faced with an immediate threat of danger and need to take rapid physical action, many of the immune system's response mechanisms are transiently diminished in order to conserve energy for the more immediate activities required by the body. Thus, through a variety of connection pathways within our bodies, the nervous system and the immune system operate coherently with one another to generate and maintain the integrity of ourselves in relation to our environments.

5   Consciousness, self-reflection, and the mind

The environment in which we maintain the integrity of ourselves as humans consists of many 'non-self' things, both non-living and living. Particularly crucial among these are the other humans with whom we live. We maintain a complex network of relationships with other humans using our biological senses to coordinate our activities together in an intriguing way. This involves ascribing meaning to particular sensations, behaviours, and contexts, giving rise to the phenomenon that we know as communication. Communicative interactions are ways in which we coordinate our activities with other people.

As such, the meanings denoted by communicative acts must therefore be understood similarly by each party—they require consensual agreement. In order to develop such a consensus we have to live cooperatively with other people for some time so that we can develop and learn recurrent forms of meaningful interaction.

Over many millions of years of living cooperatively in this way, humans have developed a particularly rich communicative domain that we call language. Coherently with this process, the human body has evolved to facilitate ever more subtle and rich linguistic communications. We are born with an enormous potential for linguistic development and during early childhood we quickly learn to live in a language of consensual coordination with other humans. In fact, modern humans live so totally immersed in linguistic interactions with other humans that it is almost impossible for us to conceive of living in any other way. Three crucial related phenomena arise during this process; they are 'consciousness', 'self-reflection', and 'mind'. Let us briefly explore how this happens.

As children we learn to coordinate our living with others through a variety of gestures and indications. We learn to 'make sense' of particular sequences or patterns of behaviours and sensations, and to associate them with particular meanings. In doing so, we learn to distinguish objects and after a time we learn to distinguish one special object that we each call 'myself'. When a 'self' object arises for us, we become aware of it as distinct from 'other' objects—we become 'self-conscious'—and we conceptually associate it with our own bodies. Furthermore, we can reflect upon the distinctions we have made and become aware that the object we have designated as 'self' is also the very thing that is doing the distinguishing. We become conscious that it is 'us' who are paying attention to our distinctions and the meanings we are ascribing to them. That conscious, attentive process is something we label as 'thinking' (minding) and we create a conceptual object in which to locate it that we call the 'mind'.

Notice that all this arises in us in the context of our linguistic coordinations with other people. In learning to live in human society, we learn to ascribe meanings to forms of communication and we make sense of those meanings with relevance to our 'selves'. As we learn to live in language with others, 'self', 'other', 'consciousness', 'reflection', and 'mind' arise in us. 'Mind' and what we term psychological processes therefore evolve out of the ways we coordinate our living together consensually with other people. They depend on how and what we are biologically sensitive and receptive to and, like any other sensory perturbations, they modulate and are moderated by our bodily structure.

6 Body and mind—domains of self-expression

We have seen how, as biological organisms, we continually generate biological 'selves' and maintain them as entities distinct from the environments in which we exist. We have discussed how, as living things, we are sensitive to various features of our environments and how the structure of our biological selves alters and adapts in response to changes in those features to maintain an adequate relationship for living. We have also briefly explored the nature of the interactions that occur between humans living cooperatively in social communities and how a new domain of 'self'—the psychological self—arises through recurrent linguistic interactions. The psychological domain is clearly distinct from the biological domain. The psychological self is not the biological self but influences it. For example, when I see someone whom I love, many aspects of my nervous system and other parts of my body change as a result of the psychological meaning and value that such a visual experience has for me. The psychological domain provides a semantic layer conditioning my senses and modulating my biological response to them. We call this effect 'emotion'—a disposition of our bodies to act in a certain manner associated with a particular psychological perception. Conversely, the biological self is not the psychological self but influences it also. For example, when I have a respiratory infection such as a cold, I feel differently about myself and about the people I live with, and I perceive and interpret my world differently. The biochemical changes generated by my immune response to the respiratory virus alter my neurochemistry and so affect my psychological perceptual processes.

Biological and psychological are therefore distinct but mutually influential domains. The biological self is generated out of the biological processes that maintain a living body as distinct from but adaptively coordinated with its physical environment. Biological sensory experiences trigger changes in the structure of the biological body that maintain a relationship between the biological 'self' and 'non-self'. Those changes depend on the nature of the sensory experience, as well as the structure and history of the body at the time. In a similar manner, the 'psychological self' is generated out of the linguistic processes that maintain our identities as distinct from but adaptively coordinated with our social environments. Here, it is not biological sensory experiences *per se* that affect the psychological processes but the *semantic connotation of those sensory experiences*. These, too, are conditioned by the structure and history of the biological body of the person experiencing them, and also by the psychosocial 'structure' and history of that individual. Because of this, we can consider body and mind as distinct but interactive domains of self-expression that work in concert to generate that which we each discern as our personal identity.

7   Meaning, purpose, and existence—the spiritual domain

As we interact with the things and people about us, we generate a domain of experiences and perceptions that have meaning and value for us, both biologically and psychologically. Through these, we distinguish and express ourselves as unique individuals. Beyond these, as we reflect upon the flow and content of our lives as individuals and in concert with others, we generate a third level of self-expression—the spiritual realm. It is here that questions and concerns about the nature of our existence *per se* and the reasons for our experiences are embedded. The spiritual realm is where we make sense not simply of our sensations and perceptions, but of the patterns of our own life experience in the context of life as a whole. It gives ultimate meaning, purpose, and value to the uniqueness of our existence as individuals and to our place in the scheme of existence—human and otherwise. Religions and religious practices comprise some of the rituals through which we seek to structure our spiritual experience and share it with others.

Just as the psychological domain requires biologically sentient humans and arises out of recurrent linguistic cooperative interactions among them, so the spiritual realm requires self-reflective, psychological 'selves' and arises out of the social and cultural conversations in which they participate. Our participation in the spiritual domain requires us to be biologically living (i.e. biological beings), conscious of our selves (i.e. psychological beings), and conscious of our relationships with the people and things about us. Spiritual questions therefore pertain to how each person fits his or her individual existence and experiences meaningfully into a variety of contexts; the context of other human lives (present, past and future), the more general context of all living processes, and the overarching framework of existence as a whole.

8 Patterns that shape us—coherence among domains of self-generation

Each human life travels its own unique path shaped by an interplay of biological, psychological, and spiritual factors. At the biological level we have seen that we are all self-generating entities that maintain a dynamic relationship with our environments by continually changing our structure in response to environmental perturbations. At any moment, the options available to us for biological changes are therefore a consequence of our current biological make-up, which is shaped by our history of biological interactions and changes. Our biological selves are shaped by the patterns of our biological life experiences.

When we learn to generate psychological selves through the recursive processes of linguistic communication with others, we become aware of another journey—that of our psyches. Our psychological selves are moulded by our interactions with others and with the world around us and, in turn, shape the manner of those interactions. Moreover, because the interactions that generate our psychological selves require a biological body as a vehicle for their expression, our psychological selves are constrained and conditioned by their embodiment. What happens in our bodies affects us psychologically. Lose an eye and you see the world differently. Conversely, through the meanings and values that we attach to events and experiences in our lives, we generate emotions that affect how our bodies work. Emotions are the biological changes that arise as a result of psychological perturbations and they dispose our bodies to certain sets of actions. For example, I may become paralysed by an emotion of fear simply by imagining standing on the edge of a high cliff. Thus, through our psychological selves, we are sensitive to the linguistic domain of our social milieu. We are sensitive to the *meanings* that events, experiences, and concepts have for us. Consequently, those meanings have the capacity to affect our bodies through our emotions in ways that are very similar to purely biological sensory perturbations. Psychological processes also shape us biologically through interwoven linguistic and emotional processes.

The spiritual domain pertains to life's purpose. Yet before we can reflect upon the purpose of our lives we have to be self-conscious. This means that spiritual issues are predicated on the psychological domain and correspondingly will be influenced by psychological processes (which, in turn, are affected by biological processes). How we determine our spirituality, therefore, will be affected by our experiences of biological, social, and cultural milieux. Conversely, how we find meaning and purpose in the flow of our lives, and what things, people, and relationships are of value to us (in other words, our spirituality), will affect how we interpret our experiences and, accordingly, how we generate our psychological selves, and in turn our biological selves. The meaningful framework of our existence—our spirituality—modulates our psychobiological flow. In the words of David Aldridge: 'like a piece of jazz music, we are constantly improvised to meet the internal and external demands of our daily lives. Each of us has a theme that is our identity and a repertoire of being that we use to adapt biologically and existentially' (3). Thus, there is a coherence and interdependence among these levels of self-generation (4–6)—biological, psychological, and spiritual—yet we are truly aware of this only at the psychological level because it is only at this level that consciousness and self-awareness arise.

9   Psychospiritual healing—re-solving ourselves

Psychotherapy involves conversations between a therapist and a patient/client with the intention of understanding and/or altering aspects of the patient's behaviour or construction of his or her psychological self. Because each person is living in a biological body and because of the interplay between psychological and biological domains through language and emotions, psychotherapeutic conversations always result in biological changes; some relatively transient, others more long-lasting. Healing occurs when the patient recognizes changes that bring his or her life into alignment with what he or she considers to be a healthy existence. Healing, therefore, comprises a restoration of health and is dependent on the context of what is considered healthy. In some circumstances, certain behaviours, ways of thinking, or manners of living might be considered unhealthy, while in other circumstances they might be deemed healthy. For example, habitually having to undertake a long list of menial tasks might be seen as boring, futile, and soul-destroying by someone with other interests, while they might be perceived as essential, responsible, and life-affirming by someone devoted to a life requiring that kind of service.

What we experience as we live our lives and how we are sensitive to those experiences depend on our present make-up and on what has gone before. For example, when we label an experience as trivial, profound, ugly, or beautiful, we do so in terms of our particular sets of values, meanings, and perspectives that comprise our spiritual outlook. In other words, our spirituality determines our aesthetic sense—what we are moved by and how it moves us. It shapes and colours our relationships with the world beyond ourselves by affecting our linguistic and emotional responses to that world. In doing so, it also shapes and colours how we construct ourselves socially, psychologically, and biologically.

The spiritual domain, as a framework of overall meaning and purpose for the psychological and biological flow of a person's life, provides a container for the narrative through which each person makes sense of his or her existence. Because of this, psychological and biological events and experiences are ultimately interpreted in terms of a spiritual context. Indeed, whether overt or covert, there is a spiritual framework underpinning all psychotherapeutic conversations. Finding a solution to troubling aspects of life necessitates either removing or reframing them, or revising our understanding and construction of a life path and its dimensions of meaning. This is essentially a spiritual quest and so it is not surprising that willingness to address spiritual dimensions of cancer has been reported to enhance therapeutic relationships and the efficacy of psychosocial interventions (7).

10   A framework for integrating spirituality with psychoimmunology

Because the immune system within our bodies comprises a particularly significant facet of our biological self/non-self discriminatory capacity, it is often viewed as a system that not only defends us against external pathogens but also monitors and censors errant internal cellular behaviour (such as tumour cell development). Taken together with the extensive cross-talk between the immune and nervous systems in the human body, it is tantalizing to propose that psychological processes affect immune system behaviour to a degree that might influence the course of cancer progression and even cancer initiation. This proposition underlies much of the research into the psychoimmunology of cancer. To date, there are indications that the proposition has substance but with two caveats. The first is the difficulty of attributing causal factors in cancer initiation without undertaking long-term prospective studies.

The second concerns the problem of identifying immune mechanisms active in cancer and demonstrating that they are affected in relevant ways by psychological processes. Immune processes are many and varied, and what we observe as an immune response to a particular substance is part of the continuous self-evaluating and self-defining process of biological adaptation. While a variety of immune effector mechanisms have been shown to destroy cancer cells in culture, it has proven more difficult to demonstrate definitively that these effectors are instrumental in cancer recovery *in vivo*. Moreover, we are limited in what human immune material we can sample. Lymphocyte populations in blood, for example, are relatively easy to sample but comprise less than 10 per cent of the lymphocytes in the body and are not necessarily representative of the total lymphoid pool. Because neither the immune system nor immune function is a deductively determined process, some immune measures are highly correlated with one another while others are more or less independent. In addition to this, immunity is not a unidimensional variable and the immune system undergoes continual change. In effect, therefore, a change in any particular immune measure does not necessarily correlate with enhanced or diminished immunity as a whole, because there is no representative measure of immune behaviour. In fact, the notion of a representative measure of the immune system is essentially meaningless.

Bearing in mind these qualifications, how might we integrate spirituality with psychoimmunology? As we have discussed, the biological, psychological, and spiritual domains are interwoven aspects of human existence. Our biological selves can be considered to stem from our need to maintain our integrity in the context of an ever-changing environment. Our psychological selves, on the other hand, can be conceived as arising out of inter-human relationships mediated by our recurrent linguistic interactions. This identity is borne out of the social and cultural immersion in which we live and it conditions how we respond biologically to much of our sensory experience. The spiritual realm comprises that through which we make sense of our individual existence in terms of the ebb and flow of life events and the contexts in which we live. It shapes our experiences by assigning them value or meaning for us. It is through our spiritual perspective that we perceive the beauty and majesty and purpose in our world; how we apprehend that which is beyond ourselves. It governs our aesthetic sense.

In order for our lives to have coherence from moment to moment, there must be a degree of alignment among the self-generative processes through which we construct ourselves in the biological, psychological, and spiritual domains such that they are in purposeful harmony with one another; they are

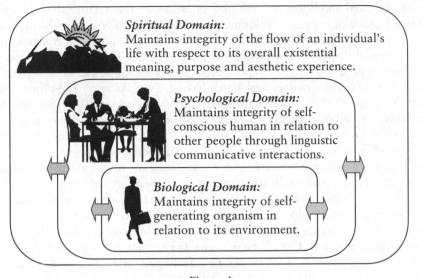

Spiritual Domain:
Maintains integrity of the flow of an individual's life with respect to its overall existential meaning, purpose and aesthetic experience.

Psychological Domain:
Maintains integrity of self-conscious human in relation to other people through linguistic communicative interactions.

Biological Domain:
Maintains integrity of self-generating organism in relation to its environment.

Figure 1

teleologically coherent (4–6). Given that the spiritual domain could be regarded as a superset of the other two (see Figure 1), the manner of relationship between our psychological and biological domains is shaped by spiritual considerations. Our spiritual perspectives give our experiences particular aesthetic values that modulate the manner in which our languaging and emotioning are braided. By articulating ultimate value, meaning, and purpose within a human life, the spiritual realm provides a form or framework for psychoimmune self-expression. In effect, the interactions between psychological and immune processes are constrained to be consistent with the dimensions of meaning and purpose that a person might identify within his or her spiritual domain. Some spiritual perspectives may promote healing, while others may impede it in some people. As a consequence, recognizing the pivotal nature of an individual's spiritual concerns might be a most effective means of influencing the psychoimmune axis in cancer.

11 Psychospiritual disharmony and cancer

If the manner in which our psychology and biology are affected by events in our lives is conditioned by spiritual factors then it is conceivable that these factors might also influence the development and course of illness. As will be discussed in the next section, evidence is accumulating that spiritual factors can have a profound impact on the health and possibly the longevity of people with cancer. This suggests that the course of the illness is amenable to psychospiritual modification, but the question of the relationship between spiritual issues and cancer development is much less readily answerable. During the 1980s there was considerable interest in the possibility of a constellation of personality factors predisposing people to cancer. This so-called 'Type C' or cancer-prone personality represented the polar opposite of the hostile, easily angered, competitive, and hard-driving Type A (coronary-prone) pattern (8). Type C people are characterized by behaviour patterns that include suppression of emotions such as anxiety and anger (9), being overly cooperative, unassertive, conforming, and compliant (10), and having a tendency to develop feelings of hopelessness, helplessness, and depression (11). It was suggested that people with these characteristics are 'pathologically nice' and live continually under stress as a result of the disparity between their outward appearance and their inner feelings. Consequently, they have constant autonomic arousal and concomitant immune depression, which weakens their natural resistance to carcinogenic influences and facilitates the development of cancer (12).

In essence, it is not Type C behaviours *per se* that are important here but rather the discrepancy between people's feelings and actions; a discrepancy between what is meaningful to them and how they consider they ought to act. In other words, a Type C pattern could be viewed as one in which there is a particular kind of spiritual disharmony in which the 'inner' self of an individual is in conflict with the 'self' whom they purport to live through and display to others in social interactions. Such ambivalent living would foster corresponding biological disharmony within the body of the individual. Moreover, if we accept that the immune system is intimately involved in generating and maintaining a coherent biological 'self', we might speculate that the physiological milieu characteristic of Type C spiritual disharmony would be one in which self-regulation would be difficult to maintain and, as a result, uncontrolled pathological growth (i.e. tumours) would occur more readily. Interestingly, a study of medical students 40 years after completing questionnaires about habits, emotions, and relationships revealed that those who developed cancer displayed psychological traits 40 years earlier characterized by a lack of closeness to parents and ambivalent attitudes to life and human relationships (13).

Today, there is less enthusiasm for Type C behaviour patterns as influences in the development of cancer, largely because of the paucity of supporting data due to the difficulty of proving causal associations without long-term prospective studies. Nevertheless, the concept is useful and can lead to powerful insights into what psychospiritual changes might need to be considered in the lives of cancer patients in order to arrest the development of their condition.

12   Spiritual factors in cancer therapy

The aims of cancer therapies, psychospiritual or otherwise, are threefold—remission of overt pathological illness, improved quality of life, and life extension.

While there is considerable optimism (14, 15) about the possibility of psychologically-based (i.e. cognitive behavioural, psychosocial, or psychospiritual) interventions positively affecting remission and life extension based on the findings of some research (16–19), other studies have failed to support this (20, 21). Also, for the methodological and conceptual reasons discussed earlier, ascribing the effects of any such interventions to beneficial changes in immune function is proving a difficult challenge. Although there is little direct evidence for a relationship between psychospiritual experience, immune changes, and cancer control (17, 22), a recent study hints at a relationship in HIV-infected people (23), giving grounds for further investigations in cancer patients. The study examined the relationship between religiosity and the affective and immune status of HIV seropositive, symptomatic gay men. There were two distinct aspects to religiosity—religious coping and religious behaviour. Religious coping (e.g. placing trust in God, seeking comfort in religion) was significantly associated with lower depression scores, but not with specific immune markers. On the other hand, religious behaviour (e.g. service attendance, prayer, spiritual discussion, reading religious literature) was significantly associated with higher T-helper-inducer cell (CD4) counts and higher CD4 percentages, but not with depression (23).

In contrast with the paucity of data relating psychospiritual factors to remission or life extension in cancer patients, there is considerable evidence linking spirituality and quality of life. Psychoeducational and psychotherapeutic programmes for cancer patients are well known to produce improvements in both mood and quality of life (24–26). Cunningham has organized the types of therapies into a hierarchy involving increasingly active participation, from providing information, through emotional support, behavioural training in coping skills, and various kinds of psychotherapy, to spiritual/existential therapy (27). He suggests that although it is the least studied to date, spiritual/ existential therapy can have the most profound effects on some patients (28). Part of the explanation for this may lie in the decreased anxiety reported to be associated with spiritual well-being in adults diagnosed with cancer (29). More broadly, it might benefit patients by helping them make connections among previously discordant aspects of their lives, making sense of their illness, and integrating their life experiences into a more coherent and acceptable whole.

Other facets of spiritual well-being such as faith, hope, meaning, loneliness, support, coping style, and the type of spiritual domain in which a person's spiritual experience exists are clearly germane to psychospiritual healing as well. Patients classified as intrinsically religious were found to have significantly higher spiritual well-being scores than did those classified as extrinsically religious (30) and high intrinsic religiosity was associated with hope and positive mood states (31). In a comparison of terminally-ill patients with either AIDS or cancer, AIDS patients reported significantly lower spiritual well-being than did patients with cancer and the best predictors of spiritual well-being overall were social support and loneliness, which together explained 47 per cent of the variance in spiritual well-being (32). Spiritual experience has been categorized not only as either intrinsic or extrinsic but also in other studies into three types: religious, existential, and non-spiritual. Chronically ill patients in the non-spiritual group reported significantly lower levels of quality of life than did patients in the religious or existential groups (33). A majority of cancer patients reported that their religious belief had been of support to them after they became ill from cancer and many patients viewed spirituality as a bridge between hopelessness and meaningfulness in life (34). Those who had found meaning in their disease thought they had a better quality of life than before the diagnosis (35). Using a brief spiritual beliefs inventory containing two principal factors, one measuring spiritual beliefs and practices, the other measuring social support related to the respondent's religious community (36), Baider and colleagues (37) found a significant positive correlation between spiritual beliefs and active-cognitive coping style in a group of cancer patients with malignant melanoma.

Moreover, the type and manner of spiritual experience affect its impact on cancer-related variables. In a comparison between Catholic and Evangelical Hispanic women in treatment for early-stage breast cancer, Alferi and colleagues (38) found that among Catholic women, greater religiosity tended to be associated with more distress throughout the year. In contrast, among Evangelical women, greater religiosity tended to be associated with less distress throughout the year. Religious coping tended to have divergent effects in the two groups as well. Among Catholics, church attendance at 6 months predicted greater distress at 12 months, while among Evangelical women, obtaining emotional support from church members at 6 months predicted less distress at 12 months (38). Another recent study assessed differences in how patients describe their spiritual or religious life in relation to their illness. Those identifying themselves as 'spiritual' described recovery and healing as happening *through* them whereas those identifying themselves as 'religious' were more likely to say it happened *to* them (39).

The importance of psychospiritual factors in healing is exemplified by what patients who survive cancer beyond a 'terminal' diagnosis attribute the reasons for their survival. For example, in one study of cancer survivors there were almost twice as many spiritual, attitudinal, and behavioural attributions as there were medical or treatment-related attributions. More than half the patients attributed their healing to a spiritual and existential shift in their perspectives about life (40). Another study reported that all long-term survivors of a 'terminal' diagnosis were actively involved in the healing process. Following diagnosis, survivors reported a strong incentive to make the changes that they thought were essential for continued life although the nature of these changes varied greatly (41). This suggests that patients must discover what is life-giving for themselves in a manner that is coherent with their own spiritual context. Thomas and Retsas (42) sum it up in discussing a grounded theory of the spiritual dimensions of people with terminal cancer. They suggest that patients with terminal cancer develop a spiritual perspective that strengthens their approaches to life and death. Moreover, the discovery of spiritual meaning through a process of transacting self-preservation incorporates three phases: taking it all in, getting on with things, and putting it all together. As people with terminal cancer move through these phases they generate self-preservation by discovering deeper levels of understanding themselves (42).

13 Summary

Does psychospiritual healing affect immune function and cancer cell growth? Clearly there are relationships between psychospiritual healing and unexpected recovery from 'terminal' cancer and there are some studies indicating associations with certain immune changes. However, there are few such studies and so the psychoimmune connections must be regarded as relatively tenuous as yet. Nevertheless, if healing is defined as becoming more aligned with what is considered to be a healthy existence, then psychospiritual therapies promote healing in cancer patients by facilitating 'peace of mind', diminishing fear and anxiety, and engendering hope, purpose, and meaningful existence. As such, therefore, they are of considerable benefit.

14 Acknowledgements

I am most grateful to Linda Cameron and Joanna Booth for helpful insights, discussions, and encouragement.

15 References

1. Varela, F. G., Maturana, H. R., and Uribe, R. (1974). Autopoiesis: the organization of living systems, its characterization and a model. *Curr. Modern Biol.*, 5, 187–196.
2. Maturana, H. R. and Varela, F. J. (1987). *The Tree of Knowledge: The Biological Roots of Understanding.* Shambhala Publications, Boston.
3. Aldridge, D. (1998). Life as jazz: hope, meaning, and music therapy in the treatment of life-threatening illness. *Adv. Mind Body Med.*, 14, 271–282.
4. Booth, R. J. and Ashbridge, K. R. (1992). Teleological coherence: exploring the dimensions of the immune system. *Scand. J. Immunol.*, 36, 751–759.
5. Booth, R. J. and Ashbridge, K. R. (1993). A fresh look at the relationship between the psyche and immune system: teleological coherence and harmony of purpose. *Adv. Mind Body Med.*, 9, 4–23.
6. Booth, R. (1996). New directions in psychoneuroimmunology. *Adv. Mind Body Med.*, 12, 12–16.

7. Potts, R. G. (1996). Spirituality and the experience of cancer in an African-American community: implications for psychosocial oncology. *J. Psychosoc. Oncol.*, **14**, 1–19.
8. Temoshok, L. (1987). Personality, coping style, emotion and cancer: towards an integrative model. *Cancer Surv.*, **6**, 545–567.
9. Greer, S. and Watson, M. (1985). Towards a psychobiological model of cancer: psychological considerations. *Soc. Sci. Med.*, **20**, 773–777.
10. Baltrusch, H. J., Stangel, W., and Waltz, M. E. (1988). Cancer from the bio-behavioral perspective: the Type C pattern. *Act. Nerv. Super.*, **30**, 18–21.
11. Eysenck, H. J. (1994). Cancer, personality and stress: prediction and prevention. *Adv. Behav. Res. Ther.*, **16**, 167–215.
12. Baltrusch, H. J., Stangel, W., and Titze, I. (1991). Stress, cancer and immunity. New developments in biopsychosocial and psychoneuroimmunologic research. *Acta Neurol.*, **13**, 315–327.
13. Thomas, C. B. (1988). Cancer and the youthful mind: a forty-year perspective. *Advances*, **5**, 42–58.
14. Spiegel, D. (1995). How do you feel about cancer now? Survival and psychosocial support. *Public Health Rep.*, **110**, 298–300.
15. Spiegel, D. *et al.* (1998). Effects of psychosocial treatment in prolonging cancer survival may be mediated by neuroimmune pathways. *Ann. N. Y. Acad. Sci.*, **840**, 674–683.
16. Spiegel, D. *et al.* (1989). Effect of psychosocial treatment on survival of patients with metastatic breast cancer. *Lancet*, **2**, 888–891.
17. Fawzy, F. I. *et al.* (1990). A structured psychiatric intervention for cancer patients. II. Changes over time in immunological measures. *Arch. Gen. Psychiatry*, **47**, 729–735.
18. Fawzy, F. I. (1995). A short-term psychoeducational intervention for patients newly diagnosed with cancer. *Support. Care Cancer*, **3**, 235–238.
19. Maunsell, E., Brisson, J., and Deschenes, L. (1995). Social support and survival among women with breast cancer. *Cancer*, **76**, 631–637.
20. Gellert, G. A., Maxwell, R. M., and Siegel, B. S. (1993). Survival of breast cancer patients receiving adjunctive psychosocial support therapy: a 10 year follow-up study. *J. Clin. Oncol.*, **11**, 66–69.
21. Cunningham, A. J. *et al.* (1998). A randomized controlled trial of the effects of group psychological therapy on survival in women with metastatic breast cancer. *Psycho-Oncology*, **7**, 508–517.
22. Richardson, M. A. *et al.* (1997). Coping, life attitudes, and immune responses to imagery and group support after breast cancer treatment. *Altern. Ther. Health Med.*, **3**, 62–70.
23. Woods, T. E. *et al.* (1999). Religiosity is associated with affective and immune status in symptomatic HIV-infected gay men. *J. Psychosom. Res.*, **46**, 165–176.
24. Cunningham, A. J. *et al.* (1995). A randomised comparison of two forms of a brief, group, psychoeducational program for cancer patients: weekly sessions versus a 'weekend intensive'. *Int. J. Psychiatry Med.*, **25**, 173–189.
25. Spiegel, D. (1995). Essentials of psychotherapeutic intervention for cancer patients. *Support. Care Cancer*, **3**, 252–256.
26. Spiegel, D. (1997). Psychosocial aspects of breast cancer treatment. *Semin. Oncol.*, **24**, S1–47.

27. Cunningham, A. J. (1995). Group psychological therapy for cancer patients. A brief discussion of indications for its use, and the range of interventions available. *Support. Care Cancer*, **3**, 244–247.

28. Cunningham, A. J. and Edmonds, C. V. (1996). Group psychological therapy for cancer patients: a point of view, and discussion of the hierarchy of options. *Int. J. Psychiatry Med.*, **26**, 51–82.

29. Kaczorowski, J. M. (1989). Spiritual well-being and anxiety in adults diagnosed with cancer. *Hospice J.*, **5**, 105–116.

30. Mickley, J. R., Soeken, K., and Belcher, A. (1992). Spiritual well-being, religiousness and hope among women with breast cancer. *Image J. Nurs. Sch.*, **24**, 267–272.

31. Fehring, R. J., Miller, J. F., and Shaw, C. (1997). Spiritual well-being, religiosity, hope, depression, and other mood states in elderly people coping with cancer. *Oncol. Nurs. Forum*, **24**, 663–671.

32. Pace, J. C. and Stables, J. L. (1997). Correlates of spiritual well-being in terminally ill persons with AIDS and terminally ill persons with cancer. *J. Assoc. Nurs. AIDS Care*, **8**, 31–42.

33. Riley, B. B. *et al.* (1998). Types of spiritual well-being among persons with chronic illness: their relation to various forms of quality of life. *Arch. Phys. Med. Rehabil.*, **79**, 258–264.

34. Ringdal, G. I. (1996). Religiosity, quality of life and survival in cancer patients. *Soc. Indicators Res.*, **38**, 193–211.

35. Fryback, P. B. and Reinert, B. R. (1999). Spirituality and people with potentially fatal diagnoses. *Nurs. Forum*, **34**, 13–22.

36. Holland, J. C. *et al.* (1998). A brief spiritual beliefs inventory for use in quality of life research in life-threatening illness. *Psycho-Oncology*, **7**, 460–469.

37. Baider, L. *et al.* (1999). The role of religious and spiritual beliefs in coping with malignant melanoma: an Israeli sample. *Psycho-Oncology*, **8**, 27–35.

38. Alferi, S. M. *et al.* (1999). Religiosity, religious coping, and distress: a prospective study of Catholic and Evangelical Hispanic women in treatment for early-stage breast cancer. *J. Health Psychol.*, **4**, 343–356.

39. Woods, T. E. and Ironson, G. H. (1999). Religion and spirituality in the face of illness: how cancer, cardiac, and HIV patients describe their spirituality/religiosity. *J. Health Psychol.*, **4**, 393–412.

40. Berland, W. (1995). Unexpected cancer recovery: why patients believe they survive. *Adv. Mind Body Med.*, **11**, 5–19.

41. Roud, P. C. (1989). Psychospiritual dimensions of extraordinary survival. *J. Humanist. Psychol.*, **29**, 59–83.

42. Thomas, J. and Retsas, A. (1999). Transacting self-preservation: a grounded theory of the spiritual dimensions of people with terminal cancer. *International J. Nurs. Stud.*, **36**, 191–201.

5

Can psychosocial interventions extend survival? A critical evaluation of clinical trials of group and individual therapies

K. CALDE, C. CLASSEN, AND D. SPIEGEL

1 Introduction

Does living better mean living longer? A small number of studies published over the last two decades have examined the provocative question of whether or not providing psychotherapeutic support can increase survival time for cancer patients. While initially such an effect would seem implausible, it must be borne in mind that there are two components to the equation that can account for variance in cancer progression: (a) the tumour's characteristics; and (b) host resistance. The former is largely determined by genetic damage— the tumour's anaplasty, loss of contact inhibition, ability to induce a vascular supply, and tendency to metastasize. The latter involves the host's ability to respond to tumour invasion, including physiological systems subject to neural control. These include behaviour, adherence to medical treatment, and the endocrine, immune, and autonomic nervous systems. It is thus not entirely mysterious (if also not well understood) how participation in various psychotherapeutic programmes could affect survival time with cancer.

To date, five of eleven trials show such an effect, which is surprising given the inherent difficulty of conducting such studies and the low likelihood of finding such a pronounced effect of psychotherapy that it can be measured in months of survival. Below we review the strengths and weaknesses of extant studies, suggest commonalities among them, and pose questions remaining for future research.

2 Studies reporting life-extending effects of treatment

2.1 SPIEGEL ET AL.

In 1989 Spiegel *et al.* published a study examining the effects of group therapy on the survival of 86 women with metastatic breast cancer (1). Researchers randomized the women into either a treatment ($n = 50$) or a control group ($n = 36$), with all study participants receiving regular medical care.

The treatment group met weekly for 90-minute sessions for 1 year. The therapy sessions were co-led by either a psychiatrist or a social worker, together with a therapist who had breast cancer in remission. The researchers used a supportive–expressive therapy model, utilizing the creation of a supportive environment where participants were encouraged to face their problems, strengthen their relationships, and find meaning in their lives. More specifically, the group therapy content included: (a) building bonds of new social support, (b) venting emotions, (c) talking about how they were managing their treatment, (d) finding meaning in their lives through helping others, (e) facing existential concerns, including grieving the deaths of fellow group members, (f) improving support from family, (g) improving communication with physicians, and (h) the teaching of self-hypnosis for purposes of pain control (1, 2). A major purpose of the therapy sessions was to create a close-knit group that would serve to counter feelings of isolation. 'The group format also allows patients to give unique support to one another, providing an expanded social network, role models for coping with various aspects of the illness, and an opportunity to enhance self-esteem by providing concrete help to others in a similar situation' (2). Leaders kept members focused on issues central to their diagnoses of metastatic breast cancer, and on facing and grieving their losses.

Subjects completed a pre-randomization set of psychological inventories, as well as follow-up questionnaires every 4 months thereafter throughout the initial year of the study. The psychological tests specifically measured locus of control, mood (anxiety, depression, anger, vigour, fatigue, and confusion), self-esteem, coping responses, phobias, and a measure that describes a person's method of coping with problems (1).

The original intent of this study, when it was conducted in the 1970s, was to examine the effects of group therapy on breast cancer patients' quality of life. It was not until 10 years following the conclusion of the study that survival was examined. Spiegel did not expect to find a difference in survival time between the two groups. In fact, Spiegel's intent when examining the survival numbers was to discount the often overstated belief that the mind can influence disease and disease progression (3). He found no difference in survival time during the time of treatment. It was not until 20 months after the beginning of the study that there was a divergence in survival time; the participants in the treatment group lived, on average, 18 months longer than those in the control group, a statistically significant difference favouring the intervention sample. Researchers also found in the treatment group a significant improvement in quality of life, which increased steadily throughout the intervention and reached levels that were significantly different from the control group at 1 year. More specifically, tension-anxiety, fatigue, confusion, maladaptive coping responses, phobias, and depression decreased, while vigour increased (4).

It is certainly possible that the participants in the experimental group were a group of highly motivated subjects who took extra steps to ensure their prolonged survival. It is also possible that those in the control group were special in that they died at a faster rate. However, the fact that the study was randomized makes either of these two possibilities unlikely. What is more problematic is that the study was not originally designed to test for a survival effect, and the study's sample size was small. Study replication is necessary to confirm or refute its findings.

2.2 RICHARDSON ET AL.

In the 1980s, Richardson *et al.* (5) examined the relationship between treatment adherence and survival in 94 lymphoma and leukaemia patients. This prospective study examined how an intervention designed to increase adherence to medical treatment might also increase patients' survival time. Study participants were recruited using a cohort design, and were assigned to one of four groups—one control ($n = 25$) and three experimental groups ($n = 69$)—depending on the period of time when they were admitted to the study.

The subjects in the control group received regular care from the same medical staff providing treatment to the experimental groups. Those in the experimental groups were assigned to one of three groups: (a) an educational and shaping group ($n = 23$), (b) an educational and home-visit group ($n = 22$), or (c) an educational, home-visit, and shaping group ($n = 24$).

The educational component consisted of a nurse giving an interactive slide and tape presentation, including a description of 'the specific disease, its treatment, the expected side effects of treatment, and the patient's responsibility in compliance and self-care' (5). The nurse would stop the presentation at the end of each section to answer any questions the patient might have had, and to discuss the presented material.

The same nurse who conducted the educational presentation also conducted the pill-shaping component of treatment. This interactive process involved the nurse offering explanations of the medications, the patient repeating this information back to the nurse, the patient notifying the nurse when it was time to take his or her medication, and the patient assuming responsibility for self-administering his or her medication after successfully completing the other steps in the shaping process.

The home visit was conducted within 1 week of the patients' discharge from the hospital. The nurse helped the patient with a pill-taking schedule, designed to help the patient to remember to take his or her medication. The nurse also involved at least one family member in this process to help support the patient in his or her self-care responsibilities. Finally, a poster was left at the home to reinforce the educational component the patient previously received.

The psychological factors that the researchers measured were depression, locus of control, and coping. All study subjects were measured at baseline, and again 6 months later (6). Survival data were assessed 2 to 5 years after participants entered the study.

The results of the study indicate that treatment adherence, disease severity at diagnosis, and assignment to any of the three treatment groups were predictive of better treatment adherence, as originally predicted, as well as longer survival times. It is especially interesting that the intervention effects on survival time remained significant even after Richardson *et al.* controlled for treatment effects on adherence. Psychological measures showed no correlation with increased survival times (6).

Richardson *et al.* (5) speculated on the causes of this positive survival effect. An obvious possibility is that the participants learned other behaviours that may have enhanced survival, such as drinking plenty of fluids, keeping appointments, and going to the hospital for a fever or other side-effects. The experimental group participants also learned skills that may have increased their sense of control over their situation, reducing their levels of fear and anxiety. A placebo effect has been found to occur in other treatment compliance studies (7, 8), and may have been occurring here. Whatever the reason might be for the increased survival effect, this study showed that an intervention can have a positive effect on patient adherence behaviour, and ultimately on the patients' survival time, independent of effects on adherence.

2.3 FAWZY ET AL.

Fawzy *et al.* published a study in 1993 that examined the effects of a group psychosocial intervention on malignant melanoma patients (9). The researchers randomized the 68 participants with stage 1 or stage 2 cancer to either a treatment group ($n = 38$) or a control group ($n = 28$). The treatment group consisted of 7–10 participants who met on a weekly basis for 90 minutes at a time for 6 weeks. Attendance was close to 100 per cent. The sessions were co-led by Fawzy I. Fawzy, MD, a psychiatrist and director of the study, and Norman Cousins, a fellow researcher and adjunct professor at UCLA Medical School. The group leaders used a highly structured cognitive-behavioural approach, and included the four following elements in the group meetings: (a) education about melanoma and nutrition, (b) teaching stress awareness and stress management techniques, (c) teaching of coping skills, and (d) a supportive environment. Those randomized to control received the same medical treatment that the others received, which was surgical removal of their primary tumours. Some members in each group also had local nodes surgically removed.

Fawzy and Fawzy *et al.* (10) provided a structured intervention as described in their treatment manual. The health education component involves teaching about the specifics of melanoma, its treatment, and good follow-up routines. Patients are given information from the American Cancer Society and the National Cancer Institute. This information is discussed in the group sessions.

The stress awareness and stress management components are more involved. Participants are first taught how to identify sources of stress, and then how to identify their own physiological, psychological, and behavioural reactions to it. The group members learn how to manage stress by problem solving, changing their own perception of the stressor, and using relaxation techniques to change their physiological response to stress. Patients are encouraged to practice the relaxation techniques each day, as well as apply them in actual stressful situations.

Before presenting specific coping methods, group participants are taught the elements of good coping skills: optimism, practicality, flexibility, and resourcefulness. After this step the group learns about different coping methods, both beneficial and detrimental: active-behavioural, active-cognitive, and avoidant. 'The patients are then taught five steps of problem solving: relaxation, identification of the problem, brainstorming for possible solutions, selection and implementation of an appropriate potential solution, and evaluation' (10). Finally, the participants apply the skills they learned to specific situations.

The supportive environment element of the model underlies the entire intervention. The group has structured conversations about their specific situations in living with cancer, and they discuss various scenarios. As they do so, they share their feelings and their stories.

Five to six years after participants entered the study, researchers analysed survival data. Those in the intervention group were significantly more likely than control patients to have survived (3 vs. 10 deaths). Natural killer (NK) cell activity was also higher in those who participated in the experimental group, 6 months after the intervention, indicating that the intervention had a specific physiological effect on an aspect of immune function known to be salient to cancer.

Another predictor of survival was baseline scores of distress. Higher levels of distress were indicative of subjects' motivation levels, so that subjects with higher distress at baseline were actually more likely to survive than those with low distress, regardless of whether they were in the treatment or the control group. Those with strong coping skills at baseline were also in a good position to survive at the 5–6-year follow-up period, again regardless of their group. All of those in the treatment group measured significantly lower distress skills compared with those in the control group after the intervention, and these differences were even greater 6 months later (10). Fawzy *et al.* say that these results help us to understand why we must assess cancer patients' psychological state of mind at the time of diagnosis so that we can tailor their treatment according to their needs (9).

2.4 KUCHLER *ET AL.*

A randomized controlled trial conducted by Kuchler *et al.* (11) examined the effects of psychotherapeutic support on the survival of patients with gastrointestinal cancer. Two hundred and seventy-one men and women diagnosed with cancer of the oesophagus, stomach, liver/gallbladder, pancreas, or colon/rectum were stratified by gender and assigned to either control ($n = 136$) or intervention ($n = 136$) groups; those in the control group received routine medical care and those in the treatment group received psychotherapeutic support in addition to standard medical care. All were assigned to a surgical ward dependent on the characteristics of the cancer and received their care while in hospital.

Two therapists, one male and one female, were assigned to the treatment group. Both had been formally trained in behavioural and analytical psychotherapy and had considerable experience working in the field. In preparation for the study they received additional training in understanding the challenges specifically encountered by those with gastrointestinal cancer. The therapists were supervised by a psychotherapist who was not a part of the research team. The therapists' general goal was to offer support in order to help the patients cope with their disease and related surgery.

Each patient in the control group was assigned to a surgeon who was in charge of the patient's care. Nurses tended to the patients' general medical and emotional needs, helping them cope with their disease as well as their experiences at the hospital. If needed, some patients received physical therapy, and others requested the assistance of a social worker to aid them with discharge planning.

Patients in the experimental group received the care as described above as well as psychotherapeutic services. The intervention was provided during the hospital stay, both prior to and following the surgery, and was tailored to each individual following an interview used to assess the patient's disease, emotional and psychological status, coping skills, and amount of available emotional support. Along with establishing a supportive relationship with each patient in the intervention group, prior to surgery the therapists aimed to reduce the patients' anxiety and help them build hope and confidence. Post-surgery they offered 'support for coping with the psychological and physical consequences of surgery' (11, p. 324). They met with the patients once every two days, if not more frequently. The mean number of days spent in hospital was 27 for the experimental group, and 23.4 for the control group. Patients were followed for up to two years or until death.

It is important to note that during the post-operative period, by their own request, 10 participants in the experimental group were transferred to the control group, and 34 participants in the control group were transferred to the experimental group. Participants remained in their originally assigned groups for the analysis, which may have diminished the effects of the intervention.

At the two-year follow-up, it was found that patients in the experimental group lived longer than controls, and that females in the experimental group had an added survival advantage. Although the number of patients was too small to reach significant conclusions, it appears that those with cancer of the stomach, liver, and colorectal regions also tended to live longer. At the end of the follow-up period, 69 of the 136 experimental group patients, as opposed to 45 of the 135 control patients, were still alive. When genders were compared, 66 per cent of the women in the intervention group survived, compared to 41 per cent of the men; in the control group, 39 per cent of the women and 29 per cent of the men were alive after the two-year follow-up period. Kuchler et al. notes that the 'women in the study received somewhat more therapy in terms of frequency and duration' (p. 334), which may account for the gender differences. No psychosocial outcome data was reported.

Kuchler et al. speculates that the individualized nature of the psychotherapy may have reduced the participants' stress levels. As Fawzy et al. (9) theorize, reducing stress levels in cancer patients may enhance the immune system enough to influence survival in a positive direction. Kucher *et al.* also posit that the effect of the intervention may have been increased by delivering the intervention early in the course of the disease.

2.5 RATCLIFFE *ET AL.*

Ratcliffe *et al.* (12) examined the effects of hypnosis and relaxation training in patients with Hodgkin's disease and non-Hodgkin's lymphoma. Of the 63 patients that were recruited, the intervention group ($n = 36$) received relaxation training with or without hypnosis to examine whether or not chemotherapy side-effects could be prevented or ameliorated. Apparently the intervention was provided to the patients in groups but no additional information about the intervention is provided. All patients received chemotherapy appropriate for their diagnosis and controls were given an antiemetic review procedure to control for the effects of receiving medical attention by the staff. The authors do not indicate whether patients were randomized to each condition. Personality, anxiety, and depression scales were administered to patients for a 5-year follow-up period.

Hypnosis reduced treatment-related anxiety significantly, and relaxation training reduced nausea. Because the incidence of side-effects was low, so was compliance. Ratcliffe *et al.* were therefore surprised to find an effect on survival; those receiving the intervention had a 33 per cent reduction in the risk of dying by the end of the study.

3   Studies reporting no life-extending effects of treatment

3.1 LINN *ET AL.*

Linn *et al.* (13) studied the effects of counselling on quality of life, level of physical functioning, and survival time. One hundred and twenty men diagnosed with cancer were recruited from a Veterans Administration Hospital and randomized to a treatment ($n = 62$) or a control ($n = 58$) group. Patient diagnoses included a range of cancer types, such as lung, pancreatic, leukaemia, skin, lymphoma, and bone. All study participants had end-stage cancer, and had been given 3 to 12 months to live.

The therapists received training from Dr Kubler-Ross on working with dying patients, and also came to the study with experience in counselling the dying and working with hospice patients. They aimed to establish close relationships with the patients and their families. This closeness fostered open communication, which allowed the patients to trust their counsellors. The therapist helped the participants find meaning in their lives, share their feelings, plan for those they would leave behind at the time of their deaths, adopt a realistic view of their prognosis, and yet maintain a sense of hope. Most importantly, the therapist was intended to be a supportive presence, listening to the patient and serving as an understanding confidant. Members of the family would also take part in the counselling sessions when the patient chose.

The counsellors included in their assessment of quality of life 'depression, self-esteem, life satisfaction, alienation, and locus of control' (13). The five areas, along with a measure of functional status, were assessed at baseline, and then at five subsequent periods throughout the 1 year of the study.

At the conclusion of the study, no difference in survival between treatment and control groups was found. Functional status was also not affected, but quality of life did show a significant improvement for the treatment group. All the psychological areas improved in the experimental group compared with the control group, although the difference in depression only reached statistical significance during the third month of the intervention. Depression scores during the third and sixth month were moderately correlated with death during the subsequent follow-ups at the sixth and ninth months, respectively. Because half of the sample was composed of lung cancer patients ($n = 65$), researchers analysed this group separately. Although the numbers were smaller, the trends observed for the overall group held.

Linn *et al.* had hypothesized that if patients' quality of life improved, their physical functioning would also improve, resulting in increased survival time. However, their subjects' disease had progressed to the point where, as the researchers said, any psychosocial intervention would be likely to have little or no effect on the body. There was a high attrition rate throughout this study due to patient death, and, consistent with the initial prognosis, almost the entire sample died within the initial year of the study. This reduced the likelihood of any possible intervention effect on survival time.

3.2 GELLERT *ET AL.*

Gellert *et al.* (14) examined the effects of a psychosocial treatment developed by Bernard Siegel on the survival rate of breast cancer patients. One hundred and two cancer patients who took part in the Exceptional Cancer Patients (ECaP) programme were matched to 34 patients selected from local hospital tumour registries who had not participated in the programme. Patients were diagnosed between the years 1971 and 1980, and were followed until 1991. ECaP participants were matched to non-participants 3:1 on the basis of 'race, age at histologic diagnosis (± 2 years), stage of disease (localized, regional involvement, or distant), surgery (positive or negative history), and sequence of the malignancy (single primary cancer, primary cancer with one subsequent cancer, or secondary cancer with at least one previous cancer)' (14). The original study ended in 1981, but researchers extended the study another 10 years to assess survival data.

The ECaP participants met weekly in groups of 8–12 cancer patients for 90 minutes. Friends and relatives were invited to attend. The sessions were unstructured, but had the goal of getting patients to take control of their lives, accept responsibility for their disease, and still maintain a sense of hope. Specific activities included the use of mental imagery, meditation, and discussion of patient issues. The number of sessions attended by each treatment group participant varied.

The results showed no statistically significant relationship between ECaP participation and survival. The results held when comparing number of sessions attended. The only benefit that was detected was for women who entered the programme soon after diagnosis; however, the numbers of women in this category were too small to reach statistical significance.

Gellert *et al.* collected their death-rate information from the Connecticut tumour registry. Forty-six of the patients were not reported in the registry as deceased at the time of the latest follow-up in 1991. This could mean that the 46 subjects were still alive, but it could also mean that if any or all of them relocated and died in another state, the information on these participants may not have been included in the registry. This brings the final numbers into some question.

Researchers also acknowledged possible problems in drawing conclusions from a non-randomized study. The study participants self-selected to attend or not attend the therapy group, and therefore there was a bias in their selection. For example, those who chose to attend the group may have done so because they felt they were worse off. However, it is also important to note that the bias could have been in the opposite direction, favouring individuals with the motivation, energy, and resources to learn about and participate in the programme.

3.3   ILNYCKYJ *ET AL.*

In 1994 Ilnyckyj *et al.* (15) reported the finding of their study of survival effects of group therapy. This randomized, prospective study of 127 participants was originally designed to study the psychological effects of group therapy. The study was not limited by type of cancer, with the most common diagnoses among them being breast, lymphoma, colon, and ovarian cancer. After subjects were stratified based on gender, performance status, and disease status, they were randomized to either a control group ($n = 31$) or one of three treatment groups: (a) a group ($n = 31$) that was professionally led, (b) a group ($n = 30$) that was professionally led for the first 3 months and then self-led for the remaining 6 months, and (c) a group ($n = 35$) that was self-led for the entire 6 months. An additional group of 21 patients was later admitted to the programme and was assigned to the unled group for the last 3 months of the intervention.

The groups that had professional leadership were run by a social worker with experience in facilitating groups. However, the social workers were not told to structure the groups by applying any specific therapeutic model; rather, they were encouraged to give information and be supportive. For the group without professional leadership, a social worker attended the first meeting to instruct them on logistics and to let them know that they could do anything they wanted during the times they were to meet. All treatment groups met weekly for 60 minutes for 6 months.

The psychological instruments that the researchers used measured depression, anxiety, and locus of control. These measures were administered prior to randomization, and at regular intervals throughout the study.

This study did not produce any results that would indicate a survival effect from any of the treatment groups. Although many of the group participants reported enjoying the groups, no psychological benefits were found. Analysis was done with and without the group of 21 patients who joined the unled group for the last 3 months, but still no treatment effect was found.

Ilnyckyj *et al.* postulated a number of possible explanations for the negative findings, including the heterogeneous composition of the groups, the qualifications of the group leaders, the absence of the teaching of pain management techniques, and the high attrition rate (only 55 per cent of the original 127 participants completed the study). They noted that the highest attrition rate was in the group without professional leadership. They also noted that those who withdrew from the study had a poorer prognosis and disease status, and more advanced disease progression. We suggest that the high attrition in the unled groups may indicate that those participants were the most dissatisfied with the intervention.

3.4   CUNNINGHAM *ET AL.*

Cunningham *et al.* (16) conducted a study to examine the effects of a psychosocial intervention on mood, quality of life, and survival time of metastatic breast cancer patients. The 66 participating women were randomized to either a treatment ($n = 30$) or a control group ($n = 36$). All participants received routine oncological care.

The intervention consisted of three components: (a) 35 weekly group therapy sessions (with the option to continue for an additional 15 sessions) that combined supportive–expressive group therapy with cognitive-behavioural therapy, (b) a 20-week course of cognitive-behavioural homework assignments, and (c) an intensive workshop focused on coping skills, to be held over the course of one weekend. The sessions were each led by a psychologist with extensive experience in group psychotherapy and with cancer patients, and either a doctoral candidate or a social worker, both of whom also had many years of experience. Each group included approximately eight participants. The weekly group sessions consisted of mutual support, problem solving, facing the likelihood of one's own death and the death of other members, emotional expression, as well as a spiritual component. The average attendance was 21.9

sessions with a range of 7 to 50. The homework assignments consisted of monitoring and modifying maladaptive thoughts and behaviours and developing a more balanced lifestyle. These assignments were discussed in the group sessions. On average, 7.7 assignments were completed. In the coping skills training course, subjects learned relaxation, mental imagery for healing and stress control, and positive affirmations and goal setting. Nineteen of the 30 treatment group participants actually attended the course. Those in the control group also received the materials covered in the weekend workshop, which contained a workbook and two audiotapes with instructions in relaxation and mental imagery.

Participants were assessed on the following psychosocial dimensions: (a) mood disturbance, (b) quality of life, (c) functional social support, (d) psychological adjustment to cancer, (e) rational versus emotional defensive styles, (f) social desirability, and (g) defensive repression. Measures were administered at baseline, and at 4, 8, and 14 months following study entry. Survival was also assessed 5 years after the entry of the first participant.

Cunningham and colleagues found no effect of the intervention on either survival or psychosocial factors, with the exception of an increase in anxious preoccupation and a decrease in helplessness over time among the intervention group compared with the control group. A *post hoc* analysis showed that those intervention participants who also attended outside support groups showed significantly longer survival time compared to all other participants. The results of the study surprised the researchers, and they speculated on possible reasons for the negative outcome. They considered six different areas, including: (a) sensitivity of the instruments they used, (b) whether or not the specific population of patients could show gains on psychometric tests, (c) the competence of the therapists, (d) whether or not there were important differences between the two groups, (e) whether or not there was variation in treatment compliance, and (f) whether or not the sample was of adequate size to detect differences. The researchers concluded there may be a small number of highly motivated patients that make sufficient changes in their lives to ultimately effect their survival, and that a correlative experimental design may be needed to show any effect in this small group.

It is unclear how to interpret the results of this study. The psychosocial results showed limited benefit (a decrease in helplessness) and some detriment to participants (an increase in anxious preoccupation). There was no improvement in mood, quality of life or other, or social support. Although there was no survival advantage for the intervention group, a subset of participants in the intervention group who also sought additional therapy outside of the study were found to live significantly longer. Because this was a *post hoc* analysis, the findings should be interpreted with caution. However, one possible interpretation is that their intervention was insufficient to affect mortality rate but when combined with other unknown psychotherapies may have contributed to longer survival. Another possibility is that those individuals who sought additional psychotherapy were highly motivated and engaged in behaviours that enhanced their survival or they were healthier and therefore had the energy to pursue other groups.

As noted by Cunningham and colleagues, there are several differences between their study and that of Spiegel and his colleagues (1, 4). These differences are substantial and may account for the failure to find a survival effect. The intervention itself was quite different, consisting of a combination of supportive–expressive group therapy and cognitive-behavioural therapy, a 20-week cognitive-behavioural course, and a weekend workshop. While it is clear that these additional components were intended to strengthen their intervention, it is also possible that they did not. The group support was shorter—35 versus a minimum of 52 weeks in the Spiegel trial, although some individuals received 15 additional sessions for a total of 50 weeks. The shorter time frame might not be adequate to address the emotionally challenging issues faced by metastatic patients. Furthermore, the sample was smaller (66 vs. 86 in the original Spiegel *et al.* (1) study). A null finding in a smaller group than the original study leaves open the question of what would have happened in a larger sample. This limited power to detect a difference was further reduced by the fact that the control group was an active treatment group. This is likely to have diminished the effect size, and thus decreased the power.

Cunningham's report on survival may also be premature due to inadequate follow-up time. They report on survival 5 years after the commencement of the study, while Spiegel and colleagues' survival effect was found 10 years after the intervention (1). It also appears that the participants in the Cunningham study were healthier than participants in the Spiegel study. Four years after the study all control participants had died in the Spiegel study and at 5 years 20 per cent of controls were still alive in the Cunningham study. Given the better health of Cunningham's participants, this suggests that Cunningham might need to wait even longer than 10 years before determining whether there is an effect on survival.

A final notable difference is the context in which each of these studies occurred. The Spiegel study occurred at a time when psychosocial support was not readily available to cancer patients. Furthermore, the Spiegel study was not designed to assess the impact on survival and patients were not led to believe that the intervention might increase survival. The Cunningham study, on the other hand, occurred at a time of ample resources available to patients as was illustrated by the fact that approximately 25 per cent of the sample participated in other support groups. Furthermore, participants were informed that the study was designed to see whether the intervention would result in longer survival. It is possible that both the knowledge of the potential benefits of support groups and the accessibility of outside support groups resulted in more participants seeking additional support groups, thereby making it more difficult to show a treatment effect.

3.5 EDELMAN ET AL.

A 1999 study by Edelman *et al.* examined the effects of Cognitive Behavioral Therapy (CBT) on the survival time of women with metastatic breast cancer (17). One hundred and twenty one women were randomized to either control ($n = 61$) or treatment ($n = 60$) groups. The treatment component consisted of 8 weekly sessions and a family night. Three subsequent monthly sessions were designed to help participants maintain the skills they learned in previous sessions.

The group leaders in the Edelman *et al.* study were both therapists, at least one of whom was a registered psychologist and had a background in CBT; both therapists had experience working with cancer patients and leading groups (18). The intervention group met for twelve 2-hour sessions and consisted of 7 to 9 participants in each group (19).

Edelman *et al.* describe 3 main elements of the CBT intervention: (a) cognitive restructuring, (b) behavioural strategies, and (c) self-expression (19). More specifically, skills the women were taught included 'thought monitoring, cognitive restructuring, use of coping statements, effective communication, goal setting, and relaxation' (17). Participants were also given weekly homework assignments and discussed any questions that arose from the assignments during the weekly sessions. Homework assignments consisted of weekly thought-monitoring exercises and occasionally included exercises that focused on specific topics addressed in the group session. An educational component was included and addressed topics such as self-esteem and depression management.

Along with survival, mood and self-esteem were assessed and the medical status of participants was tracked. Questionnaires were completed at baseline, 3 months, and 6 months. Survival analysis was done between 2 and 5 years after recruitment, depending on when each participant entered the study.

No survival advantage was found for the intervention group. Both mood and self-esteem were reported to have improved immediately following the intervention for the treatment group, but the effects were not sustained at the 6-month follow-up. Further analyses were conducted to deal with the potential confounding effects of drop-outs and participation in outside groups. Similar to their original analysis, only medical prognostic variables predicted survival.

Edelman and colleagues consider some of the possible reasons for the lack of a survival effect. These include the timing of the survival analysis, type of intervention, length of the intervention and the lack of a sustained improvement in psychological outcome. They argue against the effect of any of these factors on survival outcome.

3.6 GOODWIN ET AL.

Goodwin *et al.* (20) conducted a multi-center trial designed to replicate Spiegel's study (1) described above. Although Spiegel *et al.*'s original research question focused on quality of life issues and only later examined the intervention's effect on survival, Goodwin *et al.*'s primary question was whether or not supportive-expressive group therapy prolongs survival in metastatic breast cancer patients; psychosocial status was a secondary outcome.

The 235 women who participated in the study were randomized to treatment ($n = 158$) or control groups ($n = 77$). All participants were determined to have at least 3 months to live. Those in the control group continued to receive standard medical care and educational materials. The experimental group received the same care and materials but also participated in weekly, 90-minute sessions of supportive-expressive group therapy for at least one year. The groups were led by psychiatrists, psychologists, social workers, or nurse clinicians, at least one of whom was female. The leaders were to follow the manual written by Spiegel *et al.* (21) and received training in supportive-expressive therapy.

At baseline and every 4 months thereafter for one year, patients' completed questionnaires addressing their mood states, pain and suffering, social support, and demographics. The medical status of each participant was also collected on this schedule.

During the 12-month follow-up period it was found that the women who were distressed at study entry and were in the intervention group were less distressed. It was also found that for those whose baseline scores of pain were high, women in the experimental group reported less of an increase of pain at the 12-month follow-up period. Self-hypnosis/relaxation exercises were part of the intervention, and Goodwin *et al.* speculate that this could account for these results; also, the group leaders discussed the benefits of pain management and encouraged participants to discuss pain management with their physicians.

Although the intervention was shown to have psychosocial benefits, no survival benefit was found for the intervention group. Goodwin *et al.* make the reasonable argument that given psychosocial benefits were detected, the intervention was delivered effectively. On the other hand, despite randomization, the treatment group differed from the control group by being significantly younger at diagnosis, more distressed at study entry, with more positive lymph nodes, more being progesterone positive and having received more adjuvant chemotherapy. Controlling for these variables did not affect the survival results.

4   A study looking at disease progression

4.1   DE VRIES *ET AL.*

de Vries *et al.* (22) conducted a study assessing the effects of psychosocial treatment on tumour progression. The purpose of the study was to investigate in a phase II study the effects of a psychosocial counselling programme on the disease progression in patients with advanced cancer. Although survival was not the dependent variable in this case, the aim of the study was similar to the above reviewed studies.

Ninety-six patients with a histologically confirmed diagnosis of malignant neoplasm and no options for further medical treatment agreed to participate in the study. Only 35 of the original 96 participants were included in the analyses. The other 61 patients were considered not evaluable, because they either withdrew from the study, their health deteriorated too rapidly, they died, they had tumours that were immeasurable, or they received some other form of medical treatment. The tumour sites with the highest incidences were colorectal, pancreas, stomach, and ovary. Participants were offered 12 weekly sessions of individual psychosocial counselling, each session lasting between 1.5 to 2 hours. They also attended a support group every 10 days, each lasting 2.5 hours. Partners of the patients were also invited to attend both the individual group sessions. Patients needed to attend a minimum of 12 sessions for their data to be included in the study analysis. Therapists were selected not by their qualifications in any specific treatment model, but rather by their maturity, experience, and ability to carry out time-limited psychotherapy with advanced-stage cancer patients. Supervision was used to align their diverse training backgrounds.

There were four overall themes in the programme: (a) helping the patients to experience their needs and to realize their aims and potentials in life, (b) encouraging active exploration of problems and helping them learn coping skills, (c) promoting autonomy while accepting social support, and (d) encouraging patients to express their feelings. The programme combined two therapeutic models, existential and experiential. The existential elements were said to be in line with the model used by Spiegel *et al.* (1). In the experiential model the focus is on the person's feelings, needs, aims, and potentials, which may eventually help the patient to become aware of inconsistencies between his or her cognitive and behavioural schemata and his or her feelings and needs. It is the hope of the therapists that awareness of these inconsistencies will bring about congruence. 'Central to the existential approach is the development of an honest, realistic and personal attitude towards one's life situation, including both what is happening now and how one chooses to live one's life in the future' (22). Patients are encouraged to face the likelihood of their own death. Also important in the group format is the promotion of group cohesion, which counters social isolation.

The psychological tests that the researchers gave the participants measured depression, loneliness, purpose in life, autonomy and social relationships, and locus of control. Natural killer cell activity (NKCA) was also measured. Participants were assessed at study entry, after 6 and 12 therapy sessions, and at 6 and 12 months following study entry. However, materials from the last two follow-up sessions were omitted from the analyses because the number of evaluable participants dropped too low.

In five of 35 patients, tumour growth stopped for a period of 3 to 9 months ($n = 4$) or 2 years ($n = 1$) during or immediately following therapy. Participants showed a significant increase in the purpose in life scores, although the magnitude of the increase was small. No increases in depression, locus of control, or loneliness were measured. There was no significant change in NKCA, and no significant correlations between NKCA and scores on any of the psychological measures. After a qualitative analysis was done, using questionnaires from all available interviews and session reports, it was found that the five patients with slowed tumour growth showed a good to excellent psychological change. They also showed evidence of having healthier coping styles from the start. Although the timing of the slow-down of the tumour growth in relation to the counselling suggests that the counselling may indeed have had an impact on tumour growth, it also may have been due to spontaneous arrest.

The study is important to review because it assessed the impact of a psychosocial intervention on the body, and because disease progression is linked to survival. The outcome suggests that a mild therapeutic effect may have occurred. However, as stated by de Vries and colleagues, because this was a phase II study no conclusions can be drawn about causal relationships. Thus, we cannot classify the study as having either a positive or negative outcome, because no control group was used to compare against the treatment group. The number of study participants was also small. Given the study's method of research and the researchers' goal of measuring tumour progression as opposed to survival, it is difficult, if not impossible, to compare this study with the aforementioned studies.

5   Elements shared by the positive outcome studies

It is impossible to know with any certainty which elements of the studies may account for the different outcomes, whether it is a combination of elements that are needed to produce an effect, or whether it is some other variable that accounts for the differences. Nonetheless, based on the research that has been completed thus far, we identify the shared aspects of the studies that showed a beneficial survival effect. Specifically we will look at (a) education; (b) homogeneity of the treatment groups; (c) the definition of the therapy; (d) the supportive environment; (e) the teaching of coping skills and stress management techniques; and (f) the psychosocial outcomes.

5.1   EDUCATION

In four of the five studies the participants learned behaviours that not only aided them in their treatment compliance but also were likely to have contributed to feelings of increased control. Information can be a powerful antidote to disease-induced helplessness, since acquiring information is among the top three priorities for cancer patients (2). In the Richardson *et al.* (6) study the educational component was very structured; patients were given information about cancer and were instructed in behaviours thought to help them with treatment compliance. The researchers speculated that the educational component, combined with the supportive aspect of the programme design, was indeed responsible for increased survival times in the treatment group participants. Similarly, in the Kuchler *et al.* study (11), therapists provided information related to the hospital, diagnostic procedures, and treatment issues (under the guidance of the primary surgeon). In Fawzy's study the group specifically learned about melanoma, nutrition, risk factors, and warning signs. They were also provided with booklets from the American Cancer Society and the National Cancer Institute on nutrition as well as the immune system (23). In the Spiegel study the participants learned from one another. Through talking about their experiences and encouraging one another to seek treatment, the participants learned effective coping skills and behaviours.

5.2 HOMOGENEITY OF GROUPS

The three intervention studies that used a group support model used assembled groups that were homogeneous for disease type (1, 9, 12) and two were homogeneous for disease stage (1, 9). Many group members in the Spiegel study reported that their friends and family had withdrawn from them because they were either afraid of catching the cancer or afraid of the strong anxiety associated with the death of someone close to them (4). Therefore, building relationships with those in similar situations may be extremely beneficial to the patient, and ultimately beneficial to their families and friends. One function that group therapy serves is to bring together a group of people who have something in common, helping them to feel less isolated. When treatment groups are homogeneous, the issues and concerns that they have are likely to be similar. For example, lymphoma patients tend to have more concerns about treatment and have a high level of concern about feeling different; breast cancer patients, on the other hand, tend to be focused on issues of sexuality and body image (24). If patients with these two cancers formed a support group, they may not find much in common with one another. 'Homogeneity contributes to the social support and group cohesiveness as the experience of women with recurrent and metastatic breast cancer is quite different than that of women with primary breast cancer' (25). Not only does a homogeneous group help to alleviate the feeling of being 'the only one', but it also helps participants to problem-solve with one another, learn from the experiences of others, and provide empathic support to other group members.

   The participants in the Gellert *et al.* (14) study had different stages of breast cancer, and friends and family were invited to attend the sessions; this could have affected not only the patients' feelings of emotional safety, but it also may have interfered with the focus of the group. In Ilnyckyj's (15) study, the group was composed of patients with a range of different types of cancers, limiting the similarities among group members.

5.3 CLEARLY DEFINED INTERVENTION

All the studies showing a beneficial survival effect used either a specific model to direct the content of the treatment (1, 9) or had clearly defined goals and treatment strategies (5, 11, 12). The Spiegel study based its intervention on Irvin Yalom's well-defined models of group therapy (26) and existential therapy (27). In the Fawzy et al. (9) study, the leaders applied a highly structured and manualized cognitive-behavioural model. In both the Richardson (5) and Kuchler (11) studies, the project nurses or therapists who met with the patients had clear agendas—regarding the information and support they were to provide their patients. In Ratcliffe's study (12) the goal of the groups was clearly defined as providing relaxation training either with or without hypnosis.

In the study by Ilnyckyj et al. (15) only one group had professional leadership, and the leaders were not trained to apply any particular therapeutic model. The Cunningham study, on the other hand, used well-trained therapists but applied an intervention that involved several components that may or may not have been well integrated or compatible (16).

Having a well-defined intervention is crucial when trying to replicate the study. When an intervention is ill-defined, it is difficult to identify the variables that may have come into play in the original study, making it impossible to duplicate those variables and include them in a replication study. Both Fawzy and Spiegel have created manuals that can be used to standardize replications of their studies (10, 21).

5.4 SUPPORTIVE ENVIRONMENT

In four of the studies the participants received support from group members, their leader, or both (1, 5, 9, 11, 12). (Insufficient information is provided on the Ratcliffe study for us to draw this conclusion (12)). This is an explicit component of the model Spiegel used, where patients give support to one another and the therapist serves as an additional source of support. Participants regularly talked openly about their feelings, and could even plan their memorial services with one another. Family and friends of the terminally ill tend to find this talk morbid, and downplay the seriousness of the illness (25). In the Fawzy study the therapist talked to the group specifically about the importance of having support structures in their lives (10). The patients quickly formed a cohesive group, and they received a great deal of social support; they were able to express their feelings freely to the understanding and sympathetic group (9). In both the Richardson (5) and Kuchler (11) studies the format was different. Although the patients did not have the support of a group, they received one-on-one attention from a nurse or therapist who had the explicit purpose of being helpful to the patients. In addition, in the Richardson study, several of the interventions were intensified by being conducted in the patients' homes.

These studies are in stark contrast to the Ilnyckyj *et al.* (15) study, which had one of the group leaders leave one of the groups half way through the intervention. The group without the leader did not have anyone to guide them in supporting one another in living with their disease. Also, because the groups were not homogeneous, they may have found it more difficult to find common ground on which to base their relationships and to offer mutual support. In the peer-led group there was also a high attrition rate which suggests that the departing members did not get the support they needed. In addition, their departure may also have been experienced as unsupportive by the remaining group members.

5.5 COPING SKILLS AND STRESS MANAGEMENT

Coping skills reduce harmful environmental conditions, enhance prospects of recovery, help patients tolerate and adjust to negative events and realities, and help them maintain satisfying relationships with others (25). In both the Richardson *et al.* (5) and Kuchler (11) studies the patients learned about their disease and how to treat it. This helped the patients cope with their fears and anxiety levels and increased their feelings of control. In the Spiegel study the patients learned coping mechanisms from one another. Group problem-solving reduced participants' anxiety levels and increased their feelings of control (4). Emotional expression was another way to cope with their distress, which served to help patients manage the intensity of their feelings. Lessons in self-hypnosis for pain control may have helped the patients endure difficult medical procedures, which in turn may have had an effect on their survival. For instance, Ratcliffe *et al.* (12) found that teaching hypnosis and relaxation to patients with Hodgkin's disease and non-Hodgkin's lymphoma had a positive effect on survival. In Fawzy's study the instruction in coping skills was more formal. After learning about different kinds of coping skills, they integrated them with their stress management techniques and applied them to specific scenarios. The stress management skills involved problem-solving, attitude modification, and relaxation exercises (23).

It is interesting that teaching coping skills was an explicit and major component of the Cunningham intervention and in the Spiegel study coping skills were not explicitly taught but instead were learned informally. This suggests that learning appropriate coping strategies may not be sufficient for affecting survival.

5.6 PSYCHOSOCIAL IMPROVEMENT

Three of the five studies that reported increased survival time also reported significant increases in quality of life scores (1, 5, 9). Unfortunately, the Kuchler (11) and Ratcliffe (12) studies do not report whether the intervention resulted in any psychosocial improvement. Although the studies by Linn *et al.* (13), Cunningham and colleagues (16, 28), Goodwin *et al.* (20), and Edelman *et al.* (18) found an improvement in quality of life among those who received the intervention, there were no survival benefits.

In Linn's study quality of life was improved (13). Although the participants in therapy did not live longer, the participants were all diagnosed with Stage IV cancer, and were judged to have between 3 and 12 months to live. Although counselling was shown to reduce their level of depression and sense of alienation, and improve their levels of life satisfaction, self-esteem, and sense of internal control (13), it could be that at this late stage psychosocial interventions have no effect on survival. This theory is further supported by the Spiegel study, where it was not until 20 months after participants entered the study that a divergence of survival time was found.

The Cunningham study showed limited impact on psychosocial variables and was not suggestive of clear benefits from the intervention (28). In the Cunningham study the intervention did not seem to improve the overall quality of life for the participants, and their anxiety levels were actually increased. This gives support to the theory that psychosocial benefits are necessary in order for survival time to be affected. Also, Cunningham reported that the patients' distress scores at baseline were low. If we accept Fawzy's theory (9) that baseline distress scores must be somewhat elevated for patients to be motivated to actively engage in their treatment, then we must consider this as another possible reason for the lack of a treatment effect in Cunningham's study.

Goodwin's study (20) demonstrated a reduction in distress and the experience of pain as a result of participating in the supportive-expressive group therapy suggesting they had an effective intervention. Nevertheless, they were unable to demonstrate a survival benefit. While there were differences between the treatment and control groups despite randomization, controlling for these variables did not affect the results, making it unlikely that they explain the absence of survival effects (29). It is possible that they were unable to replicate Spiegel's original study (1) because of cohort effects (29). There have been significant improvements in medical treatment for breast cancer and there is a much greater availability of psychosocial support than existed 20 years ago.

Edelman and colleagues found improvement in distress scores immediately after their brief cognitive behavioral group intervention compared to the control condition but these changes were not sustained at the 3 and 6 month follow-ups (18). The brevity of the psychosocial benefit calls into question the effectiveness of the intervention.

6   Possible mediators for psychosocial treatments

The general methods by which psychosocial treatments may affect disease course are improved patient self-care behaviour, increased patient compliance with medical treatment (5, 30), and influenced activity in biological pathways of disease and resistance (31). We have recently found abnormalities in the diurnal variation of cortisol among metastatic breast cancer patients that predicts early mortality (32). These patients show a loss of normal diurnal variation which involves a peak in the morning. Patients with shorter sub-sequent survival had either flat curves or peaks later in the day. These patterns were associated with lower natural killer cell cytotoxicity, and were associated with stressors such as widowhood, divorce, or sleep disruption. Creuss and colleagues (33) found that participation in group therapy results in lower mean cortisol levels among breast cancer patients. In a study of prostate tumour tissue, Feldman's group (34) identified a type of prostate cancer whose growth is stimulated by cortisol activation of androgen receptors. Thus there is increasing evidence that the hypothalamic–pituitary–adrenal axis as well as the immune system (and their interactions) may mediate stress- and support-related effects on cancer progression. These areas may be central to how psychosocial interventions may lead to a physical effect, and are discussed at length in other chapters.

7   Opportunities for future research

There is considerable opportunity and need to increase our understanding of the effects of psychosocial interventions. Currently, Spiegel and colleagues are conducting a replication trial of the Spiegel *et al.* (1) study. This study consists of a sample of 125 metastatic breast cancer patients (35–7). This trial is especially important in the light of the findings from the Goodwin group (20).

There remain many questions about the efficacy of psychosocial treatment, and before we can conclusively say that psychosocial treatment indeed prolongs survival, we need to examine a number of variables, including biological pathways, diet, exercise, cancer type, and demographics.

Further study of the immune, endocrine, and other potential biological mechanisms will help us understand how psychological treatment may affect the body and disease progression. Along similar lines, psychotherapeutic effects on diet and exercise may also tell us something about cancer and its progression.

Type of cancer may be crucial; for example, breast cancer patients and lung cancer patients may differ in the etiology of their disease, their psychological response to their condition, and their sociodemographic characteristics (38). Psychosocial issues specific to breast cancer are different from those for lung cancer, prostate cancer, or leukaemia. Furthermore, the tumours themselves differ, some being, for example, hormone sensitive (e.g. breast cancer).

Hormone-sensitive tumours may respond more to psychosocial interventions which could affect hormone levels although this was not bourne out in the Goodwin study (20). In addition, the fact that positive intervention effects on survival have been observed in lymphoma (5, 12) and melanoma (9) suggests that hormone sensitivity is not a necessary criterion (although these tumours may have some hormone sensitivity not yet identified).

Before we can conclude that psychosocial interventions extend survival in cancer patients, we need to explore these other areas and their associated issues. It may be that these different diseases require different kinds of psychosocial interventions, tailored to the unique needs of the participants.

Another complex area that needs further research is in the area of patient characteristics. Demographic variables such as age, gender, socio-economic status, education level, race, and culture could influence the efficacy of a psychosocial intervention. African-Americans have the highest incidence rates for cancer in the United States (39), yet there is a dearth of information available on effective treatments for this population. There is also sufficient evidence to indicate that certain groups are disadvantaged in relation to their access to preventive screening, treatment, surgery, and psychosocial interventions, including those who are poor, unmarried, living in disadvantaged neighbourhoods, non-English speaking, or non-white (40). While it is challenging to recruit subjects from various backgrounds, it is important that we strive to offer these interventions to all cancer patients. Whereas the subjects in the study by Richardson et al. (5) spoke either English or Spanish, and were mostly of lower SES, those in both the Fawzy and Spiegel studies were of middle to high SES and were English speaking. Therefore, it is important to apply the successful interventions to under-researched populations to determine whether or not group therapy would be as successful with them.

8   Conclusion

Can psychosocial interventions prolong life? There are currently eleven studies that attempt to answer this question. Although the results of those studies showing a beneficial survival effect are compelling, the literature is clearly divided, and we cannot yet definitively conclude that survival can be prolonged by psychosocial interventions. Replication studies must offer us more data by which we can make our final judgements. What the studies provide us with is useful information about what is likely or unlikely to produce a survival effect. Education, homogeneous groups, clearly defined interventions, a supportive environment, coping skills, and stress management may contribute to a positive outcome. The existing research suggests that an improvement in psychosocial outcome may be necessary before a survival effect can be found.

If nothing else, these studies have made the examination of the relationship of quality and quantity of life among cancer patients a respectable scientific question. They challenge us to systematically examine the interaction of mind and body, and to determine the specific aspects of therapeutic intervention that are most effective, specific populations most likely to benefit, and mediating physiological mechanisms which could account for an effect of psychosocial support on disease progression. Such research will help us discover with certainty the extent to which living better means living longer.

9 References

1. Spiegel, D. *et al.* (1989). Effect of psychosocial treatment on survival of patients with metastatic breast cancer. *Lancet*, 2, 888–891.
2. Spiegel, D. (1999). Psychotherapy for cancer patients. In *Efficacy and Cost-effectiveness of Psychotherapy* (ed. D. Spiegel). American Psychiatric Press, Inc., Washington, DC.
3. Spiegel, D. (1993). *Living Beyond Limits: New Help and Hope for Facing Life-threatening Illness*. Times Books/Random House, New York.
4. Spiegel, D., Bloom, J. R., and Yalom, I. (1981). Group support for patients with metastatic cancer. A randomized outcome study. *Arch. Gen. Psychiatry*, 38, 527–533.
5. Richardson, J. L. *et al.* (1990). The effect of compliance with treatment on survival among patients with hematologic malignancies. *Am. Soc. Clin. Oncol.*, 8, 356–64.
6. Richardson, J. L. *et al.* (1990). Psychosocial status at initiation of cancer treatment and survival. *J. Psychosom. Res.*, 34, 189–201.
7. Pizzo, P. A. *et al.* (1983). Oral antibiotic prophylaxis in patients with cancer: a double-blind randomized placebo-controlled trial. *J. Pediatr.*, 102, 125–133.
8. Epstein, L. H. (1984). The direct effects of compliance on health outcome. *Health Psychol.*, 3, 385–393.
9. Fawzy, F. I. *et al.* (1993). Malignant melanoma. Effects of an early structured psychiatric intervention, coping, and affective state on recurrence and survival 6 years later. *Arch. Gen. Psychiatry*, 50, 681–689.
10. Fawzy, F. I. and Fawzy, N. W. (1994). A structured psychoeducational intervention for cancer patients. *Gen. Hosp. Psychiatry*, 16, 149–192.
11. Kuchler, T., *et al.* (1999). Impact of psychotherapeutic support on gastrointestinal cancer patients undergoing surgery: Survival results of a trial. *Hepato-Gastroenterology*, 46, 322–35.
12. Ratcliffe, M. A., Dawson, A. A., and Walker, L. G. (1995). Eysenck personality inventory L-scores in patients with Hodgkin's disease and non-Hodgkin's lymphoma. *Psycho-Oncology*, 4, 39–45.
13. Linn, M. W., Linn, B. S., and Harris, R. (1982). Effects of counseling for late stage cancer patients. *Cancer*, 49, 1048–1055.
14. Gellert, G. A., Maxwell, R. M., and Siegel, B. S. (1993). Survival of breast cancer patients receiving adjunctive psychosocial support therapy: a 10-year follow-up study. *J. Clin. Oncol.*, 11, 66–69.
15. Ilnyckyj, A. *et al.* (1994). A randomized controlled trial of psychotherapeutic intervention in cancer patients. *Ann. R. Coll. Physicians Surg. Can.*, 27, 93–96.

16. Cunningham, A. J. *et al.* (1998). A randomized controlled trial of the effects of group psychological therapy on survival in women with metastatic breast cancer. *Psycho-Oncology*, 7, 508–517.

17. Edelman, S., *et al.* (1999). Effects of group CBT on the survival time of patients with metastatic breast cancer. *Psycho-Oncology*, 8, 474–81.

18. Edelman, S., Bell, D. R., and Kidman, A. D. (1999). A group cognitive behaviour therapy programme with metastatic breast cancer patients. *Psycho-Oncology*, 8, 295–305.

19. Edelman, S. and Kidman, A. D. (1999). Description of a group cognitive behaviour therapy programme with cancer patients. *Psycho-Oncology*, 8, 306–14.

20. Goodwin, P. J., *et al.* (2001). The effect of group psychosocial support on survival in metastatic breast cancer. *New England Journal of Medicine*, 345, 1719–26.

21. Spiegel, D. and Spira, J. (1991). *Supportive/Expressive Group Therapy*. A treatment manual of psychosocial intervention for women with recurrent breast cancer. Stanford University School of Medicine.

22. de Vries, M. J., *et al.* (1997). Phase II study of psychotherapeutic intervention in advanced cancer. Psycho-Oncology, 6, 129–137.

23. Fawzy, F. I., Fawzy, N. W., and Canada, A. L. (1998). Psychoeducational intervention programs for patients with cancer. *American Society of Clinical Oncology*, 396–411.

24. Harrison, J. *et al.* (1994). Concerns, confiding and psychiatric disorder in newly diagnosed cancer patients: a descriptive study. *Psycho-Oncology*, 3.

25. Leszcz, M. and Goodwin, P. J. (1998). The rationale and foundations of group psychotherapy for women with metastatic breast cancer. *Int. J. Group Psychother.*, 48, 245–273.

26. Yalom, I. (1995). *Theory and Practice of Group Psychotherapy*. Basic, New York.

27. Yalom, I. D. (1980). *Existential Psychotherapy*. Basic, New York.

28. Edmonds, C. V. I., Lockwood, G. A., and Cunningham, A. J. (1999). Psychological response to long term group therapy: a randomized trial with metastatic breast cancer patients. *Psycho-Oncology*, 8, 74–91.

29. Spiegel, D. (2001). Mind matters—group therapy and survival in breast cancer. *New England Journal of Medicine*, 345, 1767–8.

30. Kogan, M. M. *et al.* (1997). Effects of medical and psychotherapeutic treatment on the survival of women with metastatic breast carcinoma. *Cancer*, 80, 225–230.

31. Spiegel, D. *et al.* (1998). Effects of psychosocial treatment in prolonging cancer survival may be mediated by neuroimmune pathways. In *Neuroimmunomodulation: Molecular Aspects, Integrative Systems, and Clinical Advances* (eds S. McCann *et al.*), pp. 674–683. New York Academy of Sciences, New York.

32. Sephton, S. E. *et al.* (2000). Diurnal cortisol rhythm as a predictor of breast cancer survival. *J. Natl. Cancer Inst.*, 92, 994–1000.

33. Creuss, D. G. *et al.* (2000). Cognitive-behavioral stress management reduces serum cortisol by enhancing benefit finding among women being treated for early stage breast cancer. *Psychosom. Med.*, 62, 304–308.

34. Zhao, X.-Y. *et al.* (2000). Glucocorticoids can promote androgen-independent growth of prostate cancer cells through a mutated androgen receptor. *Nat. Med.*, 6, 703–706.

35. Classen, C. *et al.* (1996). Coping styles associated with psychological adjustment to advanced breast cancer. *Health Psychol.*, 15, 434–437.

36. Spiegel, D. (1996). Psychological distress and disease course for women with breast cancer: one answer, many questions [editorial; comment]. *Journal of the National Cancer Institute*, **88**, 629–31.
37. Koopman, C. *et al.* (1998). Social support, life stress, pain and emotional adjustment to advanced breast cancer. *Psycho-Oncology*, **7**, 101–111.
38. Compas, B. E. *et al.* (1998). Sampling of empirically supported psychological treatments from health psychology: smoking, chronic pain, cancer, and bulimia nervosa. *J. Consult. Clin. Psychol.*, **66**, 89–112.
39. Meyerowitz, B. E. *et al.* (1998). Ethnicity and cancer outcomes: behavioral and psychosocial considerations. *Psychol. Bull.*, **123**, 47–70.
40. Cwikel, J. G., Behar, L. C., and Zabora, J. R. (1997). Psychosocial factors that affect the survival of adult cancer patients: a review of research. *J. Psychosoc. Oncol.*, **15**, 1–30.

6

Psychological factors and cancer progression: involvement of neuroimmune pathways and future directions for laboratory research

B. GARSSEN AND K. GOODKIN

1   Introduction

Psychological factors may exert their influence on tumour processes through various pathways. One possible pathway is through an effect on health behaviour, and will be discussed in the next chapter. Another more studied, but not necessarily more likely, pathway is via changes in the endocrine and immune systems, and is discussed in this chapter (see also reviews in 1–6). The influence on the immune system can be exerted along two roads. One is directly via the nervous system; the second is through nervous system modulation of the endocrine system, which in turn can regulate immunological activities. In some types of cancer, especially breast cancer and endometrial cancer, tumour growth can also be influenced by hormone levels, which represent a more direct, potential pathway for the effect of psychological factors.

This broad outline of psycho–neuro–endocrine–immune–tumour (PNEIT) pathways was for a long time seen as an adequate explanation for the possible relationships between psychological factors and tumour initiation and progression. Nowadays, it is considered as too simple and in some aspects even misleading. The present situation is that the possible pathways can be described accurately, but that there is also more uncertainty than in earlier days about the clinical relevance of the model. This holds especially for the last step in the chain of physiological events: the supposed influence of immunological factors on cancer progression.

The PNEIT relationships, depicted in Figure 1, are complicated for several reasons. First, there is not one endocrine system, nor is there one immune system, but a multitude of interacting endocrine and immunological subsystems. Second, the response of immune cells to hormonal stimulation may vary, and depends on previous hormonal exposure of these cells. Third, systems on the various levels form complicated feedback loops. A well-known neuroendocrine feedback loop is exemplified by the influence of augmented cortisol levels, leading to an inhibitory effect on corticotrophin-releasing hormone (CRH) secretion from the hypothalamus. This inhibitory effect of cortisol is executed either directly on the level of the hypothalamus or via an effect on the hippocampus, and results in a decreased release of adrenocorticotropic hormone (ACTH), which in turn dampens the cortisol production. Immunological factors can also modulate the activity of the nervous and endocrine systems. Fourth, the role of endocrine and immunological systems will be different over the course of carcinogenesis; that is for initiation of cancer, growth of solid tumours, and metastatic spread. It will also differ, depending on the type of cancer. Fifth, a solid tumour may itself influence the level of activity of the endocrine and immune systems.

The relationships between the various steps in the PNEIT pathway will be discussed in this chapter. Less attention will be paid to the first steps, because they concern relationships that are well known or discussed elsewhere in this book, while we will elaborate more on relationships involving carcinogenesis

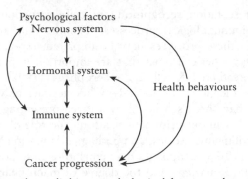

Figure 1 Possible pathway linking psychological factors and cancer progression.

and cancer progression. We will first discuss briefly why the immune system is expected to have an effect on tumour cells, and which immune cells might be involved.

2 Which immune cells might be important in cancer processes

The function of the immune system, relevant to this chapter, is to protect from pathogenic microorganisms and carcinogenic agents. The major way for immune cells to recognize a foreign cell or a host cell infected by viruses is by detecting deviant protein fragments (antigens) on their cell walls. This occurs through contact of immune cells with membranes of the foreign or infected cells, or through contact with specialized antigen-presenting cells (APCs), such as macrophages. All proteins of a cell, including antigenic viral proteins, are sooner or later broken down into their peptide fragments. These peptides bind to a site on so-called 'major histocompatibility complex' (MHC) molecules (in humans these are called human leukocyte antigens or HLAs). The complex formed by the peptide bound to the MHC molecule is then transported to the cell membrane, where it is presented to circulating lymphocytes. One type of 'cell killing' immune cells, the cytotoxic T lymphocyte (CTL)—an MHC class 1 cell—is activated by antigens that are thus presented on the cell membrane of an antigen-presenting cell. Other cytocidal cells, such as Natural Killer (NK) cells and macrophages, use different methods for detecting 'non-self' material.

Generally speaking, tumour cells are atypical cells and immune cells are expected to recognize and destroy such cells. Tumour cells may develop because of mutations in DNA sequences, defective repair of DNA breaks, or other DNA 'defects'. DNA 'information' is used in protein synthesis, and in the case of DNA damage, protein synthesis may be disturbed. Protein synthesis requirements may be exceeded or unfulfilled, or abnormal proteins may be formed, whose fragments might present as antigens on the cell membrane. In this way, tumour cells potentially form a target for cytotoxic T lymphocytes. However, the description of MHC-peptide presentation, recognition, and cell destruction applies to what occurs in normal immunological processes. Tumour cells are atypical cells and various steps in these processes may be impaired, especially the antigen-presentation process. Other cell types that are important in preventing tumour development and spread are NK cells and macrophages (7–9).[1]

Cytotoxic T cells (the $CD8^+CD11a^+$ T lymphocytes) are only able to destroy cells to which they have been sensitized by antigen-presenting cells, while NK cells can destroy cells without prior sensitization. The role of NK cells is more compelling in controlling metastases, and perhaps in initiation, than in containing tumour growth (10). Macrophages may constitute an important part of the tumour mass—up to a quarter—and the degree of macrophage infiltration of the tumour correlates directly with a favourable diagnosis (1). Some cytokines[2] may also play a direct role in the destruction of cancer cells, especially the interferons, tumour necrosis factor (TNF) alpha and beta, and interleukin (1, 2, and 12). Interferons affect tumour cells, slowing down the cycling time of cell division and altering the cell surface, leading to cell death (1). Other immune cell types that may be involved because of their modulating influence are T-helper (CD4 lymphocytes) and T-suppressor cells (CD8 and CD11a lymphocytes).

3   The influences of psychological factors and the nervous system on the endocrine system

The intricate relationship between the nervous system and the endocrine system has been unravelled since the beginning of this century. There is also a long research tradition which has shown that psychological factors can modulate the activity of almost all hormones (11, 12). Numerous studies have demonstrated that this in fact occurs continually in normal life, at least for CRH, ACTH, cortisol, dehydroepiandrosterone (DHEA), catecholamines (epinephrine and norepinephrine), prolactin, thyroid-releasing hormone (TRH), thyroid-stimulating hormone (TSH), triiodothyronine (T_3), testosterone, 17-beta oestradiol, growth hormone, endorphin, and enkephalin, which are most important in PNEIT relationships.

4   Influences of the nervous system on immunological variables

The discovery that the nervous system communicates with the immune system implied a major change in ideas about the control of this system. The earlier

---

[1] Monocytes circulate in the blood and are the precursors of macrophages, which are found in tissues.
[2] Cytokines are messenger molecules by which the immune cells communicate.

conception was that the immune system operates independently, while more recent discoveries indicated the potential of the immune system to adapt its activity level in anticipation of behavioural requirements.

One important step leading to this conceptual change was the neuroanatomical finding that nerves of the autonomic nervous system have endings in the lymphoid organs: the thymus, the spleen, and the lymph nodes (13). Next, it was demonstrated that the nervous system had the capacity to modulate the immune system's activity (14). Lymphocytes and macrophages have receptors that are sensitive to neurotransmitters and hormones, which allows the nervous and endocrine systems to communicate with the immune system. These neuroendocrine messenger – lymphocyte receptor interactions are not fixed, as receptor density of immune cells is variable and may change within a time span of minutes.

5   Influences of hormones on immunological variables

Hormones, especially hormones of the limbic hypothalamic–pituitary–adrenal (LHPA) axis, catecholamines, and endorphins can modulate immunological activities. The relationships between the systems are complicated. The diversities of the immune system and the existence of feedback loops between neuro-endocrines and the brain have already been mentioned. The lymphocytes themselves can also secrete neuroendocrines, which interact with neuro-endocrine receptors and with the brain. In addition, the magnitude and even the direction of responses of immune cells to a certain hormone depend on pre-exposure of these cells to other hormones.

The most intensely studied link between the nervous, endocrine, and immune systems is the LHPA axis. When this axis is activated, the hypothalamus produces CRH, which triggers the pituitary gland to release ACTH. ACTH in turn stimulates the adrenal glands to secrete cortisol. Although most of the effects of ACTH and its releasing factor CRH on immunity are mediated by the release of cortisol and its endogenous antagonist DHEA, both hormones can also act directly on the immune system (15). The predominant effects of cortisol on the body are immunosuppressive.

Activation of the LHPA axis accompanies both acute and chronic stress reactions, as well as major depressive disorder. The sympathetic adrenomedullary (SAM) system is shown to be more involved in acute stress reactions. One should realize that this is a schematic view, because both systems are often engaged in stress response patterns. The SAM system is engaged most strongly in connection with fear and anger, as well as other acute emotional states such as excitement, while activation of the LHPA axis is thought to occur during threats appraised as more overwhelming and that are less readily coped with (16). Activation of the SAM system may start with excitation of sympathetic centres of the brain stem and nervous outflow along the sympathetic ganglia.

When these impulses reach the medulla of the adrenals, catecholamines are released. Catecholamine release results in a redistribution of NK cells from storage pools (e.g. the walls of peripheral blood vessels) into the circulation—leading to an increase in NK cell count in the blood—an increase in suppressor T (CD8$^+$) cells, and a reduction of functional efficacy of T cells. Injection of norepinephrine has been shown to increase NK-cell cytotoxicity (16). The stimulatory role of catecholamines on NK-cell cytotoxicity has also been demonstrated in animal studies (17), although this is not always the case, particularly in the setting of chronic stressors (18).

The expected short-term immune responses to acute hormonal stimulation can be summarized as follows.

Acute (up to a few days) activation or subacute (a few days to a month) activation of the LHPA axis generally leads to a decrease in number of NK cells and cytotoxic T cells and to a diminished functional capacity of these cells.

Acute activation of the SAM system generally leads to an increase in number of NK cells and cytotoxic (CD8$^+$) T cells, an increase in NK-cell cytotoxicity, but a reduction of cytotoxic T-cell activity.

6   Influences of psychological factors on immunological variables

Research into the role of psychological factors in modulating immunological activity started some 35 years ago (19). The state of the art is described in several excellent reviews (16, 20–23; see also Chapter 2). Nowadays, most researchers no longer doubt the potential influence of these factors, but it is not firmly established how far-reaching these influences are on the immune system with respect to clinical relevance. The effects are generally modest, but psychological factors may play a decisive role in those whose immune system is already compromised, for instance because of illness, such as HIV-1 infection, or medical treatment, such as systemic chemotherapy.

Chronic stressor effects on immune *function* act mainly in a negative direction (suppression of activity), whereas the *number* of immune cells may be either increased or decreased (24). Psychological conditions thought to favour immunosuppressive effects are exposure to chronic stressful conditions, a condition leading to passivity and withdrawal, and a passive, avoidant coping style. Immunosuppression has, for instance, been found shortly after bereavement (18, 25), but also with milder stressors, such as during medical school examinations (22, 26).

The response to acute stressors, such as a public-speaking task, mental arithmetic, and challenging computer games, may be different from the downregulating response found in chronic stressors and in depressive disorders.

The response to such acute stressors includes an increase in NK cells and CD8$^+$ T lymphocytes, with proliferative responses to mitogens diminished (27). Because these acute responses start quickly—of the order of a few minutes— they are probably driven by SAM activation and not by LHPA axis activation.

Herbert and Cohen (24) presented an excellent meta-analysis of 38 studies on psycho–neuro–immune (PNI) effects of exposure to different types of stressors. Stressors could be acute laboratory stressors or naturalistic stressors, such as examinations, unemployment, divorce, and bereavement. Besides statistical significance, they also determined a kind of certainty measure. 'Not certain' (our term) means a marginal, though significant, effect that needs additional confirmation. Taking all types of stressors together, an immunosuppressive effect was found for most immune measures. The number of NK cells, B cells, total T cells, helper T cells, and suppressor/cytotoxic T cells decreased with stressor exposure. Selected immunoglobulin (antibody) levels may also be diminished (salivary IgA and serum IgM). However, as may be expected, antibody titres to latent viral infections (e.g. herpes viruses, such as herpes simplex virus type 1 and Epstein–Barr virus) rise.[3] Of the functional measures, the proliferative responses of lymphocytes to mitogen and NK-cell cytotoxicity was also diminished. The changes in enumerative measures were generally 'not certain', except for the decrease in suppressor/cytotoxic T cells and the increase in herpes virus antibody titres. 'Certain' effects were found for the functional measures: lymphocyte proliferative response and NK-cell cytotoxicity. (No effect was found for number of monocytes, total number of lymphocytes, the T cell helper/suppressor (CD4/CD8) ratio, and for serum IgA and IgG.) A direct comparison between short-term and long-term stressors was only possible for some immune measures. Whereas long-lasting naturalistic stressors (lasting more than a month) were associated with a decreased number of suppressor/cytotoxic T-cells, acute laboratory stressors showed an increase in their number.

Responses to acute stressors depend on previous stressor exposure, as was demonstrated by Pike *et al.* (28) in a study on healthy subjects. Number and cytotoxicity of NK cells were increased after the acute stressor (as were levels of catecholamines, cortisol, ACTH, and β-endorphin), but the magnitude of the response was different for persons having experienced many or a few chronic life stressors. The chronic stress group showed a greater increase in number of NK cells (and of epinephrine) and a blunted response for NK-cell cytotoxicity (and β-endorphin) compared to the control group (no difference for norepinephrine, ACTH, and cortisol).

---

[3] Common infectious agents, such as herpes viruses, can remain contained for long periods of time. When the immune activity is suppressed, one expects increased viral activity and thus more specific antibodies to such latent viruses (while levels of more general immunoglobulins, such as salivary IgA, are lowered).

7   Influences of hormonal factors on tumour development and growth

Certain hormones play a role in the development of cancers in organs whose cells have receptors for hormones and respond to hormonal stimulation by cell division. This is the case for the breast, endometrium of the uterus, and prostate, and hormone-sensitive cancers may develop in these organs. Hormones that stimulate cell division are potentially carcinogenic. These include somatotropin and prolactin, secreted by the pituitary; thyroxine, secreted by the thyroid gland; and oestrogens and androgens, secreted by the ovary, testis, and adrenal cortex. Glucocorticoids from the adrenal cortex and progesterone from the ovary, on the other hand, generally inhibit cell replication, although these hormones seem to promote cancer development and growth under certain conditions (29). Prolonged exposure to oestrogen is predictive of an increased incidence of breast cancer. Major risk factors for breast cancer are early menarche, late menopause, and having the first pregnancy late in life, which are all factors related to longer exposure to oestrogen and under-exposure to progesterone. The most important hormones in the neoplastic transformation of cells of the breast are oestrogen and prolactin, although a number of other hormones may also be involved, partly by their influence on immune functioning: progesterone, β-endorphin, ACTH, cortisol, and catecholamines (5).

8   Influences of immunological factors on tumour development and growth

Before an invasive tumour has developed, the entire process of carcinogenesis must have transpired, and the immune system will have different effects depending on the phase of carcinogenesis. The first phase of malignant transformation concerns one or some cells. After this initial phase, there is a phase of growth, leading to the development of a tumour, consisting of 10^{10} to 10^{12} cells. According to the 'immunosurveillance' hypothesis, an important function of the immune system is to detect and destroy these tumour cells.

This surveillance effect has been demonstrated in animal studies. In these studies, animals were first injected with killed tumour cells, which led to immunity against the tumour antigen. When the same animals were then injected with living tumour cells, no tumour growth occurred, in contrast to animals without earlier immunization. In humans, solid tumours are sometimes infiltrated with macrophages and lymphocytes, which also implies immuno-logical defence.

Immunosuppression will increase the chance for malignant cells to escape surveillance. Indeed, a higher incidence of leukaemias, lymphomas, cervical carcinoma, and melanoma has been found in people whose immune system is suppressed by drugs because of organ transplant. In general, the incidence is increased for cancers which are lymphoreticular in origin and of cancers associated with oncogenic viruses which are, presumably, held in check by an effective immune system (30). The mainly viral etiology of these cancers, however, may indicate that an anti-virus response is suppressed, rather than an anti-tumour response (31). According to this argument the role of the immune system may be unimportant in the initiation of these cancers, although it could still play an (additional) role in the development of virally induced tumours.

The value of the surveillance theory depends on whether tumour cells are capable of being recognized as foreign and a cytotoxic immune response induced. For several reasons, the role of the immune system in controlling tumour development seems, however, modest:

1. It has been demonstrated in animal studies that only cancers induced by viruses consistently provoke strong immune responses (32). On the other hand, spontaneously arising cancers in mice, which are likely to be more akin to many human cancers, provoke little or no immune response (33).
2. Tumour cells have a great capacity to mutate, which allows them to avoid destruction by discarding or changing their distinctive antigens. Also, the presentation of antigens (both general and tumour-specific antigens) to the T cells may be disturbed in cancer cells, resulting in a complete disarming of the T-cell defence against any potential tumour antigen. This happens, for instance, when the expression of MHC proteins is reduced, which occurs in many human tumours. The MHC proteins are necessary for the presentation of tumour peptides to the immune system. Tumour antigens can also be simply shed from the cell wall.
3. Tumour cells can directly suppress the efficacy of various immune cells (34).
4. A problem for a generalized immunosurveillance hypothesis is also that unusual types of cancers occur more often in patients on immunosuppression drugs, while the rate for the most common cancers (breast, colon, and lung) is hardly increased. The increased incidence of specific types of cancers following organ transplantation might be caused by a factor other than immunosuppression. The chronic presence of the allograft, with its foreign antigens, implies a chronic stimulation of the lymphoid tissue. This may lead to cell proliferation which can promote the development of cancer in lymphoid tissue. Indeed, animal studies have shown that repeated administration of foreign antigens causes an increased incidence of malignant lymphomas.

There are other reasons why specific tumours sometimes evade an immune response. For instance, immune reactions are less effective in the brain, where the level of immunological monitoring is low. Also, a dense tumour stroma consisting of connective tissue can shield tumour cells from immune recognition and destruction. Some tumours proliferate so quickly that the immune response is simply not efficacious enough to keep their growth in check (35).

Most of this scepticism about the value of the surveillance hypothesis is, however, levelled at the influence of the immune system on growth of established solid tumours. However, there seems to be an important role for the immune system in keeping metastatic spread in check. Most tumour cells that enter the circulation are destroyed during the first 24 hours and only a few cells succeed to extravasate and develop into metastatic foci in distant organs (7). Tumour cells enter the circulation as single cells or small clumps and are, therefore, highly accessible and more vulnerable to destruction by immune mechanisms.

The potential to kill tumour cells in the blood has been attributed to NK cells, which represent 5–10 per cent of peripheral blood mononuclear cells (PBMCs) (7), but macrophages/monocytes may also be influential. NK cells are hardly effective in reducing solid tumour growth, but can play a role in eliminating metastatic cells, metastatic foci, and early tumour nidus (10). NK cells can kill tumour cells rapidly without prior sensitization or MHC restrictions. It has been demonstrated in successfully treated malignant melanoma (36) and breast cancer (37) patients that level of NK cell cytotoxicity was predictive for the chance of later recurrence.

NK cells and macrophages/monocytes may also play a role in the long-term effect of surgery for cancer. Surgical resection of solid tumour provides a major opportunity for cure in many patients. However, surgical procedures may also cause dissemination of tumour cells to the circulatory system (38). Radiotherapy and chemotherapy may inhibit this spreading of tumour cells. It is also believed that metastatic cells fail to survive because the immune system is successful in destroying such malignant cells. Thus, whether a curative resection will be successful may depend on the host's immune response to kill residual tumour cells. In breast cancer patients changes in degree of immunosuppression from before to 12 months after surgery were predictive for the development of metastatic disease in the next 3 years (39). It should be emphasized that the trauma of surgical resection of a tumour itself induces immunosuppression, including a decrease in NK-cell cytotoxicity (NKCC) (40) and the number of T helper cells (41), thus reducing a potentially inhibiting factor for metastatic spread.

A link between psychological factors and NKCC is substantiated in several studies. It has already been mentioned that NKCC is suppressed during chronic stress exposure in healthy persons (22, 24). In breast cancer patients a relationship with social support has been demonstrated (42); the more social support was perceived from the spouse and the doctor, the higher the NKCC was. Social support was in fact the most potent predictor for NKCC, and appeared to account for more of the NKCC variance than biological predictors (receptor status, Karnofsky index, extent of surgery, number of positive lymph nodes, tumour size, and age). Psychotherapy in melanoma patients led to an increase in NKCC in a study of Fawzy *et al.* (43). Moreover, changes in anxiety and depression were negatively related in this study to changes in NK cell measures (cell number and cytotoxicity), while anger was positively related to these immune measures. The patients who showed the greatest increase in immune activity were those who reported the greatest decrease in depression and anxiety but the most increase in anger (43). One of the few studies in the field of surgery-related PNEI research is by Tjemsland *et al.* (44). The preoperative depression level predicted postoperative immune status: a higher depression level was associated with a lower number of B cells, T-helper cells, total number of T cells, and lymphocytes, and a lower helper/suppressor ratio. Higher intrusion scores were associated with a lower number of B cells. In a regression analysis, controlling for medical and health behaviour variables, both preoperative depression and intrusion scores predicted magnitude of change in immune measures induced by surgery.

To summarize, the role of immunoregulation in carcinogenesis seems to be modest, and needs further testing for specific types of tumours. Tumours showing at least some immunogenicity are those induced by viruses, but also malignant melanoma, and certain brain and renal tumours. Immune efficacy might be modified in these specific tumours by psychological factors. Chronic stressor exposure, especially when associated with uncontrollability, low social support availability, and a passive avoidant coping style, might promote tumour development, because of its immunosuppressive effect. Its effect might be countered by psychological factors such as social support and an active coping style.

While immune surveillance is nowadays seen as less important in the development of most types of solid tumours, the role of the immune system is probably considerable in limiting early tumour development and late-stage metastatic spread.

9 The influence of angiogenesis and apoptosis on tumour growth

There are other mechanisms, besides the classical PNEI pathway, that possibly mediate between psychological factors and tumour growth, namely a cytokine effect on angiogenesis and apoptosis.

A tumour needs an adequate blood supply for further development; a major factor in the growth of solid tumours is their ability to form their own microcirculation. This process, called *angiogenesis*, is one of the crucial steps in a tumour's transition from a small, harmless cluster of mutated cells to a large, malignant growth, capable of spreading to other organs throughout the body (45). Angiogenesis is a normal physiological process, which is important in ovulation, menstruation, embryogenesis, and wound healing. Normally, there is a strict period of angiogenesis, followed by an inhibition of blood vessel formation, but this regulation is disturbed in growing tumours. Several cytokines, including interferon-α, tumour necrosis factor-α (TNF-α), angiostatin, endostatin, angiogenin, interleukin 8 (IL-8), and growth factors (vascular endothelial, fibroblast, and epidural growth factor; VEGF, FGF, and EGF), regulate this process.

Tumour cells can also secrete growth factors themselves. These factors act as chemical signals, stimulating endothelial cells to migrate, divide, grow, and form new blood vessels in the tumour mass. Tumour cells are genetically unstable and enormously varied, and therefore difficult to attack, as was discussed before. However, the basis of angiogenesis, namely the endothelium of blood vessels, consists of stable and uniform cells. This may even imply a more obvious anti-tumour psychosocial mechanism than any direct immune effect on tumour growth. If levels of these cytokines can be modified through psychosocial factors, an alternative pathway is implied for the effect of these factors on tumour progression.

Programmed cell death, 'cell suicide', or *apoptosis*, is a fundamental biological process that occurs in all normal tissues (except in the neural tissue of adults). Every second, thousands to millions of cells are newly formed, and a similar number of cells are destroyed. Cell death is thus an important aspect of life. Programmed cell destruction means that the cell contents are broken into fragments in an orderly way, whereas cell death by necrosis begins with the destruction of the cell membrane.

Apoptosis is regulated by a genetic programme. This programme can be started by external factors, namely (lack of) growth factors, cytokines— especially IL-2, TNF-α, TGF-β (transforming growth factor), anti-Fas[4], and certain hormones (e.g. cortisol) (46). The programme can also be started through internal factors. This occurs in the case of DNA damage that cannot be repaired. Apoptosis thus prevents cells with DNA damage from remaining intact and eventually developing into a tumour. One of the most reproducible inducers of apoptosis is mild oxidative stress (47).

An important route of programmed cell death is initiated by the p53 gene. This gene has been altered in many human cancers, though not in all. Tumour cells with an intact response mechanism are probably more vulnerable to external factors leading to cell-cycle arrest or to apoptosis. For instance, tumours having retained a functional p53 gene or Bcl-2 gene, which is another gene involved in the apoptotic process, are often better targets for medical treatment than similar tumours with a functional p53 or Bcl-2 gene mutation. (The same diversity in vulnerability might apply for psychological factors, implying a possible differentiation in patients in whom psychological factors can have, or do not have, an effect on tumour progression.) Selected cytokine

---

[4] Fas is a membrane protein with a cytoplasmic anchor, which has a structural homology with the TNF-α receptor.

stimulation might increase the apoptotic rate in tumour cells, especially in tumour cells with more or less intact apoptotic intracellular mechanisms.

Cytokines have a regulating role in both angiogenesis and apoptosis. As some studies have demonstrated an effect of psychosocial factors on cytokine production (26, 48), there is an alternative, though speculative, pathway for the influence of psychological factors on tumour growth. This should not be surprising, as cortisol level has been associated with a shift in cytokines—a shift from cytokines produced by T helper 1 cells (IL-2, interferon-α, and IL-12) to cytokines produced by T helper 2 cells (IL-4, 5, 6, 10, and 13)—and with increases in apoptosis (49). One study suggested an effect of stressor exposure, in the form of examination stress, on apoptosis (50).

10 Influences of psychological factors on tumour growth: involvement of neuroimmune pathways in animal studies

A series of animal studies has substantiated the relationship between psychosocial factors and tumour development. These studies indicated that exposure to stressful conditions may enhance or suppress tumour growth. In particular, lack of control over a stressful situation seems to promote the development of tumours. Sklar and Anisman (51) found that mice subjected to inescapable shocks developed tumours at a faster rate and died sooner than mice subjected to escapable shocks after implantation of breast tumour cells.

Metastatic spread after injection of breast tumour cells was studied by Ben-Eliyahu *et al.* (10). Exposure to an inescapable stressor led to twice as many lung metastases compared to control animals which had been given the same injection with tumour cells. NKCC activity to the same breast tumour cells was also measured, and appeared to be suppressed in stressed rats compared to half of that of non-stressed control rats. When NK cells were blocked with an antiserum to NK cells or a selective NK antibody, lung metastases grow enormously, reaching a 100-fold increase. This suggested that stressors reduced NKCC, which appeared to be the main reason for the increased rate of lung metastases.

Exposure to stressful conditions does not always lead to tumour enhancement. Some animal studies even reported suppression of tumour growth with stressor exposure. Justice (32) discussed in his review these contradictory findings and tried to explain them in terms of timing effects and type of tumours. When stressors were applied after an injection of virally induced cancer cells, an increase in size and number of tumours would occur. However, when stressor exposure had ended before tumour injection, tumour growth and incidence would be inhibited. The latter response was explained by Justice as a rebound effect. In non-viral tumours the timing pattern would be just the opposite. When discussing Justice's suggestion, Hilakivi-Clarke *et al.* (52) concluded that his 'rule' explained many contradictory findings, but that a number of results still did not fit into the framework. They suggest as additional explanatory concepts (un)controllability and acute vs. chronic exposure to stressors. Acute stressors generally facilitate tumour growth and shorten survival, whereas chronic exposure to the same stressors inhibits carcinogenesis (51, 53).

In another animal model the role of social relationships is studied, especially aggressive confrontation between animals. An 'intruder' animal is placed in a cage with other animals having established social relations. The intruder is attacked by the 'resident' animals, sooner or later leading to submissive behaviour of the intruder. Stefanski and Ben-Eliyahu (17) studied the degree of lung metastasis in rats after injection of breast tumour cells, using this social confrontation model. Compared to control animals, which were also given this injection, the intruder showed a threefold increase in lung metastasis. Injection of a β-adrenergic antagonist reduced the metastasis–inducing effect of social confrontation by 50 per cent, while removal of the adrenal medulla abolished its effect. These findings support the role of the sympathetic adrenomedullary system, including catecholamine secretion, in the tumour-enhancing effect of social confrontation, possibly mediated through an increased activity of NK cells (16).

Housing conditions—living individually, or in groups of animals—is another social variable that has been related to tumour growth. In mice, a change from group to individual conditions induced larger tumour growth rates following tumour cell injection, compared to rehousing from an individual to a group condition. With stable housing conditions, tumour growth rate was intermediate, although smaller in group-housed animals than in individually housed animals (54, 55).

These animal studies have clearly demonstrated the possible role of psychological factors on growth of tumours and on metastatic spread. Controllability and predictability of a stressful condition sometimes appeared to be far more important factors than their physical aspects. Timing of stressful conditions and type of tumour (virally induced or not) also seemed of influence, and variations in these factors might explain reported discrepancies in stress effects on tumour growth. The role of social factors in enhancement or reduction of cancer development was also demonstrated. Psychological influences on tumour processes seemed to be mediated in some studies by catecholamine activity and in others by β-endorphin activity. These animal studies also substantiated the role of NK cells in limiting metastatic spread.

11   The effects of psychological factors on hormonal and immunological variables in human psycho-oncology studies

11.1   INTERVENTION STUDIES

Only two intervention studies to date with an adequate methodological design and a long-term follow-up have documented the effect of therapy on survival for patients with cancer, namely those of Spiegel *et al.* (56) and Fawzy *et al.* (36). Both studies found longer survival in patients receiving therapy. Fawzy *et al.* (43) also measured immunological variables, which were determined before and after therapy and at 6-month follow-up. Patients were excluded if they were undergoing immunotherapy, chemotherapy, or radiotherapy, or if they were receiving medication that could affect their immune function. We will restrict the discussion to their follow-up data, which were corrected for baseline values.

Compared to the control group, the therapy group showed an increase in number and interferon-augmented cytotoxicity of NK cells, though not in number of suppressor/cytotoxic T cells. There was also an unexpected decrease in helper T cell counts. Thus, at least NKCC changed as expected from the 'intervention–PNI–cancer' hypothesis. Changes in anxiety and depression were negatively related to changes in NK-cell measures (number and cytotoxicity), while anger was positively related to these immune measures. This association is also in accordance with the intervention–PNI hypothesis. Unlike with distress levels, changes in coping were unrelated to changes in immune measures.

In the later publication by Fawzy *et al.* (36), the relationships of psychological and immunological variables to recurrence and survival were studied. The predictor variables in the analyses were both baseline values and magnitude of changes from baseline to 6-months follow-up. Significant predictors for a *disease-free interval* appeared to be NKCC, distress level, and active-behavioural coping at baseline. Higher NKCC, higher distress levels, and more active coping at baseline were related to lower chance for recurrence. Change scores of these measures were not related to recurrence. Significant predictors for *survival* were distress level and active-behavioural coping baseline values, and changes in coping. Higher distress, more active coping, and a greater increase in active coping were related to better survival.

Thus, with regard to NKCC the following effects were found: (a) therapy induced an increase in number and cytotoxicity of these cells; (b) the magnitude of these NK changes was related to the magnitude of psychosocial changes; and (c) the psychological intervention led to a longer disease-free interval and longer survival. The most interesting test was whether the intervention effects on disease outcome were mediated by changes in NKCC. While most of the findings of Fawzy *et al.* supported the evidence for a relationship between psychological variables and cancer progression, this test of the specific intervention–PNI–cancer progression hypothesis was, however, not confirmed: changes in NKCC were not related to recurrence or survival.

The following three pilot studies described here did not evaluate disease progression, but assessed therapy outcome with respect to immunological variables. Schedlowski *et al.* (57) studied immunological outcome in a small number of breast cancer patients, using a waiting-list control design. Their intervention consisted of 10 sessions of 2 hours each, and included relaxation, information about 'body–mind' relationships, health education, and enhancement of coping skills. Measurements at the beginning and end of therapy included illness-related coping, plasma levels of cortisol, and white blood cell counts. No effect on coping was demonstrated, but cortisol decreased and the number of lymphocytes increased in the therapy group, and did not change in the control group. A decrease in cortisol is expected with a decrease in chronic distress, reducing the immunosuppressive effects of cortisol.

Elsesser *et al.* (58) compared the effect of structured, individual therapy with a waiting-list control condition in a small number of patients with various types of cancer. Their therapy consisted of anxiety management training, which involved relaxation training and learning to apply these skills in everyday stressful situations, and cognitive restructuring, which included learning to recognize 'worrying cognitions' and to substitute them with anxiety-reducing formulations. Psychological and immunological variables were measured before, during (midway), and after therapy. Anxiety and number of somatic symptoms decreased and quality of life increased in the therapy group, compared to the control group. No significant, differential effects were found for depression, blood injury phobia, and locus of control. Immunological variables included number of T helper (CD4) cells, suppressor/cytotoxic (CD8) T cells, B cell, total lymphocytes, and the CD4/CD8 ratio. The number of CD4 cells increased more in the therapy group than in the control group, while the other immunological variables showed no significant, differential effect. The relationships between changes before and after treatment in psychological and immunological variables were also determined. Quality of life was related to number of CD4 cells, total lymphocyte number, and CD4/CD8 ratio. The more the quality of life had increased, the larger were the increases in these immunological variables. Decreases in anxiety, somatic symptoms, and phobias and increases in quality of life were associated with decreases in B-cell counts. There were also relationships with locus of control, but these were inconsistent with regard to direction.

Hersh and Kunz (59) studied a small sample of 13 women with early-stage breast cancer. There were seven women in the intervention and six in the waiting-list control group. The structured intervention consisted of relaxation training, guided imagery, and EMG-feedback. The design is not clearly described: the intervention, given in groups and individually, appeared to include 15 sessions over 9 weeks and a unknown number of monthly follow-up sessions. The control group started their therapy after 6 months. The measurements included NKCC, lymphocyte proliferative response to concanavalin A (Con A), proliferative response in mixed lymphocyte culture, lymphocyte IL-2 production, plasma titres of IgG, IgA, and IgM, total white cell count, and cortisol. They found higher levels of total white cell count, response to Con-A, mixed lymphocyte responsiveness (MLR), and plasma IgG titre, and lower plasma cortisol levels in the intervention group compared to the control group. It is surprising how many significant findings could be demonstrated with the small number of participants in this study, especially given the generally found modest effect sizes and the need for control variables to be considered.

11.2 NON-INTERVENTION STUDIES

In a series of reports, Levy and colleagues (37, 42, 60, 61) described the relationships between psychosocial variables and NKCC, both cross-sectionally and prospectively, in women with early-stage breast cancer. The procedures in these four reports look similar, and the reports are probably based on the same group, to which more participants were added in successive reports. There were measurements some days after surgery, and at 3 and 15 months follow-up.

In the earlier reports (60, 61), the relationships between psychosocial baseline measures and NKCC at 3-month follow-up were determined, controlling for NKCC level at baseline. The relationships were significant in cross-sectional analyses at baseline and at 3-month follow-up for adjustment as rated by an observer, scores on the fatigue subscale of the Profile of Mood States (POMS), and perceived social support. There were, however, no significant relationships in the longitudinal analysis, using the conventional α-level of 0.05.

In their 1990 publication (42) the focus was on the cross-sectional relationship between social support measures and NKCC, measured at baseline. The more social support was perceived from the spouse and the doctor, the higher NKCC was. Social support was in fact the most potent predictor for NKCC, and accounted for more of the NKCC variance than biological predictors (oestrogen receptor status, Karnofsky index, extent of surgery, number of positive lymph nodes, tumour size, and age). No significant relationships were found for coping or mood.

In the most recent report (37) the relationship between NKCC, distress, and later recurrence in early-stage breast cancer patients was investigated. NKCC was determined shortly after surgery and 15 months later. It was found that the higher NKCC was at 15 months, the lower was the chance for later recurrence. This is an expected outcome, because NK cells are able to destroy metastatic cells (10). Curiously, there was an opposite relationship for baseline NKCC—higher NKCC at baseline predicted a larger chance for disease recurrence.

NKCC and distress were predictors for different aspects of disease outcome. At 15-months follow-up, NKCC, but not distress, predicted the *chance of recurrence* in the total sample. However, within the subgroup of women having a recurrence, distress, but not NKCC, predicted the *duration of the disease-free interval*.

Levy *et al.* also determined whether NKCC was related to distress. The cross-sectional relationship was not significant at 15-months follow-up, nor at other measurement points. Higher distress at baseline showed a trend, however, to be associated with lower NKCC at 15-months follow-up ($p < 0.06$).

To summarize the findings of Levy *et al.*, substantial and interesting cross-sectional relationships were demonstrated for NKCC and psychosocial variables, which hold for various time points. However, knowing the tight relationship between NKCC measures over time, the psychological variables did not contribute to the explained variance of NKCC in longitudinal analysis, once baseline NKCC was taken into account. Interesting relationships between distress and disease progression have also been found in Levy *et al.*'s studies. However, the direct test that this relationship was mediated by the immune system was not convincingly demonstrated.

11.2.1 *Receptor status*

Breast tumours are sensitive to specific hormones, and may or may not have receptors for oestrogen and progesterone. If tumours have receptors for these hormones (oestrogen and/or progesterone receptor positive), prognosis is more favourable. Razavi *et al.* (62) studied the relationship between receptor status and psychosocial correlates. They found that patients with negative receptor status for oestrogen and/or progesterone scored higher on anxiety, phobic anxiety, and 'paranoid ideation' as measured with the SCL-90 than patients with a positive receptor status. No differences in receptor status were found with respect to number of life events and the repression/sensitization dimension. Ramirez *et al.* (63) have criticized this study, because the receptor-negative group included relatively more patients who received chemotherapy than the receptor-positive group. Somatic symptoms induced by chemotherapy might have led to the higher SCL-90 scores. Their own case-control study seemed to indicate that relapse in breast cancer occurred more frequently if women had experienced a severe life event, compared to no severe life event, at least among women with oestrogen receptor-positive tumours. There was no such difference among women with oestrogen receptor-negative tumours. These findings support the hypothesis that the effect of psychosocial variables on breast cancer is mediated via an endocrine mechanism. Also in response to Razavi *et al.*'s article, two research groups reported that they had reanalysed their data sets to see whether receptor positive and negative breast cancer patients differed in psychological measures. Neither group could demonstrate any difference (64, 65). Tjemsland *et al.* (66) only found one out of 14 psychological variables to be significantly associated with receptor status, namely the life-event category 'Having experienced a serious illness/accident/hospitalization' (the present illness was not included). Other life-event categories, emotional control, neuroticism, social support, adjustment to cancer, and psychological distress were not related to receptor status. The one significant relationship may be a spurious finding. This study does not support the suggestion that receptor status is associated with psychosocial variables (but does not undo the interesting finding of Ramirez *et al.* with respect to later relapse).

To summarize, immunological effects have been found in four therapy studies. In two of these studies the total number of lymphocytes increased (57, 59). The two other studies determined changes in subsets of lymphocytes. They found no change in suppressor/cytotoxic T cell counts and a decrease in T helper cell counts (43), or an increase in T helper cells (58). An increase in number and cytotoxicity of NK cells has also been found (43).

The NK-cell changes in Fawzy *et al.*'s study were related to changes in mood, and the T- and B-cell changes in Elsesser *et al.*'s study were related to quality of life, mood, and psychiatric symptoms. NK cell cytotoxicity also predicted a lower likelihood of disease progression (36, 37). Therapy-induced changes in NKCC, however, did not mediate the positive effects of a psychological intervention on disease outcome (36).

12 Influences of tumour cells on endocrine and immune functions

A last point to be discussed is the possible influence of tumour cells on endocrinological and immunological functioning. Endocrinological assays have shown differences between healthy persons and persons with cancer, depending on the phase of the disease. These relationships are probably explained by an effect of the developing tumour on the endocrine system. In advanced cancer patients who had stayed symptom-free for a long time, catecholamine levels have been found lowered and platelet serotonine levels increased, as compared to healthy control subjects. However, in patients with short-term symptom-free periods, or in patients whose disease state exacerbated, catechol levels and cortisol levels were increased and platelet serotonine levels decreased. In terminal patients, the pattern reversed again, leading to extremely low levels for catecholamines and cortisol. Platelet serotonine also showed very low levels (67). The extreme reactions in terminal patients could possibly be interpreted as the exhaustion phase of an overstimulated adrenal medulla and cortex. In a study from our own institute, breast cancer patients with and without metastasis, receiving only tamoxifen as a treatment, were compared to healthy women (68). Baseline levels of cortisol, ACTH, and prolactin were measured, as well as the endocrinological responses to a behavioural challenge. Cortisol baseline levels were higher in the breast cancer patients than in healthy women; similar to what was found in advanced cancer patients in the previous study. Metastatic breast cancer patients had higher cortisol levels than early stage-breast cancer patients. No group differences were found for ACTH and prolactin. The behavioural challenge induced a significant increase in ACTH and prolactin, but an unexpected decrease in cortisol. The metastatic breast cancer patients showed lower post-challenge values for cortisol and prolactin than the other two groups.

A treacherous effect of tumours is that they can suppress immune functions (34). *In vitro* experiments, for instance, have shown that the cytolytic action of lymphocytes can be blocked by the addition of sera of tumour-bearing individuals. It has also been demonstrated in animal studies that tumour-bearing subjects accept transplants more readily and are also more susceptible to bacterial infections, which are both signs of immunosuppression. The immuno-suppressive effects can be simply demonstrated by a hypersensitivity test. Its response is often inhibited in tumour-bearing persons. The magnitude of this response is even related to the extent of the tumour burden (34). The immuno-suppressive effects have been shown most consistently in patients with metastatic disease, but some impairments may also occur among patients with localized disease, as was demonstrated by Mandeville *et al.* (69). The hyper-sensitivity response was not different for healthy subjects and non-metastatic breast cancer patients, but a lower number of persons with a positive hyper-sensitivity response was found among breast cancer patients with metastasis. The lymphocyte response to phytohaemagglutinin (PHA) and Con A was lowered in all patient groups they studied, including a group of patients with benign breast disease. The response to PHA, though not to Con A, showed, however, a gradual decline with advancing stage of the disease. The number of patients with a diminished number of T cells was greater in all patient groups compared to healthy controls, but excessively so in the group with metastatic breast cancer. This study also demonstrated that the hypersensitivity response and the PHA response as determined at diagnosis were predictive for sur-vival and disease-free interval 5 years later (69). Lechin *et al.* (67) also showed a decrease in immune function—number of total lymphocytes and natural cell cytotoxicity—with more advanced stages; from normal values in advanced patients who had been symptom-free for a long period, to lowered values in patients who showed exacerbation, and to extremely low values in terminal-stage patients.

To summarize, cancer patients show an overactive functioning of the LHPA axis and SAM system, and immunosuppression, but more so in more advanced stages than in early stages. Patients in an early stage may show an endocrinological and immunological pattern similar to that seen in healthy persons. It is not certain how these endocrinological and immunological changes are functionally related. It is suggested that tumour cells activate immune systems, which subsequently leads to production of cytokines, which in turn may influence neuroendocrine mechanisms (68).

13   Discussion

It would be a large step forwards in the study of the role of psychological factors in cancer initiation and growth if the mediating pathways were known. Generally speaking, there are two possible pathways: first, variations in health behaviours may be the linking factor. Second, the mediating pathway may be a psychophysiological mechanism. The first possibility is rarely studied, most likely because there are so many potential behaviours involved, that refuting this possibility seems a thankless task. One may also speculate that this area is seen as less challenging than the second one, which has a certain appeal for researchers. The second possibility of a psychophysiological mediating process was extensively discussed in this chapter.

In earlier days the PNEIT pathway seemed evident, and it was supposed that future research would yield detailed, experimental confirmation of this model. Indeed, some of the links in this PNEIT chain have been clearly substantiated by empirical data. This applies to the influence of psychosocial factors and nervous regulation on endocrine activity (PN→E); the endocrine regulation of immune activity (E→I); the influence of psychosocial factors and nervous regulation on immune functions (PN→I); and the role of endocrines on initiation and progression of some tumours (E→T).

The model appeared more complicated than initially thought. Psycho–neuro–endocrine–immunological (PNEI) research has revealed the complexity of various links, including feedback loops, though one may conclude that there exists nowadays at least a basic understanding of these interacting processes. The most difficult step, however, appeared to be the demonstration of the clinical relevance of these PNEI effects with respect to disease processes. Among psychologists and psychophysiologists the idea has long persisted that the immune system plays a major role in detecting and destroying tumour cells (I→T), while the overall applicability of the immunosurveillance hypothesis was already seriously questioned among immunologists.

Indeed, the role of the immune system in keeping in check tumour growth is probably the weakest link in the chain connecting psychological factors to cancer progression. In general, the role of immunoregulation in carcinogenesis seems to be modest, but needs further testing for specific tumour–immune interactions. Cancers in which viral factors are etiologically important, such as lymphoma and cervical carcinoma, should be especially considered in future PNEI research, because virally induced cancers are, in general, antigenic. Viral load, virus-specific antigen expression in tumour tissue, and antibody levels to such viral proteins may then appear to be an interesting measure in psycho-oncological research. The role of the high-risk human papillomavirus (HPV) types in cervical carcinoma has now generally been acknowledged. It has also been demonstrated that the Epstein–Barr virus and human T-cell lymphotropic virus type 1 (HTLV-1) may influence the development of some types of lymphoma (33, 70). A major problem is, however, the limited knowledge about which viruses play a role in which types of tumour. Breast cancer is also important when studying the role of psychosocial factors, because stressor-sensitive endocrines can influence its development and growth.

Acknowledging the generally modest role of immunosurveillance in carcinogenesis, it has been suggested that immunity against developing tumours is only a by-product of resistance against viruses, bacteria, and parasites. In this line, Kripke has speculated that infectious diseases are significant in terms of evolution, because they threaten the survival of species, while cancer represents a threat to individuals beyond their reproductive years (71). The suggestion is that the immunity against cancer is not well developed because it is not of primary evolutionary importance. Refocusing on the primary role of the immune system, Beverley (31) speculated that immunologists' most direct contribution to the reduction of cancer mortality might be through immunization against tumour-inducing viruses, as is now under investigation, using HPV high-risk-type peptides for a vaccine against cervical carcinoma.

Knowledge in the field of tumour immunology is, however, still too limited to draw any definite conclusions. A recent trend is to focus on local immunity, because the anti-tumour activity in the tumour mass may differ from and prove more directly relevant than the activity of the same type of immune cells obtained from the spleen or bloodstream (71). Moreover, besides the classical immunosurveillance pathway nowadays seen as less important in non-viral human cancers, there are other potential pathways for the influence of psychosocial factors on growth of solid tumours, namely through cytokine-associated angiogenesis and apoptosis. Findings in one study suggest that exposure to the stressor of a medical school examination may induce physiological changes inhibiting the ability of immune cells to initiate apoptosis (50). Both angiogenesis and apoptosis are regulated by cytokines, which may in turn be influenced by psychosocial factors (26, 48). The study of angiogenesis and apoptosis may open new avenues in the field of psycho-oncology.

One important point has often been overlooked in this discussion. Studies on the role of psychosocial factors in cancer progression rarely focus on growth of solid tumours, to which most of the scepticism about the value of the surveillance hypothesis applies. Instead of focusing on growth of solid tumours, these studies often tried to predict recurrence of cancer, implying the occurrence of metastases, second primaries, or regrowth at sites of reduced tumour burden. The role of the immune system in holding metastatic spread in check is fairly well established.

The message of this chapter is that one should abandon the general PNEIT model, and formulate hypotheses that are specific with respect to the endocrine and/or immunological factors involved in specific types of cancer by organ, grade (degree of differentiation), and cell type, and in specific stages of tumour development.

14   References

1. Pettingale, K. W. (1985). Towards a psychobiological model of cancer: biological considerations. *Soc. Sci. Med.*, **20**, 779–787.

2. Goodkin, K., Antoni, M. H., Sevin, B., and Fox, B. H. (1993). A partially testable model of psychosocial factors in the etiology of cervical cancer. 1. A review of biological, psychological and social aspects. *Psycho-Oncology*, 2, 79–98.

3. Goodkin, K., Antoni, M. H., Sevin, B., and Fox, B. H. (1993). A partially testable model of psychosocial factors in the etiology of cervical cancer. 2. Bioimmunological, psychoneuroimmunological, and socioimmunological aspects, critique and prospective integration. *Psycho-Oncology*, 2, 99–121.

4. Andersen, B. L., Kiecolt-Glaser, J. K., and Glaser, R. (1994). A biobehavioral model of cancer stress and disease course. *Am. Psychol.*, 49, 389–404.

5. Pompe, G. v., Antoni, M. H., Mulder, C. L., Heijnen, C., Goodkin, K., Graeff, A. d. *et al.* (1994). Psychoneuroimmunology and the course of breast cancer; an overview. The impact of psychosocial factors on progression of breast cancer through putative immune and endocrine mechanisms. *Psycho-Oncology*, 3, 271–288.

6. Fife, A., Beasley, P. J., and Fertig, D. L. (1996). Psychoneuroimmunology and cancer: historical perspectives and current research. *Adv. Neuroimmunol.*, 6, 179–190.

7. Hanna, N. (1985). The role of natural killer cells in the control of tumor growth and metastases. *Biochim. Biophys. Acta*, 780, 213–226.

8. Borysenko, M. (1987). Area review: psychoneuroimmunology. *Ann. Behav. Med.*, 9, 3–10.

9. Adams, D. O. (1994). Molecular biology of macrophage activation: a pathway whereby psychosocial factors can potentially affect health. *Psychosom. Med.*, 56, 316–327.

10. Ben-Eliyahu, S., Yirmiya, R., Liebeskind, J. C., Taylor, A. N., and Gale, R. P. (1991). Stress increases metastatic spread of a mammary tumor in rats: evidence for mediation by the immune system. *Brain Behav. Immun.*, 5, 193–205.

11. Cannon, W. B. (1967). *The Wisdom of the Body*. Norton, New York.

12. Mason, J. W. (1972). Organization of psychoendocrine mechanisms. In *Handbook of Psychophysiology* (eds N. S. Greenfield and R. A. Sternbach), pp. 3–91. Holt, Rinehart, Winston, New York.

13. Felten, D. L., Overhage, J. M., Felten, S. Y., and Schmedtje, J. F. (1981). Noradrenergic sympathetic innervation of lymphoid tissue in the rabbit: further evidence for a link between the nervous system and immune systems. *Brain Res. Bull.*, 7, 595–612.

14. Milles, K., Quintans, J., Cheimicka-Scherr, E., and Armason, B. G. W. (1981). The sympathetic nervous system modulates antibody response to thymus-independent antigens. *J. Neuroimmunol.*, 1, 101–105.

15. Zanker, K. S. (1994). Correlation of psychological, endocrine, and immune parameters in cancer patients: the WITTEN study. In *The Psychoimmunology of Cancer. Mind and Body in the Fight for Survival* (eds C. E. Lewis, C. O'Sullivan, and J. Barraclough), pp. 320–335. Oxford Medical Publications, Oxford.

16. O'Leary, A. (1990). Stress, emotion and human immune function. *Psychol. Bull.*, 108, 363–382.

17. Stefanski, V. and Ben-Eliyahu, S. (1996). Social confrontation and tumor metastasis in rats: defeat and beta-adrenergic mechanisms. *Physiol. Behav.*, 60, 277–282.

18. Goodkin, K., Blaney, N. T., Tuttle, R. S., Nelson, R. H., Baldewicz, T., Kumar, M. *et al.* (1996). Bereavement and HIV infection. *Int. Rev. Psychiatry*, 8, 201–216.

19. Solomon, G. F., Armkraut, A. A., and Kasper, P. (1974). Immunity, emotions and stress. *Ann. Clin. Res.*, 6, 313–322.

20. Dorian, B. and Garfinkel, P. E. (1987). Stress, immunity and illness—a review. *Psychol. Med.*, **17**, 393–407.
21. Kiecolt-Glaser, J. K. and Glaser, R. (1995). Psychoneuroimmunology and health consequences: data and shared mechanisms. *Psychosom. Med.*, **57**, 269–274.
22. Kiecolt-Glaser, J. K. and Glaser, R. (1987). Psychosocial moderators of immune function. *Ann. Behav. Med.*, **9**, 16–20.
23. Daruna, J. H. and Morgan, J. E. (1990). Psychosocial effects on immune function: neuroendocrine pathways. *Psychosomatics*, **31**, 4–12.
24. Herbert, T. B. and Cohen, S. (1993). Stress and immunity in humans: a meta-analytic review. *Psychosom. Med.*, **55**, 364–379.
25. Schleifer, S. J., Keller, S. E., Camerino, M., Thornton, J. C., and Stein, M. (1983). Suppression of lymphocyte stimulation following bereavement. *J. Am. Med. Assoc.*, **250**, 374–377.
26. Glaser, R., Rice, J., Sheridan, J., Fertel, R., Stout, J., Speicher, C. *et al.* (1987). Stress-related immune suppression: health implications. *Brain Behav. Immun.*, **1**, 7–20.
27. Herbert, T. B., Cohen, S., Marlsland, A. L., Bachen, E. A., Rabin, B. S., Muldoon, M. F. *et al.* (1994). Cardiovascular reactivity and the course of immune response to an acute psychological stressor. *Psychosom. Med.*, **56**, 337–344.
28. Pike, J. L., Smith, T. L., Hauger, R. L., Nicassio, P. M., Patterson, T. L., Mcclintick, J. *et al.* (1997). Chronic life stress alters sympathetic, neuroendocrine, and immune responsivity to an acute psychological stressor in humans. *Psychosom. Med.*, **59**, 447–457.
29. Mainwaring, W. I. P. (1991). Hormones and cancer. In *Introduction to the Cellular and Molecular Biology of Cancer* (eds L. M. Franks and N. M. Teich), pp. 357–385. Oxford University Press, New York.
30. Souberbielle, B. and Dalgleish, A. (1994). Anti-tumour immune mechanisms. In *The Psychoimmunology of Cancer. Mind and Body in the Fight for Survival* (eds C. E. Lewis, C. O'Sullivan, and J. Barraclough), pp. 267–290. Oxford Medical Publications, Oxford.
31. Beverley, P. (1991). Immunology of cancer. In *Introduction to the Cellular and Molecular Biology of Cancer* (eds L. M. Franks and N. M. Teich), pp. 406–433. Oxford University Press, New York.
32. Justice, A. (1985). Review of the effects of stress on cancer in laboratory animals: importance of time of stress application and type of tumor. *Psychol. Bull.*, **98**, 108–138.
33. Nossal, G. J. V. (1993). Life, death and the immune system. *Sci. Am.*, **269**, 20–30.
34. Somers, S. and Guillou, P. J. (1994). Tumour cell strategies for escaping immune control: implications for psychoimmunotherapy. In *The Psychoimmunology of Cancer. Mind and Body in the Fight for Survival* (eds C. E. Lewis, C. O'Sullivan, and J. Barraclough), pp. 385–416. Oxford Medical Publications, Oxford.
35. Old, L. J. (1996). Immunotherapy for cancer. *Sci. Am.*, **275**, 102–109.
36. Fawzy, F. I., Fawzy, N. W., Hyun, C. S., Elashoff, R., Guthrie, D., Fahey, J. L. *et al.* (1993). Malignant melanoma. Effects of an early structured psychiatric intervention, coping, and affective state on recurrence and survival 6 years later. *Arch. Gen. Psychiatry*, **50**, 681–689.
37. Levy, S. M., Herberman, R. B., Lippman, M., D'Angelo, T., and Lee, J. (1991). Immunological and psychosocial predictors of disease recurrence in patients with early-stage breast cancer. *Behav. Med.*, **17**, 67–75.

38. McCulloch, P., Choy, A., and Martin, L. (1995). Association between tumour angiogenesis and tumour cell shedding into effluent venous blood during breast cancer surgery. *Lancet*, **346**, 1334–1335.
39. Wiltschke, C., Krainer, M., Budinsky, A. C., Berger, A., Muller, C., Zeillinger, R. *et al.* (1995). Reduced mitogenic stimulation of peripheral blood mononuclear cells as a prognostic parameter for the course of breast cancer: a prospective longitudinal study. *Br. J. Cancer*, **71**, 1292–1296.
40. Pollock, R. E., Lotzova, E., and Stanford, S. D. (1992). Surgical stress impairs natural killer cell programming of tumor lysis in patients with sarcomas and other solid tumors. *Cancer*, **70**, 2192–2201.
41. Lennard, T. W. J., Shenton, B. K., Borzotta, A., Donelly, P. K., White, M., Gerrie, L. M. *et al.* (1985). The influence of surgical operations on components of the human immune system. *Br. J. Surg.*, **72**, 771–776.
42. Levy, S. M., Herberman, R. B., Whiteside, T., Sanzo, K., Lee, J., and Kirkwood, J. (1990). Perceived social support and tumor estrogen/progesteron receptor status as predictors of natural killer cell activity in breast cancer patients. *Psychosom. Med.*, **52**, 73–85.
43. Fawzy, F. I., Kemeny, M. E., Fawzy, N. W., Elashoff, R., Morton, D., Cousins, N. *et al.* (1990). A structured psychiatric intervention for cancer patients. II. Changes over time in immunological measures. *Arch. Gen. Psychiatry*, **47**, 729–735.
44. Tjemsland, L., Soreide, J. A., Matre, R., and Malt, U. F. (1997). Preoperative psychological variables predict immunological status in patients with operable breast cancer. *Psycho-Oncology*, **6**, 311–320.
45. Folkman, J. (1996). Fighting cancer by attacking its blood supply. *Sci. Am.*, **275**, 116–119.
46. Haanen, C. and Vermes, I. (1996). Programmed cell death in fetal development. *Eur. J. Obstet. Gynecol. Reprod. Biol.*, **64**, 129–133.
47. Hampton, M. B., Fadeel, B., and Orrenius, S. (1998). Redox regulation of the caspases during apoptosis. *Ann. N. Y. Acad. Sci.*, **854**, 328–335.
48. Glaser, R., Kiecolt-Glaser, J. K., Marucha, P. T., Maccallum, R. C., Laskowski, B. F., and Malarkey, W. B. (1999). Stress-related changes in proinflammatory cytokine production in wounds. *Arch. Gen. Psychiatry*, **65**, 450–456.
49. Clerici, M., Bevilacqua, M., Vago, T., Shearer, G. M., and Norbiato, G. (1994). An immunoendocrinological hypothesis of HIV infection. *Lancet*, **344**, 626.
50. Tomei, L. D., Kiecolt-Glaser, J. K., Kennedy, S., and Glaser, R. (1990). Psychological stress and phorbol ester inhibition of radiation-induced apoptosis in human peripheral blood leukocytes. *Psychiatry Res.*, **33**, 59–71.
51. Sklar, L. S. and Anisman, H. (1979). Stress and coping factors influence tumor growth. *Science*, **205**, 513–515.
52. Hilakivi-Clarke, L., Rowland, J., Clarke, R., and Lippman, M. E. (1993). Psychosocial factors in development and progression of breast cancer. *Breast Cancer Res. Treat.*, **29**, 141–160.
53. Sklar, L. S. and Anisman, H. (1981). Stress and cancer. *Psychol. Bull.*, **89**, 369–406.
54. Weinberg, J. and Emerman, J. T. (1989). Effects of psychosocial stressors on mouse mammary tumor growth. *Brain Behav. Immun.*, **3**, 234–246.
55. Grimm, M. S., Emerman, J. T., and Weinberg, J. (1996). Effects of social housing condition and behavior on growth of the Shionogi mouse mammary carcinoma. *Physiol. Behav.*, **59**, 633–642.

56. Spiegel, D., Bloom, J. R., Kraemer, H. C., and Gottheil, E. (1989). Effect of psychosocial treatment on survival of patients with metastatic breast cancer. *Lancet*, 2, 888–891.

57. Schedlowski, M., Jung, C., Schimanski, G., Tewes, U., and Schmoll, H. J. (1994). Effects of behavioral intervention on plasma cortisol and lymphocytes in breast cancer patients—an exploratory study. *Psycho-Oncology*, 3, 181–187.

58. Elsesser, K., Vanberkel, M., Sartory, G., Biermanngocke, W., and Ohl, S. (1994). The effects of anxiety management training on psychological variables and immune parameters in cancer patients—a pilot study. *Behav. Cognit. Psychother.*, 22, 13–23.

59. Hersh, S. P. and Kunz, J. F. (1994). Immunological responses to self-regulation training in stage 1 breast cancer patients. In *The Psychoimmunology of Cancer. Mind and Body in the Fight for Survival* (eds C. E. Lewis, C. O'Sullivan, and J. Barraclough), pp. 349–372. Oxford Medical Publications, Oxford.

60. Levy, S. M., Lippman, M., and D'Angelo, T. (1987). Correlation of stress factors with sustained depression of natural killer cell activity and predicted prognosis in patients with breast cancer. *J. Clin. Oncol.*, 5, 348–353.

61. Levy, S. M., Herberman, R. B., Maluish, A. M., Schlien, B., and Lippman, M. (1985). Prognostic risk assessment in primary breast cancer by behavioral and immunological parameters. *Health Psychol.*, 4, 99–113.

62. Razavi, D., Farvacques, C., Delvaux, N., Beffort, T., Paesmans, M., Leclercq, G. *et al.* (1990). Psychosocial correlates of oestrogen and progesterone receptors in breast cancer. *Lancet*, 335, 931–933.

63. Ramirez, A. J., Richards, M. A., Gregory, W., and Craig, T. K. J. (1990). Psychological correlates of hormone receptor status in breast cancer. *Lancet*, 335, 1408.

64. Maunsell, E., Brisson, J., and Descienes, L. (1990). Receptor status and psychological adjustment of breast cancer patients. *Lancet*, 336, 47.

65. Hislop, T. and Kan, L. (1990). Receptor status and psychological adjustment in breast cancer patients. *Lancet*, 336, 47–48.

66. Tjemsland, L., Soreide, J. A., and Malt, U. F. (1995). Psychosocial factors in women with operable breast cancer. An association to estrogen receptor status? *J. Psychosom. Res.*, 39, 875–881.

67. Lechin, F., van der Dijs, B., Vitelli-Florez, G., Lechin-Baez, S., Azocar, J., Cabrera, A. *et al.* (1990). Psychoneuroendocrinological and immunological parameters in cancer patients: involvement of stress and depression. *Psychoneuroendocrinology*, 15, 435–451.

68. Pompe, G. v., Antoni, M. H., and Heijnen, C. J. (1996). Elevated basal cortisol levels and attenuated ACTH and cortisol responses to a behavioral challenge in women with metastatic breast cancer. *Psychoneuroendocrinology*, 21, 361–374.

69. Mandeville, R., Lamoureux, G., Legault-Poisson, S., and Poisson, R. (1982). Biological markers and breast cancer: a multi-parametric study: II Depressed immune competence. *Cancer*, 50, 1280–1288.

70. Wyke, J. A. (1991). Viruses and cancer. In *Introduction to the Cellular and Molecular Biology of Cancer* (eds L. M. Franks and N. M. Teich), pp. 203–229. Oxford University Press, New York.

71. Kripke, M. L. (1988). Immunoregulation of carcinogenesis: past, present and future. *J. Natl. Cancer Inst.*, 80, 722–727.

7
Psychological factors and cancer progression: involvement of behavioural pathways

J. ANDERSON AND L. G. WALKER

1 Summary

Psychological reactions to stressful life events, mood disturbance, personality, coping styles, and compliance with medical treatment have all been implicated in altering the prognosis of individuals with cancer. Research to date has inherent methodological limitations and the evidence that psychological factors independently predict survival is inconsistent. The most compelling evidence for a causal relationship comes from prospective, randomized, controlled trials in which psychological and/or behavioural factors have been manipulated and the effects on survival evaluated. A systematic review of the literature revealed ten randomized trials comparing one or more psychological interventions with a control condition that excluded a formal intervention. Four of these studies indicated that participating in a psychological intervention resulted in a significant survival benefit. Behavioural as well as biological pathways may be involved.

The model of coping and cancer progression developed in this chapter is based on the work of Lazarus, Folkman, and Bandura (1–4). These contemporary psychologists view the process of coping as ongoing biological, psychological, and behavioural responses to a threat. How the threat is perceived, and what the individual feels can be done about it, will determine the outcome. The diagnosis of cancer poses a threat to well-being, and this model of coping explains how psychological interventions may influence the disease process and the behavioural pathways that may be involved. The model also provides a basis for understanding how patients cope with cancer and suggests a framework for timely interventions to enhance mood and quality of life and, potentially, to help patients fight their disease.

2 A cognitive-behavioural view of cancer progression

2.1 CONTEMPORARY VIEWS ON COPING

Lazarus and Folkman define coping as the 'ongoing cognitive and behavioural efforts to manage specific external and/or internal demands appraised as taxing or exceeding the resources of the person' (1, p. 141). Coping therefore involves two simultaneous processes of appraisal: an appraisal of the demand (what is the demand and is it a threat?) and an appraisal of the individual's capacity to respond to it (can a response be produced that will alleviate or reduce the threat?) (1–3).

Based on the work of Lazarus, Folkman, and Bandura, a model of coping with cancer is illustrated in Figure 1. The model highlights:

- the ongoing appraisal of the situation (what is the demand and what are its consequences?)
- physiological aspects (the stress response)
- affective responses (depression, anxiety, happiness)
- coping styles (e.g. fighting spirit, hopelessness)
- perceived self-efficacy (the extent to which the individual believes that he/she can control the outcome)

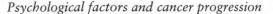

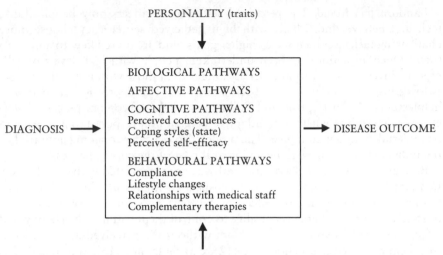

Figure 1 Coping with cancer: psychosocial, biological, and behavioural pathways that may influence survival.

- behavioural aspects (compliance with treatment, lifestyle changes such as diet, sleep habits, exercise, and healthy living, relationships with medical staff, and use of complementary therapies).

These factors, in turn, are influenced by personality variables such as extraversion, neuroticism, emotional suppression, and social conformity. Personality traits, by definition, are enduring characteristics, whereas coping styles change over time (5, 6) and are more amenable to manipulation (7, 8).

A number of studies have confirmed the benefits of social support for patients with cancer (9–11). Supportive relationships may promote healthy behaviour and encourage the early detection of symptoms. Supportive relationships may also buffer the effects of stressful life events by enhancing coping resources.[1]

2.2 PERCEIVED SELF-EFFICACY AND BEHAVIOUR

According to Bandura, certain types of behaviour are facilitated by a sense of control which he calls perceived self-efficacy: 'Perceived self-efficacy refers to beliefs in one's capabilities to organise and execute the courses of action required to produce given attainments' (4, p. 3).

---

[1] A discussion on social support is outside the scope of this chapter. The interested reader is referred to ref. 73.

Bandura has found that perceived self-efficacy affects how people think, feel, and behave. Individuals with high perceived self-efficacy choose more challenging tasks, set themselves higher goals, and are more likely to adhere to them. Once an action has been undertaken, people with high levels of self-efficacy invest more effort and persist longer than those with low self-efficacy. A low sense of self-efficacy has been associated with depression, anxiety and helplessness (4). In Lazarus and Folkman's model of coping, perceived self-efficacy determines whether an adaptive behavioural response to a threat can be undertaken and maintained. The model also considers ongoing appraisal of the individual's resources to be an integral part of the coping process.

Biological as well as behavioural pathways are associated with self-efficacy. Bandura has carried out a series of prospective studies in which self-efficacy has been manipulated and the effects on biological systems observed. Exposure to stressors with the perceived ability to control them had no adverse physical effects. However, exposure to stressors without the perceived ability to control them activated neuroendocrine (12), catecholamine (13), and opioid (14) systems, and impaired the functioning of the immune system (15).

2.3 COPING WITH CANCER

Cancer is a threat to physical and psychological well-being that makes many demands on a patient. As illustrated in Figure 1, the model of coping can be applied to how individuals cope with cancer and how this may lead to differences in survival. Most research on coping has focused on the direct relationship between coping styles and disease outcome. For example, there is some evidence that having a 'fighting spirit' towards cancer may prolong survival, whereas 'helplessness/hopelessness' may promote disease progression (16–18).

The physiological, affective, cognitive, and behavioural pathways in Figure 1 are interrelated. Changes in one aspect may induce changes in other aspects. It follows that interventions can be targeted at any of these aspects: physiological pathways (relaxation, biofeedback), affective pathways (cognitive therapy, psychopharmacology), cognitive pathways (cognitive therapy, guided imagery, developing different coping styles), and behavioural pathways (behaviour therapy to improve compliance, assertiveness, social skills). Therefore, multiple interrelated pathways may affect disease outcome. Evidence for this is the substance of the remainder of this chapter.

3 Physiological pathways

The French physiologist Claude Bernard introduced biologists and social scientists to the concept of homeostasis, which is the body's attempt to maintain the stable internal equilibrium necessary for survival. Homeostasis is a process that allows the organism to adapt to changes in the environment, thereby facilitating evolution-based survival. This concept remains central to understanding the physiological reaction to a stressful event, such as the diagnosis of cancer, which poses a significant threat. The stress response, commonly known as the 'fight–flight response', is the body's attempt to mobilize an adaptive response to the threat. It is characterized by multiple biological responses. Psychologically, it is usually associated with the perception of threat and emotions such as anger and fear.

However, the fight–flight response may become maladaptive. If it is too intense and/or prolonged, it places considerable strain on the body's ability to maintain a stable environment.

Biological mediators of the fight–flight response (stress hormones, neurotransmitters, neuropeptides, and immunopeptides) play critical roles in maintaining bodily homeostasis in the face of continually changing internal and external demands. If stress hormones such as adrenocorticotrophic hormone (ACTH), corticosteroids, catecholamines (such as adrenaline and noradrenaline), and hypothalamic hormones (such as the endorphins) are present at high levels for prolonged periods, they become immunosuppressive (19). The dynamic interplay between the neuroendocrine and immune systems and their importance in coordinating host–defence mechanisms have only been appreciated recently, as have the interaction between these biological parameters, affective reactions, cognitive pathways, and behaviour. These may have far-reaching implications for the progression of at least some cancers.

3.1 INTERVENTIONS CAN MODULATE THE IMMUNE RESPONSE TO STRESS

There is evidence that psychosocial interventions designed to enhance coping can modulate the immune response to stress in healthy individuals (20) and in patients with cancer (21).

In a prospective, randomized, controlled intervention study, Johnson *et al.* randomized 24 healthy volunteers to an experimental intervention or to a control arm (20). The experimental intervention consisted of training in progressive muscular relaxation and cue-controlled relaxation for 3 weeks plus brief hypnotic suggestions immediately prior to exposure to an experimental stressor on day 21. The stressor involved participation in a doctor–patient role-play followed by feedback. Volunteers attended on three occasions (day 1, day 21, and day 22 or 23) and samples of blood were collected on these occasions for immunological analysis. Two samples of blood were taken at the second visit (one before exposure to the experimental stressor and one immediately after).

On exposure to the stressor, volunteers randomized to the experimental intervention showed increased lymphocyte proliferation in response to a mitogen (phytohaemagglutinin) and enhanced circulating levels of the key cytokine, interleukin 1 (IL-1).

Fawzy and colleagues found that a psychosocial intervention altered host defences in patients with malignant melanoma (21). Sixty-eight patients with malignant melanoma were randomized to a group intervention or to a control condition. The intervention comprised six sessions of weekly group psychotherapy, including education about the illness, risk factors, lifestyle, and side-effects; stress management, including relaxation training; facilitation of adaptive coping strategies, and peer group and professional psychological support. At the end of the intervention, there was a significant increase in the percentage of large granular lymphocytes (CD57$^+$) in the intervention group relative to the control group. Six months following the intervention, in addition to increased CD57$^+$ cells, there was a significant increase in the percentage of natural killer (NK) cells.

These and other studies, therefore, suggest that interventions designed to enhance coping can alter host defences in healthy individuals and in patients with cancer.

4   Affective pathways

Clinically significant depression is often associated with increased synthesis and release of adrenal corticosteroids and by decreasing lymphocyte proliferation and natural killer cell activity. Depression is also associated with health-compromising behaviours such as smoking, poor sleep, poor diet, and excessive alcohol consumption. In view of these considerations, a number of studies have investigated the possibility that depression is a risk factor for the development of cancer (22–25). However, comparatively few studies have addressed the role of mood disturbance in disease progression following the diagnosis and the pathways involved.

A recent prospective clinical trial addressed the putative relationship between psychological distress and survival in women with stage II breast cancer (26). Psychological symptoms were assessed using the Symptom Check List-90 (Revised) in 280 women prior to chemotherapy. After controlling for sociodemographic variables (age, ethnicity, education, and marital status) and medical variables (lymph node status, oestrogen receptor status, menopausal status, and performance status), psychological distress did not predict length of disease-free survival or overall survival. Other studies have also found no relationship between psychological morbidity assessed before the beginning of treatment and length of survival (27–29).

However, three studies have found a positive relationship between depression and disease progression (7, 8, 30). In a study of 63 patients with Hodgkin's disease or non-Hodgkin's lymphoma, the depression score at diagnosis, assessed using the Hospital Anxiety and Depression Scale, was a significant independent prognostic factor for survival (7). Similarly, in a study of the effects of primary chemotherapy for locally advanced breast cancer, pre-treatment depression scores, again assessed using the Hospital Anxiety and Depression Scale, independently predicted pathological response to chemotherapy which is often used as a surrogate measure of survival. Higher levels of depression predicted a poorer response to chemotherapy (8).

Watson and colleagues enrolled 578 women with early-stage breast cancer in a prospective survival study. Five years after the diagnosis, 133 women had died. There was a significantly increased risk of death from all causes in women with a high depression score on the Hospital Anxiety and Depression Scale. The authors concluded that depression is linked to a significant reduction in survival, although they pointed out that this conclusion is based on a relatively small number of patients (30).

It is not surprising that studies evaluating depressive symptoms at a single time-point have yielded conflicting results. Some individuals not depressed at the time of evaluation may have been depressed previously or may have been depressed subsequently. A prospective study of 90 women with early breast cancer found that prolonged mood disturbance and level of NK-cell activity predicted disease progression (31). Mood disturbance and NK-cell activity was assessed 5 days after surgery and 15 months later, and time to recurrence was assessed during a follow-up period of between 5 and 8 years. Persistent distress after surgery predicted a shorter time to recurrence as did low NK-cell activity after surgery. Unfortunately, there was substantial attrition at the 15-month follow-up and histological grade was not controlled. It may have been that NK-cell activity simply reflected tumour aggressiveness.

Inconsistent findings have also been reported for stressful life events and cancer progression (32, 33). There are well-documented problems with the assessment of life events, particularly if they are assessed retrospectively. It is important to assess not only the occurrence of an event but also the significance of that event for the individual concerned and the individual's reaction to it (34). It may not be stressful events *per se* that promote disease progression, but rather the psychological and behavioural sequelae of chronic distress (25, 35).

5   Coping styles

The possibility that disease is affected by the way in which individuals manage taxing demands has received some attention in the literature. In a pioneering, long-term, prospective study, Greer and Morris delineated five broad categories of coping styles (16). These were: (a) Fighting Spirit (the patient accepts the diagnosis, is optimistic, determined to fight illness, and wants to participate in decisions regarding treatment); (b) Avoidance/Denial (the patient either rejects the diagnosis or minimizes the seriousness and avoids thinking about it); (c) Fatalism/Stoic Acceptance (the patient accepts the diagnosis and has a resigned, fatalistic attitude); (d) Anxious Preoccupation (the patient is preoccupied with cancer, seeks reassurance, and fears that any aches or pains indicate progression), and (e) Helplessness/Hopelessness (the patient feels overwhelmed, is pessimistic, and feels like giving up).

In stage I and II breast cancer patients, Greer and Morris found that individuals who showed Fighting Spirit or Avoidance/Denial were more likely to be alive after 5 years compared with patients who displayed Helplessness/ Hopelessness or Stoic Acceptance. These differences remained significant after 10 and 15 years (17, 18). Because the study was carried out in the 1970s, information was not available for various biological variables, for example hormone status, which have subsequently been shown to have prognostic value. Although hormone status has not been linked to coping style, oestrogen receptor negativity may be related to greater distress and shorter survival (36).

Although negative findings have been reported, associations between Fighting Spirit and good disease outcome, and between Helplessness/Hopelessness and poor disease outcome, have more commonly been found (37). The impact of the other three coping styles is less clear.

In their prospective survival study, Watson and colleagues found that there was a significantly increased risk of relapse or death in women scoring high on 'Helplessness/Hopelessness' as assessed by the Mental Attitude to Cancer Scale (30). Interestingly, 'Fighting Spirit' was not predictive of survival or recurrence. However, a number of important criticisms have been made of this latter finding (38).

An assumption underlying most studies of coping styles and disease outcome is that coping styles are stable and generalize to all aspects of the disease and its treatment. Thus, coping styles are typically measured at one time-point and disease outcome is followed over a defined period. Our model suggests this may not be an accurate representation of the coping process. Several studies have measured coping styles over time and found substantial change from one assessment to the next. In a study of 130 women with breast cancer, significant changes in internal locus of control, neuroticism, and social conformity were observed during neoadjuvant chemotherapy for breast cancer. In addition, emotional control scores were affected by mid-treatment feedback regarding clinical response (39). Another study found that social conformity and emotional suppression, commonly regarded as defining aspects of the 'Cancer-Prone' (Type C) Personality that are thought to be stable and enduring personality traits, were significantly reduced by relaxation and guided imagery (8). It is clear that patients may use a range of coping styles during treatment, disease progression, and remission (4, 5).

6   Behavioural pathways

It is recognized increasingly that individuals can make major contributions to their own health and well-being through the adoption of health-enhancing behaviours and the avoidance of health-compromising behaviours. Research into the causes of cancer has implicated behaviours such as smoking, dietary habits, high alcohol consumption, and physical inactivity. However, behavioural factors related specifically to the progression of cancer have received considerably less attention. Such factors might include:

- compliance with medical regimens (e.g. surgery, chemotherapy, radiotherapy, use of medication);
- use of professional and social resources (e.g. attendance at clinics to monitor symptoms and side-effects of treatment, developing good relationships with medical staff to facilitate active problem solving, and involving family members in treatment);
- lifestyle factors (e.g. sleep, diet, exercise, uptake of complementary therapies).

6.1 COMPLIANCE WITH MEDICAL REGIMENS

Compliance with conventional treatment is often related to the outcome of cancer. Non-compliance is a significant problem in health care generally. On average, 40 per cent of patients do not follow their doctor's recommendations. More than 75 per cent are unwilling or unable to follow recommended lifestyle changes such as exercising or eating a low-fat diet (40). In terms of disease outcome, non-compliance has been shown to be the cause of poor disease control among patients with hypertension, epilepsy, childhood asthma, post-chemotherapy fever, affective disorders, heart disease, and other health problems (41).

In studies of children and adolescents with cancer, compliance with oral medication ranges between 10 and 59 per cent. It has been suggested that not complying with medication poses a threat to the prognosis of over 50 per cent of adolescents with cancer (42). In a study of adults with haematological malignancies, more than 70 per cent did not comply with oral self-administered medication, and 30 per cent missed appointments (43). High rates of non-compliance have been reported across treatment regimens, including chemotherapy (44), radiotherapy (45), scheduled clinic appointments (43), and oral self-medication (43). However, good compliance with treatment has also been reported for children (46, 47) and for adults (48, 49). These discrepant findings may reflect a number of contextual factors, such as the quality of staff–patient communication and treatment milieu. In addition, various ways of assessing compliance have been used. Self-report typically produces higher estimates of compliance than pill counts. Electronic devices can now monitor how often bottles are opened but not that the medication is taken. Blood and urine samples give accurate estimates, although they may be expensive and impractical. Very few studies have used multiple measures.

There is a lack of research into the specific, individual determinants (personality, mood, coping styles, self-efficacy beliefs) of compliance with cancer treatments. Importantly, there is also a lack of research into the impact of non-compliance with different treatment regimens on survival.

The quality of doctor–patient communication has long been recognized as a prominent factor in the willingness and ability of patients to follow medical recommendations and may account for some of the variance in studies of non-compliance. In a recent meta-analysis of interventions designed to improve compliance (50), physician informativeness, partnership building, emotional rapport, and support were associated with improved compliance as assessed by pill counts and blood and urine sampling. Perceived self-efficacy has also been implicated: patients follow recommendations in which they believe and which they can carry out (40).

In the context of screening, studies have investigated compliance with investigations following a suspicious finding. Reported rates of compliance following an abnormal test (faecal occult blood test, mammogram, pap smear) range from 43 to 70 per cent (42). In a study of women with a family history of breast cancer, Lerman *et al.* found that, although an abnormal mammogram was distressing, this did not affect adherence to subsequent mammograms (51). Moreover, women whose breast cancer concerns had decreased following their mammogram were less likely to attend for subsequent mammograms, suggesting that they had been falsely reassured. Gilbert *et al.* found recall following a false positive mammogram was distressing, although this recall-induced distress was relatively transient (less than 5 weeks) (52). However, there is a small group of patients who do not comply with follow-up investigations. This has been associated with fear of diagnosis (53), poor communication with medical staff (54), and lack of a prompt follow-up appointment (55).

6.2 DELAYED PRESENTATION OF SYMPTOMS

Stage of disease at diagnosis is a key determinant of survival. Some individuals delay seeking treatment despite having symptoms of disease, although the factors associated with delayed presentation are not well understood. Knowledge about the disease, personal experiences of the disease, access to medical care, lower social class, and psychological distress may affect how soon an individual seeks help (42). However, there are difficulties in studying the psychosocial factors associated with patient delay. Patients who delay may be especially elusive. It is difficult to obtain baseline psychological profiles before the diagnosis and the confounding impact of the diagnosis on mood and recall is well documented (56, 57).

Another difficulty is inconsistent definitions of delay (58). A recent systematic review identified 91 studies of factors influencing the delayed presentation of breast cancer (59). The majority of studies were of poor quality. The only consistent findings were that patients who delayed seeking treatment tended to be older; were more poorly educated; had discovered abnormalities that did not take the form of a lump; and failed to disclose the discovery of the symptom to someone else. According to our conceptualization of coping, it is likely that, at least in some cases, delayed disclosure of symptoms is a behavioural response that protects against psychological distress in the face of seemingly overwhelming demands and limited coping resources.

7 Intervention studies

The most convincing evidence for the relevance to survival of the pathways already described comes from prospective and randomized, controlled intervention studies designed to manipulate these variables. A systematic review of the literature found nine randomized, controlled psychosocial intervention studies (Tables 1 and 2). Seven of these compared one or more psychological interventions with a control condition that excluded a formal intervention. Four found that the psychosocial intervention prolonged survival (Table 1).

7.1 RANDOMIZED, CONTROLLED TRIALS THAT DEMONSTRATE PROLONGED SURVIVAL

Spiegel and colleagues randomized 86 women with metastatic breast cancer to group psychotherapy plus standard medical treatment, or to medical treatment alone. The 57 women randomized to the intervention group were invited to attend 90-minute psychotherapy sessions every week for a year. These sessions were designed to elicit concerns about the disease and included peer group support, emotional expression, relaxation, and autohypnosis for pain management (60).

Ten years later, although there was no statistically significant difference in the median survival of the two groups, patients randomized to psychotherapy survived a mean of 36.6 months compared with 18.9 months in the control group. Four years after the study began, all the control patients had died, whereas a third of the intervention group were still alive. Further analyses of the data demonstrated that the results were not due to differences in initial disease stage or to the treatment received prior to or after therapy (radiotherapy, hormone therapy, or chemotherapy).

This study has been the focus of some debate. In a detailed critique (61), Fox suggested the survival curve for the control group lacked the expected right-skewed tail. He pointed out that the survival curve for those receiving the intervention bore more resemblance to local, tumour registry data than the control group. On the basis of this, he argued that the 12 longest living patients in the control group were unusual. According to local data, they should have lived even longer than they did. In response, Spiegel *et al.* pointed out that a *post hoc* interpretation of their data could not be used to invalidate the significant differences found between the treatment and control conditions within the context of a randomized, controlled clinical trial (62).

Table 1 Randomized, controlled trials which demonstrate prolonged survival

Study	Cancer	Stage	n	Follow-up	Findings
Spiegel *et al.* (60)	Breast	Metastatic	86	10 years	Women randomized to weekly supportive–expressive group psychotherapy had longer mean survival
Richardson *et al.* (63)	Mixed haematological	Mixed (newly diagnosed)	94	2–5 years	Patients randomized to any of three psychoeducational interventions designed to enhance compliance with treatment survived longer
Fawzy *et al.* (64)	Malignant melanoma	I and II	68	5–6 years	Patients randomized to a brief psychoeducational group intervention survived longer
Ratcliffe *et al.* (7)	Hodgkin's disease and non-Hodgkin's lymphoma	II, III, and IV	63	5 years	Patients randomized to relaxation and individual hypnotherapy for chemotherapy side-effects survived longer
Walker *et al.* (65)				13 years	The 13-year follow-up of this study confirmed that relaxation with, or without, hypnotherapy prolonged survival

Table 2 Randomized, controlled trials which do not demonstrate prolonged survival

Study	Cancer	Stage	n	Follow-up	Findings
Linn et al. (68)	Mainly lung	End stage (IV)	120	1 year	Patients randomized to twice weekly death counselling plus standard medical treatment or medical treatment alone. No difference in survival between the groups
Ilnycki et al. (67)	Various	Various, although mainly stage I	127	11 years	Patients randomized to one of three intervention groups or to a control group. Interventions were 1) professionally led 2) professionally led for 3 months, then peer led 3) peer led. No difference in survival compared to control group
Cunningham et al. (69)	Breast	Metastatic	66	5 years	Patients randomized to weekly group supportive therapy plus cognitive behavioural therapy or a home study cognitive behavioural package. No difference in survival between the two groups. No non-intervention control group
Edelman et al. (70)	Breast	Metastatic	121	2–5 years	Patients randomized to group cognitive behavioural therapy or to a standard care control group. No survival advantage associated with participation in the intervention relative to those who received standard care
Walker et al. (8, 71, 72)	Breast	Locally advanced	96	4–5 years	Patients randomized to relaxation and guided imagery plus standard support or to standard support alone. No survival advantage associated with relaxation and guided imagery
Goodman et al. (74)	Breast	Metastatic	235	?	Patients randomized to supportive-expressive therapy on standard care. No difference in survival in the two groups

Richardson *et al.* evaluated the effects of three interventions designed to promote compliance with oral medication and attendance at clinic appointments in 94 patients with haematological malignancies (63). Patients were randomized to one of three interventions or to a control condition. All patients randomized to an intervention received a 1-hour interactive tape and slide presentation given by a project nurse. In addition, the same nurse visited some patients at home. Some of these patients were also given a structured programme designed to enhance compliance with medication and clinic appointments. Survival data were collected 2 to 5 years after commencement of the study. Severity of the disease, compliance with medication, and assignment to any of the three interventions predicted better survival. Multivariate analysis indicated that these psychosocial interventions were associated with prolonged survival even when their beneficial effects on compliance were taken into account.

Fawzy and colleagues evaluated disease recurrence and survival in 68 patients with malignant melanoma. These patients had been randomized to a brief psychoeducational group intervention or to a no-intervention control group (64). All patients were recruited shortly after diagnosis or initial surgical treatment. The treatment group received six sessions of weekly group psychotherapy comprising: education about the illness, risk factors, lifestyle, and side-effects; stress management including relaxation training; development of adaptive coping strategies, and peer group and professional psychological support. When patients were followed up between 5 and 6 years later, 10 of the 34 control patients had died compared with three of the 34 patients who had received the intervention. Analyses of multiple covariates found that Breslow depth and being randomized to the intervention were significantly related to survival. There was also a trend for disease-free survival to be prolonged in the intervention group.

The most recent prospective, randomized, controlled intervention study to report a beneficial effect on survival was reported by Ratcliffe *et al.* (7). They randomized 63 patients with Hodgkin's disease or non-Hodgkin's lymphoma to relaxation therapy with or without hypnotherapy, or to a control condition. The trial was designed to evaluate the benefits of relaxation training and/or hypnotherapy in preventing or controlling chemotherapy-induced side-effects. Survival data have been reported 5 years (7) and 13 years (65) after the initial diagnosis. At 5-year follow-up, univariate analyses showed that survival was related to age, stage of disease at presentation, and performance status. Two psychosocial factors also predicted survival; depression scores at diagnosis (assessed using the Hospital Anxiety and Depression Scale) and L scores (assessed using the Eysenck Personality Inventory). L scores within a medical context are thought to be a measure of social conformity, a defining aspect of the 'cancer-prone' personality. Multivariate analyses showed that early stage of disease at diagnosis, low depression scores, low scores on the L scale, and having a psychological intervention were independent prognostic factors for survival. Subsequent analysis showed that the survival benefit from the intervention was greatest for patients with high L scores at diagnosis (66). The 13-year follow-up of this study confirmed that relaxation with or without hypnotherapy prolonged survival in patients with lymphoma. Thirteen years after the initial diagnosis, 35 of the 63 patients had died. Patients receiving relaxation plus hypnosis survived a mean 125.8 months, patients receiving relaxation alone survived a mean 104.5 months, compared to the control group who survived a mean 93.8 months. As found at the 5-year follow-up, high depression scores and high L scores at diagnosis were independent predictors of poorer survival.

Although none of these trials was designed to evaluate the effects of interventions on survival, the results are suggestive. They were all carried out prospectively with appropriate controls and included reasonable follow-up periods. Two trials included homogeneous groups of cancer patients (60, 64). One trial investigated patients with Hodgkin's and non-Hodgkin's lymphoma (7), and another included patients with a variety of haematological malignancies (63). The interventions were well defined and carried out by trained personnel.

The finding that a range of different psychotherapeutic interventions influenced survival can be explained using the model of cancer progression outlined earlier (Figure 1). One trial used a behavioural package designed to alter a specific aspect of behaviour, namely compliance with oral self-medication (63). Three trials incorporated relaxation training (7, 60, 64), which targeted physiological arousal and may have promoted feelings of control over the disease. Two trials used hypnotherapy which targeted physiological arousal via relaxation and cognitive pathways via positive suggestion and imagery (7, 60). One study focused on coping skills, lifestyle, and management of side-effects (64). Interestingly, all trials, regardless of the nature of the intervention, improved mood. According to the model, interventions targeted primarily at behaviour, physiological arousal, or cognitive pathways may have an effect at all other levels, including mood. Given the evidence that physiological arousal, mood, and coping have immunological correlates, it is unsurprising that psychosocial interventions affect the immune system in patients with cancer (21).

7.2 RANDOMIZED, CONTROLLED TRIALS THAT DO NOT DEMONSTRATE PROLONGED SURVIVAL

Six studies have failed to demonstrate prolonged survival (Table 2).

In one study (67), the outcome of three different interventions were combined and compared to a no-treatment control. One group met weekly for 6 months and was led by a social worker. The second group met weekly with a social worker for 3 months then continued to meet themselves for a further 3 months. The third group was peer led and met weekly without a leader for

6 months. These interventions lacked a defined protocol or purpose and it is unsurprising that, after 11 years, there were no differences in survival between the groups and the no-treatment control group.

Another study evaluated 120 patients with a variety of end-stage cancers (68). Patients were eligible if they had advanced metastatic disease and were deemed likely to survive between 3 and 12 months. Patients were randomized to intense individual counselling (based on the work of Kubler-Ross) or to a no-treatment control group. Counselling was designed to maintain hope while being realistic about the illness, to facilitate control over the environment, and to encourage patients to complete unfinished business and to find meaning in life despite the cancer. Counselling significantly reduced depression and alienation and improved life satisfaction, self-esteem, and locus of control. However, there was no significant survival benefit.

A study carried out by Cunningham and colleagues was designed specifically to test the effect of a psychological intervention on survival (69). Women with metastatic breast cancer were randomized to 35 weekly, 2-hour sessions consisting of support and cognitive behavioural therapy or a home-based cognitive behavioural package. No significant difference in survival was found 5 years after commencement of the study. However, both survival curves were similar to the survival curve of Spiegel *et al.*'s intervention group: they were unlike the curve of Spiegel *et al.*'s control group which suggests that both interventions may have been effective in enhancing survival. The lack of a no-intervention control group limits the findings, because both interventions may have had a beneficial effect.

A recently reported study evaluated the effects of group cognitive behavioural therapy on the survival time of patients with metastatic breast cancer (70). Patients were randomly allocated to an intervention group comprising 8 weekly sessions of therapy, followed by 3 further monthly sessions, or to a standard care support group. The intervention was associated with short-term benefits in mood and self-esteem. However, these were not sustained at 3-month and 6-month follow-up assessments. At the time of the survival analysis, patients had entered the study between 2 and 5 years previously. Only medical factors associated with disease severity, such as the Eastern Cooperative Oncology Group (ECOG) performance status, presence of visceral metastases, and chemotherapy treatment, significantly predicted survival time. The intervention did not prolong survival.

In a recent randomized, clinical trial, Walker and colleagues evaluated the effects of relaxation training and guided imagery on quality of life and response to primary chemotherapy in women with locally advanced breast cancer (8). Women received six cycles of primary chemotherapy, surgery, hormone therapy, and radiotherapy. In addition, they were randomized to a high level of support or to identical support plus relaxation and guided imagery. Although the groups did not differ on clinical and pathological response to chemotherapy, mood disturbance before chemotherapy was an independent predictor of both clinical and pathological response to primary chemotherapy. Multivariate analyses showed that pathological response to chemotherapy was independently predicted by tumour size and by depression (assessed by the Hospital Anxiety and Depression Scale). Anxiety and tumour size independently predicted clinical response. The lack of a significant difference between the intervention and control groups in terms of response to chemotherapy may be explained by the strikingly low incidence of mood disturbance in both groups as assessed by structured clinical interviews and by the Hospital Anxiety and Depression Scale.

This study also evaluated the effects of relaxation therapy and guided imagery on immune function. Relaxation and guided imagery increased the number and percentage of mature T cells ($CD2^+$), cells bearing the T cell receptor subunit ($CD3^+$), and activated T cells ($CD25^+$). The intervention also lowered the circulating level of tumour necrosis factor alpha and increased lymphokine-activated killer (LAK) cell cytotoxicity. Although the two groups did not differ in NK-cell cytotoxicity, self-rated imagery quality was highly correlated with natural cytotoxicity and with clinical response.

When the women were followed up for a median of 70 months, the number of patients surviving in the two groups did not differ significantly (75 and 71 per cent, respectively) (71). Multivariate analyses revealed that survival was independently predicted only by tumour size and change in the number of $CD56^+$ cells during chemotherapy. The failure of previously established prognostic factors (such as oestrogen receptor status) to predict survival suggests that longer follow-up would be appropriate (72, 73). It is interesting to note that the overall survival of 73 per cent was very high for patients with large and locally advanced breast carcinomas).

The largest study reported to date (as an abstract) was carried out in 5 centres in Canada. 235 women with metastatic breast carcinoma, with an expected survival of at least three months, were randomized to weekly supportive expressive therapy or standard care. The study was designed to replicate the finding of Spiegel *et al.* (60). Survival analyses were conducted when 86 per cent of the women had died. There were differences between the two groups at the time of randomization (i.e. before the intervention); subjects randomized to the intervention were more likely to be node positive, to be progesterone receptor positive, and to have received adjuvant chemotherapy. Multivariate analyses failed to reveal a statistically significant effect for the intervention. Although this is the largest study reported to date, a 2:1 randomization schedule was used. Although the exact figure is not reported in the abstract, this implies that the control group only contained approximately 78 women. The authors also state that all of the women received educational packages and any type of psychosocial care deemed necessary. This may have minimised between-group differences.

Most of these studies reporting no survival benefit have a number of methodological shortcomings. Two studies included diagnostically heterogeneous patients (67, 68), and one of these also included patients with different stages of disease (67). One study compared three different interventions, all of which lack a defined protocol (67). Another study lacked a no-treatment control group, comparing two cognitive-behavioural interventions that may have been equally efficacious (69). The largest study involved 7 different centres (74).

To summarise, the effects of psychological interventions on survival is currently unclear. The number of patients participating in each of the studies is so small that the effect of the intervention would have to have been very substantial to detect reliably. Also, because of small numbers, studies may find a statistically significant difference that is unreliable. The situation is further complicated by treatment heterogeneity, patient heterogeneity, disease heterogeneity and the possibility that interventions may affect survival through a number of different mechanisms, including enhanced compliance with conventional treatment, the promotion of a healthy lifestyle, direct effects on the tumour itself via a psychoneuroimmunological mechanism, and, perhaps, reducing the incidence of septic complications. It may be, therefore, that survival is only affected in selected individuals.

Perhaps the time has come to ask which patients (personality, coping, mood) with which disease (type of cancer, stage of disease) benefit from which psychosocial intervention (supportive-expressive, relaxation, imagery, existential, etc). A further consideration is that 'support' services have become much more available than previously. If 'support' itself prolongs survival, this will of course make it more difficult to demonstrate differences between an 'intervention' group and a 'control' group.

8   Conclusions

There is substantial evidence that psychological interventions are helpful in alleviating distress. There is also a growing body of evidence to suggest they may influence survival. Prospective, randomized, controlled intervention studies remain the best way to evaluate the relationship between psychological, immunological, and behavioural factors and cancer progression. Our model, based on the work of Lazarus, Folkman, and Bandura, suggests how psychological interventions may be targeted at specific aspects of the coping process. Evaluating the effects of multimodal intervention packages adds little to our understanding of the mechanisms involved. There is a need to dismantle interventions and evaluate the effects of individual psychotherapeutic components (relaxation therapy, guided imagery, hypnotherapy, cognitive therapy). Only then will the causal directions and relative importance of behavioural, psychological, and immunological pathways and their relative contributions to the disease process be understood.

9 References

1. Lazarus, R. S. and Folkman, S. (1984). *Stress, Appraisal and Coping*. Springer, New York.
2. Lazarus, R. S. (1999). *Stress and Emotion: A New Synthesis*. Springer, London.
3. Lazarus, R. S. (1993). Coping theory and research: past, present and future. *Psychosom. Med.*, 55, 234–247.
4. Bandura, A. (1997). *Self-efficacy: The Exercise of Control*. Freeman, New York.
5. Buddeberg, C., Sieber, M., Wolf, C., Landolt-Ritter, C., Richter, D., and Steiner, R. (1996). Are coping strategies related to disease outcome in early breast cancer? *J. Psychosom. Res.*, 40, 255–263.
6. Murphy, K. C., Jenkins, P. L., and Whittaker, J. A. (1996). Psychosocial morbidity and survival in adult bone marrow transplant recipients: a follow-up study. *Bone Marrow Transplant.*, 18, 199–201.
7. Ratcliffe, M. A., Dawson, A. A., and Walker, L. G. (1995). Eysenck personality inventory L-scores in patients with Hodgkin's disease and non-Hodgkin's lymphoma. *Psycho-Oncology*, 4, 39–45.
8. Walker, L. G., Walker, M. B., Ogston, K., Heys, S. D., Ah-See, A. K., Miller, I. D. *et al.* (1999). Psychological, clinical and pathological effects of relaxation training and guided imagery during primary chemotherapy. *Br. J. Cancer*, 80, 262–268.
9. Akechi, T., Okamura, H., Yamawaki, S., and Uchitomi, Y. (1998). Predictors of patients' mental adjustment to cancer: patient characteristics and social support. *Br. J. Cancer*, 77, 2381–2385.
10. Krongrad, A., Lai, H., Burke, M. A., Goodkin, K. and Lai, S. (1996). Marriage and mortality in prostate cancer. *J. Urol.*, 156, 1696–1670.
11. Waxler-Morrison, N., Hislop, T. G., Mears, B., and Kan, L. (1991). Effects of social relationships on survival for women with breast cancer: a prospective study. *Soc. Sci. Med.*, 33, 177–183.
12. Bandura, A., Reese, L., and Adams, N. E. (1982). Microanalysis of action and fear arousal as a function of differential levels of perceived self-efficacy. *J. Pers. Soc. Psychol.*, 43, 5–21.
13. Bandura, A., Taylor, C. B., Williams, S. L., Mefford, I. N., and Barchas, J. D. (1985). Catecholamine secretion as a function of perceived coping self-efficacy. *J. Consult. Clin. Psychol.*, 53, 406–414.
14. Bandura, A., Cioffi, D., Taylor, C. B., and Brouillard, M. E. (1988). Perceived self-efficacy in coping with cognitive stressors and opioid activation. *J. Pers. Soc. Psychol.*, 55, 479–488.
15. Wiedenfeld, S. A., O'Leary, A., Bandura, A., Brown, S., Levine, S., and Raska, K. (1990). Impact of perceived self-efficacy in coping with stressors on components of the immune system. *J. Pers. Soc. Psychol.*, 59, 1082–1094.
16. Greer, S. and Morris, T. (1975). Psychological attributes of women who develop breast cancer: a controlled study. *J. Psychosom. Res.*, 19, 147–153.
17. Pettingale, K. W., Morris, T., Greer, S., and Haybittle, J. (1985). Mental attitudes to cancer: an additional prognostic factor. *Lancet*, 1, 750.
18. Greer, S., Morris, T., Pettingale, K. W., and Haybittle, J. (1990). Psychological response to breast cancer and 15 year outcome. *Lancet*, I, 49–50.

254 *J. Anderson and L. G. Walker*

19. Buckingham, J. C., Gillies, G. E., and Cowell, A. (eds). (1997). *Stress, Stress Hormones and the Immune System.* New York, Wiley.
20. Johnson, V. C., Walker, L. G., Whiting, P., Heys, S. D., and Eremin, O. (1996). Can relaxation training and hypnotherapy modify the immune response to acute stress and is hypnotisability relevant? *Contemp. Hypnosis,* 13, 100–108.
21. Fawzy, F. I., Kemeny, M. E., Fawzy, N. W., Elashoff, R., Morton, D., Cousins, N. *et al.* (1990). A structured psychiatric intervention for cancer patients II: changes over time in immunological measures. *Arch. Gen. Psychiatry,* 47, 729–735.
22. Shekelle, R. B., Raynor, W. J., Ostfeld, A. M., Garron, D. C., Bieliauskas, L. A., Liu, S. C. *et al.* (1981). Psychological depression and 17 year risk of death from cancer. *Psychosom. Med.,* 43, 117–125.
23. Persky, V. W., Kempthorne-Rawson, J., and Shekelle, R. B. (1987). Personality and risk of cancer: 20-year follow-up of the Western Electric Study. *Psychosom. Med.,* 49, 435–449.
24. Zonderman, A. B., Costa, P. T., and McRae, R. R. (1989). Depression as a risk for cancer morbidity and mortality in a nationally representative sample. *J. Am. Med. Assoc.,* 262, 1191–1195.
25. Penninx, B. W. J. H., Guralnik, J. M., Pahor, M., Ferrucci, L., Cerhan, J. R., Wallace, R. B. *et al.* (1998). Chronically depressed mood and cancer risk in older persons. *J. Natl. Cancer Inst.,* 90, 1888–1893.
26. Tross, S., Herndon, J., Korzun, A., Kornblith, A. B., Cella, D. F., Holland, J. F. *et al.* (1996). Psychological symptoms and disease-free and overall survival in women with stage II breast cancer. *J. Natl. Cancer Inst.,* 88, 661–667.
27. Silberfarb, P. M., Anderson, K. M., Rundle, A. C., Holland, J. C., Cooper, M. R., and McIntyre, O. R. (1991). Mood and clinical status in patients with multiple myeloma. *J. Clin. Oncol.,* 9, 2219–2224.
28. Jamieson, R. N., Burish, T. G., and Wallston, K. A. (1987). Psychogenic factors in predicting survival of breast cancer patients. *J. Clin. Oncol.,* 5, 768–772.
29. Cassileth, B. R., Lusk, E. J., Miller, D. S., Brown, L. L., and Miller, C. (1985). Psychological correlates of survival in advanced malignant disease? *N. Engl. J. Med.,* 312, 1551–1555.
30. Watson, M., Haviland, J. S., Greer, S., Davidson, J., and Bliss, J. M. (1999). Influence of psychological response on survival in breast cancer: a population-based cohort study. *Lancet,* 354, 1331–1336.
31. Levy, S. M., Herberman, R. B., Lippman, M., D'Angelo, T., and Lee, J. (1991). Immunological and psychosocial predictors of disease recurrence in patients with early breast cancer. *Behav. Med.,* 17, 67–75.
32. Ramirez, A. J., Craig, T. J. K., and Watson, J. P. (1989). Stress and relapse of breast cancer. *Br. Med. J.,* 298, 191–193.
33. Barraclough, J., Pinder, P., Cruddas, M., Osmond, C., Taylor, I., and Perry, M. (1992). Life events and breast cancer prognosis. *Br. Med. J.,* 304, 1078–1081.
34. McGee, S., Williams, S., and Elwood, M. (1996). Are life events related to the onset of breast cancer? *Psychol. Med.,* 26, 441–447.
35. Prigerson, H. G., Bierhals, A. J., Kasl, S. V., Reynolds, C. F., Shear, K., Day, N. *et al.* (1997). Traumatic grief as a risk factor for mental and physical morbidity. *Am. J. Psychiatry,* 154, 616–623.

36. Razavi, D., Farvacques, C., Delvaux, N., Beffort, T., Paesmans, M., Leclercq, G. *et al.* (1990). Psychosocial correlates of oestrogen and progesterone receptors in breast cancer. *Lancet*, 335, 931–933.
37. Watson, M. and Greer, S. (1998). Personality and coping. In *Psycho-oncology* (ed. J. C. Holland), pp. 91–98. Oxford University Press, New York.
38. Leonard, R. C. F., Petry, J. J., and Temoshok, L. R. (2000). Psychological response and survival from breast cancer [comment]. *Lancet*, 355, 404–406.
39. Walker, L. G., Walker, M. B., Simpson, E., Heys, S., Anderson, J., Sharp, D. M. *et al.* (2001). Coping with cancer: state or trait? *Proc. Br. Psychol. Soc.*, 9, 269.
40. DiMatteo, M. R. (1994). Enhancing patient adherence to medical recommendations. *J. Am. Med. Assoc.*, 27, 79–83.
41. Richardson, J. L., Landrine, H., and Marks, G. (1994). Does psychological status influence cancer patient survival? A case still in need of evidence. In *The Psychoimmunology of Cancer* (eds C. E. Lewis, C. O'Sullivan, and J. Barraclough), pp. 228–245. Oxford University Press, New York.
42. Richardson, J. L. and Sanchez, K. (1998). Compliance with cancer treatment. In *Psycho-oncology* (ed. J. C. Holland), pp. 67–77. Oxford University Press, New York.
43. Levine, A. M., Richardson, J. L., Marks, G. *et al.* (1987). Compliance with oral drug therapy in patients with hematologic malignancy. *J. Clin. Oncol.*, 5, 1469–1476.
44. Feld, R., Rubinstein, L., Thomas, P. A., and the Lung Cancer Study Group (1993). Adjuvant chemotherapy with cyclophosphamide, doxorubicin and cisplatin in patients with completely resected stage I non-small cell lung cancer. *J. Natl. Cancer Inst.*, 85, 299–305.
45. Formenti, S. C., Meyerowitz, B. E., Ell, K. *et al.* (1995). Inadequate adherence to radiotherapy in Latina immigrants with carcinoma of the cervix: potential impact on disease free survival. *Cancer*, 75, 1135–1140.
46. Davies, H. A., Lennard, L., and Lilleyman, J. S. (1993). Variable mercaptopurine metabolism in children with leukemia: a problem of non-compliance? *Br. Med. J.*, 306, 1239–1240.
47. Lennard, L. and Lilleyman, J. S. (1993). Compliance with 6-mercaptopurine metabolism in UKALL trials. *Br. J. Haematol.*, 84(Suppl.), 19.
48. Moul, J. W., Paulson, D. F., and Walther, P. J. (1989). Refusal of cancer treatment in testicular cancer patients. *J. Natl. Cancer Inst.*, 81, 1587–1588.
49. Lee, C. R., Nicholson, P. W., Souhami, R. L., and Deshmukh, A. A. (1992). Patient compliance with oral chemotherapy as assessed by a novel electronic technique. *J. Clin. Oncol.*, 10, 1007–1013.
50. Roter, D. L., Hall, J. A., Merisca, R., Nordstrom B., Cretin D., and Svarstad B. (1998). Effectiveness of interventions to improve patient compliance: a meta-analysis. *Med. Care*, 36, 1138–1161.
51. Lerman, C., Trock, B., Rimer, B. K., Boyce, A., Jepson, C., and Engstrom P. F. (1991). Psychological and behavioural implications of abnormal mammograms. *Ann. Intern. Med.*, 114, 657–661.
52. Gilbert, F. J., Cordiner, C. M., Affleck, I. R., Hood, D. B., Mathieson, D., and Walker, L. G. (1998). Breast screening: the psychological sequelae of false-positive recall in women with and without a family history of breast cancer. *Eur. J. Cancer*, 34, 2010–2014.

53. Lerman, C., Ross, E., Boyce, A. *et al.* (1992). The impact of mailing psychoeducational materials to women with abnormal mammograms. *Am. J. Public Health*, **82**, 729–730.

54. Lauver, D. and Rubin, M. (1990). Message framing, dispositional optimism and follow-up for abnormal papanicolaou tests. *Res. Nurs. Health*, **13**, 199–207.

55. Paskett, E. D., White, E., Carter, W. B., and Chu, J. (1990). Improving follow-up after an abnormal pap smear, a randomised control trial. *Prev. Med.*, **19**, 630–641.

56. Kreitler, S., Chaitchik. S., and Kreitler, H. (1993). Repressiveness: cause or result of cancer? *Psycho-Oncology*, **2**, 43–54.

57. Servaes, P., Vingerhoets, A., Vreugdenhil, G., Keuning, J. and Broekhuijsen, M. A. (1996). Breast cancer and nonexpression of emotions. *Psychosom. Med.*, **58**, 67.

58. Caplan, L. S. and Helzlsouer, K. J. (1992). Delay in breast cancer: a review of the literature. *Public Health Rev.*, **93**, 187–214.

59. Ramirez, A. J., Westcombe, A. M., Burgess, C. C., Sutton, S. R., Littlejohns, P., and Richards, M. A. Factors influencing delayed presentation of breast cancer: a systematic review. *Psycho-Oncology* (in press).

60. Spiegel, D., Bloom, J. R., Kraemer, H. C., and Gottheil, E. (1989). Effect of psychosocial treatment on survival of patients with metastatic breast cancer. *Lancet*, **2**, 888–891.

61. Fox, B. H. (1998). A hypothesis about Spiegel *et al.*'s 1989 paper on psychosocial intervention and breast cancer survival. *Psycho-Oncology*, **7**, 371–375.

62. Spiegel, D., Kraemer, H. C., and Bloom, J. R. (1998). A tale of two methods: randomisation versus matching trials in clinical research. *Psycho-Oncology*, **7**, 371–375.

63. Richardson, J. L., Shelton, D. R., Krailo, M., and Levine, A. M. (1990). The effect of compliance with treatment on survival among patients with haematological malignancies. *J. Clin. Oncol.*, **8**, 356–364.

64. Fawzy, F. I., Fawzy, N., Hyun, L. S., Elashoff, R., Guthrie, D., Fahy, J. L. *et al.* (1993). Malignant melanoma: effects of an early structured psychiatric intervention, coping and affective state on recurrence and survival 6 years later. *Arch. Gen. Psychiatry*, **50**, 681–689.

65. Walker, L. G., Ratcliffe, M. A., and Dawson, A. A. (2000). Relaxation and hypnotherapy: long term effects on the survival of patients with lymphoma. *Psycho-Oncology*, **9**, 355–356.

66. Walker, L. G. (1998). Hypnosis and cancer: host defences, quality of life and survival. *Contemp. Hypnosis*, **15**, 34–38.

67. Ilnyckyj, A., Farber, J., Cheang, M. C., and Weinerman, B. H. (1994). A randomised controlled trial of psychotherapeutic interventions in cancer patients. *Ann. R. Coll. Physicians Surg. Can.*, **27**, 93–96.

68. Linn, M. W., Linn, B. S., and Harris, R. (1982). Effects of counselling for late stage cancer patients. *Cancer*, **49**, 1048–1055.

69. Cunningham, A. J., Edmonds, C. V. I., Jenkins, G. P., Pollack, H., Lockwood, G. A., and Warr, D. (1998). A randomised controlled trial of the effects of group psychological therapy on survival in women with metastatic breast cancer. *Psycho-Oncology*, **7**, 508–517.

70. Edelman, S., Lemon, J., Bell, D. R., and Kidman, A. D. (1999). Effects of group CBT on the survival time of patients with metastatic breast cancer. *Psycho-Oncology*, **8**, 474–481.

71. Walker, M. B., Walker, L. G., Simpson, E., Hutcheon, A. W., Sarkar, T. K., Heys, S. D. *et al.* (2000). Do relaxation and guided imagery improve survival in women with locally advanced breast cancer? *Psycho-Oncology*, 9, 355.
72. Eremin, O., Walker, M. B., Simpson, E., Hutcheon, A. W., Sarkar, T. K., Heys, S. D. *et al.* (2001). Changes in the number of natural killer, ($CD56^+$) cells, but not relaxation and guided imagery, predict survival in breast cancer. *Psycho-Oncology*, 10, 264.
73. Spiegel, D., Sephton, S. E., Terr, A. I., and Sites, D. P. (1998). Effects of psychosocial treatment in prolonging cancer survival may be mediated by neuroimmune pathways. *Ann. N. Y. Acad. Sci.*, 840, 674–683.
74. Goodwin, P. J., Leszcz, M., Koopmans, J., Doll, R., Arnold, A., Hundleby, M., *et al.* (2001). The breast expressive-supportive therapy (BEST) study: an RCT of the effect of group psychological support or survival in metastatic breast cancer. *ASCO Abstracts*, 79.

8

The state of the art: clinical implications for cancer patients and directions for future research

A. J. CUNNINGHAM

1 Introduction

This final chapter was requested as a general overview of the field, with some reference to the other papers, and some speculation on profitable directions for research, the emphasis being on clinical implications. It will thus consider broad trends rather than details. Inevitably it will be an expression of personal views, so the author's background and biases need to be acknowledged. I began doctoral training for a research career in immunology in 1964, at which time it was widely believed that control of cancer would soon be achieved through our rapidly growing knowledge of the immune system. By the early 1980s, this goal seemed as far out of reach as ever, and for this and other reasons I moved to research in health psychology, which seemed to me to have more promise for helping people with cancer. In 2001, despite many advances in knowledge of immunological mechanisms, significant deliberate control of most human cancers through this avenue is still not possible. New avenues of research show promise, and immunological research, including research on possible effects of the immune system on cancer cells, continues to have an extremely important impact on many areas, for example autoimmunity, transplantation biology, infectious disease, and general cell and molecular biology. My particular bias, however, is that the greatest potential for health promotion in many areas, including cancer, lies in better understanding of and assistance to human psychological motivation and functioning. These and other biases underlie the predictions of Table 1, which are aimed at stimulating new lines of thought.

While we do not need to comprehend all the physiological pathways through which mind acts on body in order to exert mental control over a disease process, such knowledge of mechanism would strengthen our conviction that the mind indeed has an impact, and might point to chemical analogues for some of the effects of mind. It is clear that *something* regulates many cancers, as is demonstrated by such patterns as the high incidence of precancerous lesions found in breast and prostate at autopsy, or the long periods of dormancy followed by a 'shower' of metastases in some people with breast cancer. Exactly what these mechanisms are is still subject to debate and intense investigation. The immune system is one of many candidates. A volume on *Psychoregulation of Cancer* would include a wider variety of intermediaries between mind and cancer progression; we are dealing here with a subset of these possible pathways.

2 The range of disciplines which 'the psychoimmunology of cancer' draws upon

An obvious way to arrange the fields of study covered by this subject is in a chart like Figure 1. This resembles the figure in the review by Garssen and Goodkin (Chapter 6), and the explanatory diagrams in Bovbjerg's summary chapter in the first edition of this volume (1). It embraces a number of possible intermediaries between mind and cancer progression, among them the psychoimmunological.

The aim of the psychoimmunology of cancer is to clarify all parts of this diagram involving the pathway: mind–immune system–cancer. As can be seen, many disciplines or areas of research are represented (see below). Note that

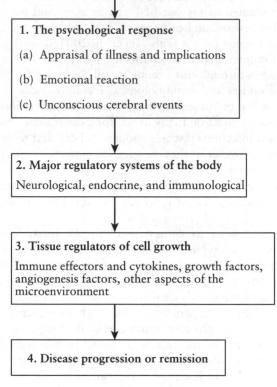

Figure 1

none is intrinsically more 'scientific' than any other; explanations for phenomena like an effect of mind on cancer can be sought at any level, and in various 'languages' (i.e. in terms of structures or of informational transductions) (2). Note also that the most popular current level of analysis in cancer research, the genetic, is not represented because it is not (yet?) suggested that it can be influenced by the mind.

3   Components of the pathway

3.1   OVERVIEWS

A newcomer to this topic could hardly do better than to read the article by Garssen and Goodkin (Chapter 6). In a balanced, critical way they have attempted to cover the whole field. While pointing to known influences of psychological and neurological factors on endocrine and immune systems, they conclude that the clinical potential for cancer is not clear; for example, there is as yet no demonstration of therapy-induced changes in immune status affecting cancer outcome. In other words, no 'three-point fix': psychological–immune–cancer. However, there is considerable evidence for linkage of the first two elements in this chain (and see Chapter 1), and some for links of psychological state to cancer outcome. They refer to the fascinating work in animal models where manipulation of perceived control over stress reliably affects rate of growth in transplanted tumours (first described by Sklar and Anisman (3)), and to recent human studies, which are taken up in more detail in Chapters 3, 5, and 7.

Booth, an immunologist, takes an Olympian stance in Chapter 4, his present topic being the logic and informational transactions involved in maintaining health. I agree with his view that we must learn to see the biological domain nested within the psychological, which is in turn encompassed by the spiritual. He would no doubt agree on the need to operationalize these concepts, for purpose of measurement and use in the clinic.

The experimental work described or referred to in this volume is usually an attempt to link events in two or three of the 'boxes' of Figure 1. The remaining chapters can be classified according to which boxes are involved.

3.2 HOW MIND AFFECTS THE IMMUNE SYSTEM

The field of psychophysiology is well-established and diverse: it relates boxes 1 with 2 and 3, describing the effects of mental change on a wide range of physiological variables (cardiovascular and endocrine, for example). Psychoimmunology is a relatively young discipline within this broad area. It can be approached from the standpoint of function, as in the brilliant experiments by Ader, Cohen, Bovbjerg, and colleagues on psychological conditioning of the immune response (4), or more from an interest in structural and biochemical relationships between the nervous and immune systems, as in Chapter 1, by Bellinger, Felten, and colleagues. Bellinger *et al.* sweep away any reservations the sceptical reader may entertain with the sheer weight of data (much of it their own excellent work) which now supports an intimate, bidirectional communication between these systems. The authors point to a need for research integrating behavioural, pharmacological, neurological, and immunological elements. This kind of work—relating multiple levels of phenomena—is extremely demanding, which means that defining the clinical implications of the basic science is likely to be slow.

3.3 HOW THE IMMUNE SYSTEM AFFECTS CANCER

Cancer immunity could be seen as part of a larger discipline that is concerned with the regulation of cell growth and differentiation. The regulation of cancer

Table 1 Comparison of views in psychoimmunology

Conventional view	Less conventional view, and predictions (for the next 15 years)
1. The immune system is a major regulator of cancer progression	1. The immune system may be a relatively minor regulator of human cancer; other mechanisms operate at the tissue level
2. The most efficient way to understand (psycho)immune regulation is by reductionist analysis (taking it apart and examining the components)	2. (Psycho)immune regulation will be best understood (i.e. in a way that will allow us to exploit it) by a more holistic, systems approach; e.g. with models derived from complexity theory
3. We will soon learn to manipulate the immune system so that it will control most cancers	3. Most cancers will continue to circumvent therapeutic attempts based on manipulating immune regulation
4. It is important to investigate mechanisms by which the mind acts on cancer via the immune system	4. It is premature to investigate this; the time to study mechanisms by which mind might affect cancer is after the normal regulators have been defined
5. Psychological factors have a very small influence on cancer progression	5. They have a large effect (a) via behaviours and (b) via attitudes, but this latter potential is only actualized in a small proportion of individuals at present
6. Psychological interventions will have no effect or a small average effect on the life span of people with cancer	6. While this may be true on average, there is potential for clinically significant effects in highly motivated individuals, and the proportion helped by psychological interventions will become larger as we better understand the changes that promote healing
7. Psychological interventions for people with cancer (and other serious disease) should be aimed only at improving quality of life	7. Setting limits to what is possible aborts scientific progress. The potential for affecting physical disease through the mind should be investigated
8. Psychological interventions aimed at prolonging life for cancer patients should be rigorously standardized; research should use RCTs and focus on the relationship between intervention and mean outcome in groups of patients	8. This is inefficient because of large inter-individual variation. Therapies should be tailored to the individual, and at the present early state of knowledge, idiographic research will be more productive, i.e. focusing on the relationship between individuals' psychological attributes, changes assisted by therapy, and outcomes
9. New ways of conceptualizing the relationship of mind to bodily health are not needed	9. They are badly needed
10. Spirituality should be left to the religious	10. Spirituality is a vital dimension of health care for the seriously ill; the potential impact of psychospiritual therapy should be investigated

growth tends to be a distinct field of study, embracing such mechanisms as inhibition of angiogenesis, regulation of apoptosis, action of cytokines, growth hormones, and other endocrines, and the general regulating effects of the tissue microenvironment on the growing tumour. Immune mechanisms are one means by which the body may regulate some cancers, and are generally studied as a branch of immunology, distinct from the analysis of other potential regulators. Chapter 2, by Szlosarek and Dalgleish, is a comprehensive look at what is known about cancer immunity, at both molecular and cellular levels. It is natural for those currently engaged in it to be optimistic, and there will no doubt be a degree of success eventually, in the sense that some tumours will become controllable by immune manipulation. The authors cite a great deal of interesting current research that may well translate into clinical benefit (although I did not find reference to the very promising research of Srivastava and colleagues (5) on heat shock proteins). It is significant that a large portion of their review is devoted to 'immunological escape', the ways in which neoplastic cells avoid or block the attentions of the immune system. The large variety of means of escape from immune surveillance offers a range of potential approaches to reversing this self-protection by tumours. Information of great value to immunology generally is being gained from this research. Nevertheless, one has to entertain doubts that immunological therapy for cancer is imminent, mainly because this field has been researched by thousands of researchers over a period of about half a century, without bringing this about.

At the end of their chapter, Szlosarek and Dalgleish make the very interesting observation that 'Both cancer and the immune system are highly complex and non-linear (chaotic) systems, whose interactions cannot be predicted from linear analysis.' Perhaps it would be valuable therefore to approach these systems in a non-reductionist way, such as by trying to define the 'attractors' or higher-order conditions that hold tumours and immune and other potential controllers in a state of equilibrium.

3.4   HOW THE MIND AFFECTS CANCER PROGRESSION

3.4.1   *Psycho-oncology as a separate discipline*

The subspecialty of psycho-oncology could be said to concern itself with two main questions: the impact of a diagnosis of cancer on mental state, and the reverse, the possible effect of mind on cancer initiation and progression. The latter has, in turn, two main divisions: the first and more practically significant is the impact of behaviours on cancer initiation; this is sometimes referred to as the 'external' loop, and studies the impact (and prevention) of smoking, diet, and exposure to other environmental hazards. The less studied although intellectually fascinating 'internal loop' is concerned with the impact of attitudes, that is, states of mind, cognitions, and emotions, on cancer progression.

Both hold promise for alleviating the impact of cancer, in prevention and therapy respectively.

The remaining three chapters fall within psycho-oncology, and seek to connect aspects of boxes 1 and 4 in Figure 1, largely bypassing the physiological intermediary mechanisms. A mechanistically inclined scientist might argue that we need to know these mechanisms, and this is certainly required for 'complete' understanding. However, from a practical standpoint, what matters most is learning to help patients, regardless of how the methods work mechanistically. If states of mind (that is, specific patterns of cognition and behaviour) can be shown to promote health, then we need to understand these patterns as fully as we can, so as to direct patients towards the healing states. Mechanisms can be elucidated later. In fact, once the intermediaries between mind and cancer are well understood, it is possible that chemical analogues will be found that mimic whatever the mind may do to retard cancer progression, thus rendering this branch of psycho-oncology obsolete!

3.4.2   *Studies on the relationship of states of mind to cancer progression, and new approaches*

Research on the relationship between personality attributes or cognitive styles and cancer incidence and progression has a long and conflicted history. Chapter 3, by Levenson and McDonald, continues this tradition. They point out that it is difficult to say what factors of this kind affect cancer, although it appears that persisting emotional repression and a helpless–hopeless orientation are risk factors, while social support in many (not all) studies is associated with living longer. The impact of depression and of stress has been frustratingly difficult to pin down in humans. Fighting spirit, thought on the basis of clinical observation and the work of Greer and colleagues (6) to be life-prolonging, did not show survival advantage in a recent large study by Watson *et al.* (7). Levenson and McDonald take a critical stance, pointing out various common flaws in the studies of this area, in particular the fact that investigators can never control for all relevant factors. They refer to the early work of Fox (8) who concluded that if stress and personality factors have an influence on cancer, it is likely to be small.

There are two broad ways of responding to the current lack of certainty in this area. The first, and easiest, is to say 'we need more studies' (of the same kind), and to proceed, in a reductionist way, to try and define elements of the psyche of cancer patients ever more precisely and comprehensively. As with the impact of immunity on cancer, the historical record leaves room for doubt that this strategy will yield much of practical value in the foreseeable future. The second is to seek a fresh approach. In considering what this might be, it helps to consider the cell biology of cancer.

When a tumour is detected, it has been growing for months or years. During that time, the population of constituent cells have been subject to variation and selection, so that what is presented in the clinic is a collection of cells that are comfortably adapted to the host microenvironment. Its rate of growth will only change if there is a change in this environment. Therapeutic changes may sometimes be brought about either by external agents (i.e. medical treatment) or internally, that is, through the development of new patterns of behaviour, cognition, and emotion initiated through the patient's mind. If the mind does not change, then, in the absence of effective external agents, there is no reason why the rate of growth of the cancer should do so. The reason for this preamble is to point out that it is of little use studying static, usually long-established psychological patterns in patients—their cancers have learned to adapt to whatever hormonal microenvironment the mind has promoted. We need, instead, to look at the relationship between *changes* in the mind and changes in the cancer's growth rate. Such change is likely to be more common in people receiving psychological therapy. So the first recommendation to be offered as a stimulant to this field of research is that we should focus on patients in therapy.

There is a second, major problem in attempting to relate states of mind to cancer progression: how to measure the former. The standard approach has been to use self-report paper-and-pencil psychometric tests. These generate numbers, on which sophisticated statistical analyses can be performed, giving an appearance of objectivity and rigour. However, as is well known, these tests provide relatively superficial information about a patient's mental processes, and may elicit invalid answers, as when the respondent pays little attention to the questions, is unable to acknowledge affect, or gives socially desirable answers. Others have pointed to the need for collecting more comprehensive and reliable data from repeated interview-style contacts (9–11). These data might then be best analysed using qualitative methods. Likewise, contextual variables are of vital importance in understanding psychological variables (12–14). We may need to attempt to characterize higher order complexes of variables, rather than becoming ever more reductionist; for example, a person's progress against cancer appeared, in an exploratory study of ours (15), to relate to a combination of their appraisal of the situation, their motivation to help themselves, and what they actually did, all being affected by factors in their social environment. The disadvantage of this kind of analysis, compared with the psychometric, is that it is much more time-consuming. This issue is discussed more thoroughly in a recent paper (16).

3.4.3 *Experimental studies on the effects of psychological therapies on cancer progression, and new approaches*

The need to relate change in psychology to outcome is potentially addressable through studies of the impact of psychological therapies on cancer progression. There is a growing number of studies of this kind, reviewed by Calde, Classen and Spiegel in Chapter 5. To my knowledge there are now (February

2001) 10, small, published trials, most with randomized controlled trial (RCT) designs. Five of these showed positive effects of psychological intervention on survival duration (17–21); five did not (22–26). Several of the authors in this volume have also offered critiques of many (not all) of these studies, and further debate seems superfluous, at least until the imminent publication of two additional larger studies, specifically aimed at testing the survival benefits of therapy. When these are available we should have a more definite idea whether one kind of therapy, 'supportive–expressive' (Chapter 5), produces a significant mean or median improvement in the survival duration of women with metastatic breast cancer. Further trials are under way elsewhere.

The form of the question posed by a controlled trial is significant: the assumption is that psychotherapy should be treated rather like a drug, administered in a standard way, and the average response of the treated group measured. This approach, while appropriate to the specific question, is not optimal for understanding the relationship between mind and cancer. Pre-morbid psychological characteristics, and the response to psychotherapy, differ enormously between patients. Many researchers in the wider field of psychotherapy outcome research have pointed out that within-subject (idiographic) techniques are likely to be much more productive than nomothetic, between-subjects research using experimental designs (12, 13, 27, 28). To put it bluntly, if we want to know how the individual's psychology, and changes in it, relate to survival outcome we need to study individuals. Such case-by-case analyses require much more effort than calculating group statistics; the psychological characterization needs to be of a detailed, qualitative kind if we are to have confidence that we truly understand the patients. In a paper already referred to (16) I have contrasted the vastly greater amount of useful information gained from applying a design of this kind in a recent study of healing through the mind with the minimal output from a concurrent RCT design. Our conclusion was that in the present early stage of the field, what is most needed is more correlational research of this kind, leading eventually to RCTs when we understand what states of mind are protective, what therapies promote these, and how to adjust our therapies to the greatly varying needs of different individuals.

3.4.4   Behavioural pathways

Finally, Anderson and Walker's contribution (Chapter 7) is nominally concerned with behavioural pathways, although in fact they have broadened their comment to include physiological intermediaries and intervention studies, justifiably, in view of Walker's own large and important contributions across this whole spectrum. In addition to the obvious unhealthy behaviours, they point to several specifically related to cancer progression: the understandable tendency of some people to delay seeking a diagnosis for suspected cancer, the surprisingly high rates of non-compliance with medical treatment, and the variable quality of doctor–patient communication.

4 Summary: where do we go from here?

Table 1 is an attempt to provoke new ways of thinking about some of the main aspects of psychoimmunology and, more broadly, psycho-oncology. The main conclusions are:

1. We need a consensus on mechanisms that are important in regulation of cancer. This appears to be many years away, and will require continuing research into many factors, including the immunological.
2. When these mechanisms are known, it will be of great interest to study how the mind can modulate them.
3. In the meantime, we can profitably investigate the direct link, mind–cancer. The temptation is to follow the model of drug research and do ever more RCTs. While this kind of study design has the potential to convince sceptics, if there continue to be some studies with positive and some with negative outcomes, the medical community as a whole is likely to remain unconvinced. Within the field of psycho-oncology, I predict that exclusive reliance on RCTs will lead only to acrimonious debate about the validity of different studies and therapies, and not to a consensus about what helps whom, and to what extent. A more informative approach for the immediate future would be idiographic, correlative studies defining how individuals change psychologically, with the help of intensive psychotherapies, and how this is related to survival outcome.

5 Acknowledgements

I thank Dr Rick Miller (an immunologist) for reading the manuscript and softening my pessimism about the possible application of immunological research to cancer control.

6 References

1. Bovbjerg, D. H. (1994). Psychoneuroimmunology: a critical analysis of the implications for oncology in the twenty-first century. In *The Psychoimmunology of Cancer* (eds C. E. Lewis, C. O'Sullivan, and J. Barraclough), pp. 417–426. Oxford University Press, Oxford.
2. Cunningham, A. J. (1995). Pies, levels and languages: why the contribution of mind to health and disease has been underestimated. *Adv. J. Mind Body Health*, 11, 4–11.
3. Sklar, L. and Anisman, H. (1979). Stress and coping factors influence tumor growth. *Science*, 205, 513–515.

4. Ader, R. and Cohen, N. (1975). Behaviorally conditioned immunosuppression. *Psychosom. Med.*, 37, 333–340.
5. Srivastava, P., Menoret, A., Basu, S., Binder, R., and McQuade, K. (1998). Heat shock proteins come of age: primitive functions acquire new roles in an adaptive world. *Immunity*, 8, 657–665.
6. Greer, S., Morris, T., and Pettingale, K. W. (1979). Psychological response to breast cancer: effect on outcome. *Lancet*, ii, 785–787.
7. Watson, M., Haviland, J. S., Greer, S., Davidson, J., and Bliss, J. M. (1999). Influence of psychological response on survival in breast cancer: a population-based cohort study. *Lancet*, 354, 1331–1336.
8. Fox, B. (1982). Endogenous psychosocial factors in cross-national cancer incidence. In *Social Psychology and Behavioral Medicine* (ed. R. Eiser), pp. 101–141. Wiley, New York.
9. Morris, T., Blake, S., and Buckley, M. (1985). Development of a method for rating cognitive responses to a diagnosis of cancer. *Soc. Sci. Med.*, 20, 795–802.
10. Temoshok, L., Heller, B. W., Sagebiel, R. W. *et al.* (1985). The relationship of psychosocial factors to prognostic indicators in cutaneous malignant melanoma. *J. Psychosom. Res.*, 29, 139–154.
11. Somerfield, M. and Curbow, B. (1992). Methodological issues and research strategies in the study of coping with cancer. *Soc. Sci. Med.*, 34, 1203–1216.
12. Seligman, M. E. P. (1995). The effectiveness of psychotherapy: the 'Consumer Reports' study. *Am. Psychol.*, 50, 965–974.
13. Tennen, H., Affleck, G., Armeli, S., and Carney, M. A. (2000). A daily process approach to coping. Linking therapy, research and practice. *Am. Psychol.*, 55, 626–636.
14. Lazarus, R. S. (2000). Toward better research on stress and coping. *Am. Psychol.*, 55, 665–673.
15. Cunningham, A. J, Edmonds, C. V. I., Phillips, C., Soots, K. I., Hedley, D., and Lockwood, G. A. (2000). A prospective, longitudinal study of the relationship of psychological work to duration of survival in patients with metastatic cancer. *Psycho-Oncology*, 9, 323–339.
16. Cunningham, A. J. (2001) Healing through the mind: extending our theories, research and clinical practice. *Adv. Mind Body Med.*, 17, 214–227.
17. Spiegel, D., Bloom, J. R., Kraemer, H. C., and Gottlieb, E. (1989). Effect of psychosocial treatment on survival of patients with metastatic breast cancer. *Lancet*, 2, 888–891.
18. Richardson, J. L., Shelton, D. R., Krailo, M., and Levine, A. M. (1990). The effects of compliance with treatment on survival among patients with hematologic malignancies. *J. Clin. Oncol.*, 8, 356–364.
19. Fawzy, F. I., Fawzy, N. W., and Hyun, C. S. (1993). Malignant melanoma. Effects of an early structured psychiatric intervention, coping and affective state on recurrence and survival 6 years later. *Arch. Gen. Psychiatry*, 50, 681–689.
20. Ratcliffe, M. A., Dawson, A. A., and Walker, L. G. (1995). Eysenck Personality Inventory L-scores in patients with Hodgkin's disease and non-Hodgkin's lymphoma. *Psycho-Oncology*, 4, 39–45.
21. Kuchler, T., Henne-Bruns, D., Rappat, S. *et al.* (1999). Impact of psychotherapeutic support on gastrointestinal cancer patients undergoing surgery: survival results of a trial. *Hepato-Gastroenterology*, 46, 322–335.

22. Linn, M. W., Linn, B. S., and Harris, R. (1982). Effects of counseling for late stage cancer patients. *Cancer*, 49, 1048–1055.
23. Morganstern, H., Geller, G. A., Walter, S. D., Ostfeld, A. M., and Siegel, B. S. (1984). The impact of a psychosocial support program on survival with breast cancer: the importance of selection bias in program evaluation. *J. Chronic Dis.*, 37, 273–282.
24. Ilnyckyj, A., Farber, J., Cheang, M. C., and Weinerman, B. H. (1994). A randomized controlled trial of psychotherapeutic intervention in cancer patients. *Ann. R. Coll. Physicians Surg. Can.*, 27, 93–96.
25. Cunningham, A. J., Edmonds, C. V. I., Jenkins, G. *et al.* (1998). A randomised controlled trial of the effects on survival of group psychological therapy for women with metastatic breast cancer. *Psycho-Oncology*, 7, 508–517.
26. Edelman, S., Lemon, J., Bell, D. R., and Kidman, A. D. (1999). Effects of group CBT on the survival time of patients with metastatic breast cancer. *Psycho-Oncology*, 8, 474–481.
27. Beutler, L. E. and Crago, M. (1991). *Psychotherapy Research. An International Review of Programmatic Studies.* American Psychological Association, Washington, DC.
28. Howard, K. I., Moras, K., Brill, P. L., Martinovich, Z., and Lutz, W. (1996). Evaluations of psychotherapy: efficacy, effectiveness and patient progress. *Am. Psychol.*, 51, 1059–1064.

Index